Safer Childbirth?

Safer Childbirth?

A critical history of maternity care

MARJORIE TEW
Formerly Research Statistician,
Nottingham University Medical School

With a new Introduction

Foreword by Sheila Kitzinger

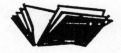

FREE ASSOCIATION BOOKS / LONDON / NEW YORK

This edition published 1998 by
FREE ASSOCIATION BOOKS LIMITED
57 Warren Street, London W1P 5PA
and 70 Washington Square South,
New York, NY 10012–1091

First published by Chapman & Hall 1990, 1995

ISBN 1–85343–426–4 pbk

A CIP catalogue record for this book is available
from the British Library

Printed in the EC by J.W. Arrowsmith Limited, Bristol

Contents

Preface to the
first edition

In all industrialized countries, the last fifty years have seen both a momentous improvement in the safety of childbirth and the completion of a momentous revolution in maternity care, with the philosophy and methods of the obstetric profession triumphant. This book tells the story of how these changes came about. It is a story urgently in need of telling, for the subject is one about which there is almost universal misunderstanding. Far from being a record of conquering idealism, the realization of an advance in human welfare through the application of scientific knowledge to improve the natural process of birth by an altruistic profession with good reason to believe in the rightness of its methods, it turns out to be a record of the successful denial and concealment of extensive and unanimous evidence that obstetric intervention only rarely improves the natural process.

The evidence is found in the impartial statistical analyses of the actual results of care, which show consistently that birth is the safer, the less its process is interfered with. The findings of statistics are in complete accord with the expectations of biology and are in turn impressively supported by the observations of critical obstetricians, evaluating particular practices.

Who should tell the story and present the accumulated evidence? It might be difficult for any obstetrician to cast aside his or her loyalty to the profession and provide a dispassionate account of the whole picture. It might be equally difficult for a midwife, whose profession lost its preeminence in maternity care, to be dispassionate or to be generally accepted as dispassionate. Partiality might be suspected also from a woman currently using the maternity service, the direction of her bias depending on whether or not she felt satisfied with the treatment she received. Partiality might be suspected also in an active crusader for women's rights. Doubt about partiality for any of these reasons does not attach to the present author. People keep asking how and why this outsider, without any obvious axe to grind, became so deeply involved in an issue perceived as being primarily of medical concern. Here briefly is the answer they seek.

I am neither a doctor nor a midwife and my personal experience of childbearing was far behind me when in 1975 I stumbled into the subject. A late re-entrant to academic life, I was teaching students in the Department of Community Health in Nottingham University's young Medical School how much they could find out about various diseases from the available official statistics. As part of these epidemiological exercises, I discovered to my complete surprise that the relevant routine statistics did not appear to support the widely accepted hypothesis that the increased hospitalization of birth had caused the decline by then achieved in the mortality of mothers and their new babies. At first it seemed hardly possible that I could be right in questioning the justification for what the medical world and everyone else apparently believed, but my further researches only served to confirm my initial discovery. My pursuit of the subject was not encouraged in the Department. My temporary contract of employment was not renewed in 1976. Fortunately, I was soon appointed as a part-time research statistician in the new Department of Orthopaedic Surgery where I have since worked happily and productively. I was able to continue my researches in maternity care, working alone on a voluntary basis in my spare time.

Medical journals were not eager to publish an article presenting the results of my statistical analyses. I was dismayed that there was such formidable resistance to discussing openly honest, well founded criticism of the basis of established policies. Against all odds, I became determined to break through the resistance and to fight against the false use of statistics to support a system that was actually harming its proclaimed beneficiaries. Daring to oppose the establishment was made easier by not being financially dependent on paid employment in the field as are most other dissidents.

After many rejections, my first article on this topic was published in 1977. It was not until then that I became aware that some doctors, some midwives and some women concerned with childbearing and with women's rights actually welcomed statistical confirmation of the apprehension their experiences raised about the benefits of the new medicalized maternity care. Otherwise preoccupied, I had been oblivious of these dissatisfactions and the protests being made on behalf of the users and some providers of the maternity service. This new source of support encouraged me to continue digging as deeply as I could to establish facts, but finding a journal willing to publish my results has continued to be very difficult. Thus when I was invited to write a book on the subject, I was eager to take the opportunity to set my statistical approaches alongside the many other factors which have contributed to the evolution of the present situation. Together they make a powerful indictment of the integrity of the forces which influence the determination and implementation of medico-social policy.

Who should read the story and ponder its implications? Safe childbirth is of intimate concern to all members of society at some stage in their lives, so insight into how it is actually achieved should not be limited to the professionals involved in providing the maternity service. It should interest all other doctors whose views make up 'medical opinion'; all those who determine and implement policies; those who have to meet the cost of what is provided; those who study how policies are in practice developed; and those who have to treat the adverse medical, social and psychological side-effects, early and late, of modern maternity care. It should be of immediate interest to those who intend to be parents, but above all it should interest those who are concerned with the welfare of mothers and babies, which should mean most people in most countries. The majority of the material used relates to English experience, but some of it is drawn from experience in other countries. The lessons to be learned from it are always the same, whatever the source. The book, therefore, should interest overseas readers as well.

Because the story hopes to appeal to readers from many different backgrounds, the language tries to be intelligible to the lay person and a glossary of technical terms is provided. Some readers will already be familiar with certain aspects of the story; frequent subheadings and cross-references are meant to help them skip quickly to the less familiar aspects. Some may indeed prefer to read the chapters on statistical methods and evaluation (6 to 9) before those on the development of the service (2 to 5). The same facts are often relevant in different contexts and these are linked up through appropriate cross-references (chapter or page number within round brackets). The many references to the writings of other authors whose work has contributed to the story are marked by numbered notes within square brackets, supplemented by the page number – (p. 00) – of the book or long article from which a precise quotation or a close paraphrase has been taken.

The first chapter of the book is a long summary, which brings together the various aspects of the story, many of which are treated in greater detail in later chapters as indicated. In the final chapter there is a brief résumé of the most crucial findings of the analysis and the implications for the future conduct of maternity care.

In my dogged lonely campaign I have been rescued from periods of despair by opportune help and encouragement from others pursuing their own campaigns. The first of these was Iain Chalmers, now

Director of the National Perinatal Epidemiology Unit at Oxford, who brought my early work to the attention of Sheila Kitzinger, the untiring champion of women's rights in childbirth, and my later work to the attention of the editor of the *British Journal of Obstetrics and Gynaecology*. I was much indebted also to Brian Watkins, who as editor of the *Health and Social Services Journal* before his untimely death in 1982, dared to publish my statistical analyses which mainstream medical journals found excuses for rejecting, and to Luke Zander, the general practitioner obstetrician who invited me to address a conference at the Royal Society of Medicine in 1980 and later to serve on the committee of the RSM's Forum on Maternity and the Newborn. I have always been glad of the warm support of several doctors, Radical Midwives and members of the Association for Improvements in the Maternity Services and the National Childbirth Trust.

When it came to the writing of this book, I relied entirely on my own statistical analyses and on other authors' published works. For information in the fields of biology and history which I have passed on, I have drawn liberally from books written by Sally Inch, Jean Donnison, Ann Oakley, Jean Towler and Joan Bramall, and I gladly acknowledge my debt to them. For specific purposes, I have made use of the work of many other researchers, not only of the observations they report but of their reference lists – helpful guides to sources of further relevant information.

Since I have used so many secondary sources, I have had to depend on Nottingham University's excellent Medical Library and I want to thank particularly Janet Mawby, the Readers' Adviser, and all the assistant librarians who have been unfailingly helpful in tracing texts for me and unfailingly friendly despite my importunities. Distanced from colleagues in relevant academic Departments with whom I should have liked to discuss my subject matter, I have turned to my husband, Brian, an academic economist with no background knowledge of medical science but with outstanding abilities in penetrating criticism, logical analysis and lucid exposition. Again and again, discussion with him has enabled me to straighten out my thoughts and arguments and so to improve the quality of my work. For this continual help and for his constant support and encouragement when I most needed it, I owe him my deepest thanks.

Marjorie Tew
Nottingham
1989

Preface to the second edition

Since the first edition went to press in 1989, there have been many important developments concerning different aspects of maternity care. To take account of these, much needs to be added to this history.

Late 1989 saw the publication of the double volume set of studies, *Effective Care in Pregnancy and Childbirth*, in which all the then existing evidence on all the associated procedures was considered and evaluated by well-informed and impartial authors representing many countries. This informative collection has since been followed by a flow of single reports of new research findings about specific subjects within the field. To incorporate the new material has involved, in particular, a considerable enlargement and rearrangement of the text and reference lists for Chapters 3 and 4, which deal with antenatal and intranatal care.

Then in 1990–1 the House of Commons Health Committee, under its chairman Nicholas Winterton, undertook a further enquiry into the maternity services in Britain. A wide range of people concerned as providers or users of the service, as well as researchers concerned to find out how well the service was meeting needs, chose to submit testimonies, written and oral. These testimonies were all later published in six volumes which offered a most valuable depiction of the maternity service from many points of view. Weighing up the submitted evidence, the committee in its report in 1992 made a series of recommendations which, if implemented, would revolutionize the organization of maternity care, for the first time making the users, the mothers and babies, the central concern, instead of the dominant providers. In response, the Department of Health set up an independent Expert Maternity Group which in its Report in 1993, *Changing Childbirth*, specifically endorsed this reorientation.

Describing these reports has occasioned a long extension to the text and reference list for Chapter 5, which deals with public involvement in maternity care. This chapter has had to become longer also to incorporate new material on voluntary organizations and on litigation.

Chapter 2, which describes birth attendants and their places of practice, has been extended to take account of recent changes reflecting the greater academic emphasis on the education of midwives and less striking changes, achieved and projected, in the education and training in obstetrics of doctors, both specialists and general practitioners. Changes also in the organization of antenatal clinics have been recorded, but imperceptibly few in the places of actual delivery, regardless of the strong evidence of the greater safety of out-of-hospital births.

Some of the new material in Chapter 7 carries forward to 1990 the official confidential enquiries into maternal deaths and once again points out how useless this type of analysis really is despite the claims made for it by obstetricians. More of the new material in Chapter 7 concerns the depressing maternal mortality in the Third World, about which more is now known.

None of the new material refutes the conclusions reached from analysis of results in the first edition – that the safety of childbirth depends principally on the good health of the mother and is more, often much more, likely than not to be prejudiced by obstetric interventions. Rather, the new evaluated material strengthens such conclusions. In Chapter 8 it is possible to present more evidence which challenges the universally accepted, but unevaluated, practice of transferring care from midwives to obstetricians when problems are anticipated, by showing how much perinatal mortality is thereby increased, not reduced. While it is now more readily conceded that obstetric management cannot make low-risk births safer, there is still not a shred of evidence to support the other universally accepted belief, also untested, that obstetric management is especially able to make safer those births, predicted on obstetricians' ever widening criteria, to be at high risk. The continued inability of obstetric management to reduce the incidence of low-weight births is noted; beliefs that neonatology can compensate for this failure and improve the healthy survival of such babies are examined.

All these recent developments have inevitably led to some changes in the summary Chapter 1 and sharpening of the conclusions in Chapter 9.

The purpose of the first edition of *Safer Childbirth?* was to make it publicly known that the organization of the maternity service has been based on obstetricians' claims of ensuring greater safety which the results of actual experience totally discredit. The revelations of the book played some part in loosening the stranglehold of wrong information and leading to the enlightened reports described in the extended Chapter 5. The purpose of the second edition is to confirm that the conclusions of the first edition are powerfully reinforced by subsequent research findings and that the reforming recommendations are fully justified.

I was encouraged to write this second edition because the first edition was so favourably received and I have to thank many people for their kind praise and interest. I have also to thank again the helpful librarians at Nottingham University's Medical Library and, most especially, my husband for his constructive criticism and constant encouragement.

Marjorie Tew
Nottingham
February 1994

Foreword

Sheila Kitzinger

Every now and again a book is published that breaks established moulds of thinking and challenges preconceptions and prejudices. This is such a book.

When *Safer Childbirth?* was first published in 1990, most people believed that hospital birth must be safer than birth at home, simply because obstetric skills and modern technology are available in an institution which are not on hand at home. Through her painstaking statistical analysis of perinatal mortality rates for hospital and home Marjorie Tew showed that this was a misconception. Statistics suggested, indeed, that for some women hospital birth might actually be more dangerous than home birth.

This was shattering information. Many professionals in the maternity services resisted it, some without bothering to read her work, and said that the study must be flawed. Most ignored it. But some began to ask searching questions. The result was subsequent research into home and hospital birth which has confirmed Marjorie Tew's initial analysis (Campbell and Macfarlane, 1994; Davies, J., 1994; Chamberlain, Wraight and Crowley, 1997; Olsen, 1997).

Home is as safe as hospital for women who are at low risk. Moreover, if low-risk women give birth in hospital they are more likely to have complicated births and be ill afterwards.

Safety is not only a matter of life or death. Indeed, though the death of a baby is an intense personal tragedy for parents, perinatal mortality rates are now so low that they are a crude measure of safety. For a woman who, as a consequence of labour and delivery, has pelvic infection after childbirth, one who cannot have sexual intercourse without pain, who is incontinent, or who becomes depressed, or is in the panic-stricken state produced by post traumatic stress disorder, or one who longs to breastfeed, but is unable to do so, birth has not been safe. Equally, for a baby who, as a result of the way in which labour and delivery were managed, is in pain, or is too stressed or sluggish because of chemical substances in its bloodstream, to relate to the mother in a satisfying way or to suckle vigorously, birth has not been safe.

Thus ways in which the management of birth is affected by the environment, and how care-givers perceive their roles in different settings, are vital elements in the study of sociology of birth. And these sociological and psychological studies need to be linked with the statistical research into birth outcomes. Quantitative research must be matched with qualitative research that enable us to develop insight into the nature of the birth experience, for both the mother and the baby, and also its impact on post-partum experience in the family. In fact, if 'post partum' means only the first six weeks after birth, it is necessary to take a longer view, we should examine how the birth experience might affect a woman's sense of personal identity, her relationships, and her interaction with her child over months – and even years.

A woman and her baby cannot be signed off and discharged from hospital after a few days as if everthing that occurred during the birth is over and done with. Far from forgetting what happened and how they were treated, as is often asserted, women remember acutely details of birth, especially positive and negative elements in the relationships with their care-givers, many years later (Simkin, 1991, 1996).

Childbirth is not simply a medical event. It is not just an incident that can be dismissed as irrelevant to everything that happens afterwards. Birth is a major life transition.

We owe a debt to Marjorie Tew for her pioneering contribution to our understanding of these issues.

REFERENCES

Campbell, R. and Macfarlane, A. (1994) *Where to be born? The debate and the evidence.* Second edition, National Perinatal Epidemiology Unit, Oxford.
Chamberlain, G., Wraight, A., Crowley, P. (1997) *Home Births: The report of the 1994 confidential enquiry by the National Birthday Trust Fund*, Parthenon, Carnforth, UK and New York Pearl River, New York, USA.
Davies, J. (1994) *Report of the Northern Region Home Birth Survey*, 1993, Northern Region Health Authority, Yorkshire.
Olsen, O. (1997) Meta-analysis of the safety of home birth, *Birth* **24**, 4–12.
Simkin, P. (1991) Just another day in a woman's life? Women's long-term perceptions of their first birth experience. *Birth* **18**, 203–10.
——— (1996) The experience of maternity in a woman's life, *Journal of Obstetric, Gynecological & Neonatal Nursing*, **25**, 3.

Introduction

The second edition of *Safer Childbirth?*, published in 1995, brought the history of maternity care up to early 1994. By then the prospect seemed set fair for the maternity service in Britain to be reorganized and henceforth to be delivered in accordance with evaluated evidence, linking treatments with beneficial outcomes for mother and baby. The impartial all-party House of Commons Health Committee under the chairmanship of Nicholas Winterton reported in 1992 the conclusions of its comprehensive inquiry into all aspects of maternity care from relevant evidence submitted by its providers and receivers at all levels and by scientific analysis of the reported results of treatments (see pp. 215–23). The Committee was convinced that, in contrast to previous practice, paramount importance should be given to the human needs of service receivers, rather than to the interests of service providers, whose professional bodies began by accepting the Committee's proposals, either immediately or, in the case of the Royal College of Obstetricians and Gynaecologists (RCOG), by the end of 1994. The RCOG's report, *The Future of the Maternity Services*, written after study of the evidence and consultation with midwives and general practitioners, acknowledged the valuable contribution certain technological interventions had made towards making birth safer, but nevertheless conceded that 'for most pregnancies and births, the application of sophisticated medical technology is totally inappropriate'.

The Department of Health's prompt response to the prospective changes in policy was to set up its own Expert Maternity Group to consider further the practical implications involved in implementing the Winterton Committee's recommendations. Following their 1993 report, *Changing Childbirth* (see pp. 223–8), implementation teams were set up in the Health Regions and they organized many pilot schemes which in due course resulted in more satisfactory outcomes for mothers and babies, and if properly organized, for midwives too. In many cases target dates were set against which improvements could be measured. It was expected that many would be reached in five years, but in the event this expectation proved overoptimistic, even unrealistic, for by then political attitudes, not only of the providers of maternity services, but also of many receivers, had reverted to their pre-Winterton state and authorities were withdrawing funds from implementation schemes, despite the probable economies of these and the much higher costs of technological obstetric treatments. The principle of the *Changing Childbirth* report could be interpreted as having been achieved if mothers were enabled to make their own informed choice of the kind of treatment they received and where it was given. The next chapter of the history of maternity care must ask the question, 'Has recent experience confirmed or otherwise that mothers have been enabled better to make an informed choice about their maternity care?'

If mothers were to have choice, they must be correctly informed about the options available and the advantages and disadvantages of each. Equally, whoever supplied this information must be correctly informed about the options available and the advantages and disadvantages of each and must be willing and able to dispense this information fairly and impartially. The first professional from whom most pregnant women will seek information is their General Practitioner (GP).

There is much evidence that before 1992 most GPs, educated as they had been in medical schools steeped in obstetricians' orthodoxy, were ill-informed about the advantages and disadvantages of different systems of antenatal and intranatal care and antenatal and intranatal therapies. Most had been persuaded of the disadvantages to themselves of home deliveries, so the advice they gave was extremely biased in favour of care and delivery in hospital. All that the action proposed in the *Changing Childbirth* report to rid the advisers of their long-standing bias amounted to was that 'Clinical practice should be based on sound evidence and be subject to regular clinical audit', but no medium was proposed how this 'sound evidence' was to be conveyed, convincingly, to GPs and how their action on it was to be audited (see p. 229); moreover, the Department of Health's advice had for many years been that every woman should be encouraged to have her baby 'in a maternity unit which can offer a range of obstetric, paediatric and supporting services necessary to cope with an emergency' – advice which accords with obstetricians' principles. So medical advisers have clung uncritically to their indoctrinated, but insupportable, belief that out-of-hospital births are dangerous, even when carefully planned, and, unlike the Winterton Committee, they remained blind to the contrary evidence which demonstrated that the danger was in fact greater in obstetrically managed hospital births.

Doctors passed on these beliefs authoritatively and, too often, harshly to pregnant women. Both reports deplored the frank hostility and deliberate unhelpfulness shown by some GPs to mothers seeking to choose the place of birth and strongly recommended that such attitudes should not continue. This harshness was confirmed in the survey of GPs' attitudes and behaviour conducted in 1993 by the National Childbirth Trust. This finding was repeated in surveys conducted by Community Health Councils in North-West England in 1994 when very few women reported that their GP discussed all possible options with them before making a booking which for most women was automatically into hospital. Frightening threats of disastrous outcomes for birth anywhere else were still being resorted to. Much publicity was given to the excruciating agony that can be suffered during an otherwise uncomplicated delivery and to the usual effectiveness of epidural anaesthesia, administration of which can only be guaranteed throughout twenty-four hours in a large obstetric hospital (see p. 175).

So either on grounds of reputed safety or facilities for pain relief, there seemed to be little confirmed evidence of widespread changes since 1992 in the advice GPs pass on to pregnant women, despite their Royal College having accepted the findings and recommendations of the Winterton Report. It was not surprising, therefore, that there was not an appreciable increase in the proportion of births taking place at home. Nor was there evidence of prompt compliance with the Winterton Report's very strong recommendation that small rural maternity units should be 'maintained as a realistically available option unless the case for closing them is overwhelming'.

Despite the already quoted principle in the RCOG report *The Future of the Maternity Services* that the application of sophisticated medical technology is inappropriate for most pregnancies, obstetricians pressed on with interventions at all stages; notably, the proportion of births delivered by caesarean section continued to increase considerably.

Certainly the competence of the surgeons had improved, leading to fewer adverse results, which encouraged them to carry out the operation for ever less convincing medical reasons, so that the percentage of deliveries by this method continued to increase, still without evaluated evidence of causing improvement in welfare for most mothers or babies.

To enable them to play their part as competent obstetric nurses, the training of midwives had to go back to emphasizing the technological aspects of their work. By the time of the Winterton inquiry, the Royal College of Midwives appeared to have been much influenced by the philosophy of the subgroup of Radical Midwives within the College and flattered that the results of applying this philosophy had so favourably impressed the Winterton Committee and the Expert Maternity Group. The College had participated enthusiastically in presenting evidence to the inquiries in favour of allowing most births to take place without technological intervention. It then elected an outstanding and inspired Radical Midwife, Caroline Flint, as its next President. But later it seems to have regretted its enthusiasm, for by 1996 it reversed its post-Winterton policy and preferred to elect as its following President a midwife whose inaugural address demonstrated that she shared the obstetricians' medicalized view of childbirth as a process always at risk of developing dangerous complications, to remedy which she favoured intervention practices in which her earlier training in the skills of obstetric nursing rather than in the arts of midwifery had experienced her.

Her inaugural address gave no indication that she was aware of the impartially analyzed results of most interventions which had so impressed the members of the Winterton Committee, and anyone else who studied them with an open mind; nor did it acknowledge the proven evidence that most complications can be overcome or avoided altogether by non-technological supportive midwifery. The training of midwives was allowed to concentrate to such an extent on the obstetric nursing aspects of their work that training in the non-intervention arts was increasingly neglected, so that they became less and less competent to conduct a home delivery, and less and less confident in so doing, without immediately accessible technology. Unless Radical Midwives happened to be in control, home births were rapidly degenerating into hospital births without equipment.

The Winterton Committee had been greatly impressed by the work of the National Perinatal Epidemiology Unit at Oxford (see pp. 222–3) which, towards the end of the 1970s had embarked on a systematic review of the effects of care, obstetric and midwifery, during pregnancy and childbirth. This resulted in a mammoth publication in late 1989 in which all the procedures were considered and evaluated by well informed and impartial authors representing many countries and also in an electronic database which has been continually updated as new evidence has become available. A summary guide to the mammoth publication was also published in 1989 and the second edition of this summary was published in 1995.

From this summary 423 conclusions can be drawn and these in turn were finally summarised in 6 tables listing the forms of care at 7 stages in the childbirth process. Effectiveness of care at these stages was graded as

1. beneficial – 39 or 9.2%
2. likely to be beneficial – 119 or 28.1%
3. partly beneficial, partly harmful – 33 or 7.8%
4. of unknown effectiveness – 95 or 22.4%
5. unlikely to be beneficial – 96 or 22.7%
6. likely to be ineffective or harmful – 41 or 9.7%.

The frequency of the word 'likely' in these categories warns against making too firm conclusions even from the best analyzed data available.

Nevertheless there is good evidence to support the contention that nearly as many common procedures are as likely to be disadvantageous (32%) as advantageous (37%), with a further group (22%) about which there is too little evidence to substantiate conclusions.

The disadvantageous interventions, which included most of the technological ones, included three which according to current practice affect most births and particularly, because of their consequent conditions, merit further study. Of these are the ones which influence or determine the mother's posture at stages during the childbearing process. By the nineteenth century, in Britain and other countries where Western medicine is practised, lying down throughout labour had come to be the policy in most maternity units and for the second stage the policy was that the mother should lie on her back with her legs raised and supported in stirrups – the 'stranded beetle' position. This position had certain conveniences for the providers of care, and this is what doctors and midwives were taught (see pp. 147 and 187).

In the light of recent experience and knowledge, changes have taken place in Britain, though less so in some other countries. Here the stranded beetle position has been virtually abandoned in routine care and the supine position has been largely replaced by the semi-recumbent position which still limits the ability of the pelvis to widen to its maximum extent to accommodate the safe passage of the fetal head. No national survey has measured the extent of changes in policy and practice regarding maternal posture, but it is obvious from television programmes of procedures in some respected hospitals that some women there are still expected to give birth confined to bed and on their backs or semi-recumbent.

Often these positions have to be resorted to make certain modern procedures and interventions, which obstetricians believe to be essential, easier or possible to implement, like electronic fetal monitoring, intravenous hydration, administration of drugs to speed up labour, and epidural anaesthesia. Certainly for television programmes the positions in bed are more discreet. And the convenience of these positions is obviously held to outweigh the associated drawbacks, for lying on the back has been found to cause a significant reduction in maternal–placental–fetal blood flow (see p. 148). Contractions are made less intense and less efficient at accomplishing cervical dilation and in compensation have to occur more frequently. Despite this greater frequency, labours last longer and cause more pain. Hence they create greater demand for pain relief.

Dependence on artificial pain relief originates from misinterpretation of the physiological role of pain (see p. 176). Pain in the various stages of labour prompts the mother to move and change her position. Painful contractions are themselves an indication that labour is becoming less efficient, for pain in fact slows labour by increasing the secretion of the body's own system of pain relief – the hormone ß-endorphin – which is the biochemical cause of uterine inertia and dystocia. Freedom to move as her body dictates helps the mother to relieve her pain and, more importantly, helps the fetus, whose efforts to be born initiate the painful stimuli, to move to the correct position in its journey and so reduce the likelihood of problems of mal-presentation and also of cephalo–pelvic disproportion if the mother adopts an upright position which allows her cervix to widen as required to accommodate the safe passage of the fetal head.

In controlled trials, the women who were asked to walk, stand, or sit upright in the first stage had shorter labours than women who stayed lying flat and this benefit was enjoyed also by those who remained upright during the second stage. They needed fewer drugs to accelerate or augment labour and they used less pain-relieving drugs or epidural anaesthesia. Thus upright positions and freedom to reduce pain by varying positions enables the mother to escape the adverse consequences that these treatments may bring. So, examining all the evidence, including that on post-partum blood loss, the up-dated *Guide to Effective Care in Pregnancy and Childbirth* could find none 'to justify forcing women to lie flat during the second stage of labour'. The balance of advantage lies strongly with upright positions. Recumbency tends not only to lengthen labour, but also to reduce the incidence of spontaneous births, to increase the incidence of abnormal fetal heart rate patterns and to reduce umbilical cord blood oxygenation.

Another increasingly favoured obstetric intervention, both in antenatal and intranatal care, is electronic fetal heart-rate monitoring, greeted by obstetricians with great enthusiasm, when it was invented in the 1970s, as a potentially life-saving intervention for the baby. Much expenditure was devoted to the ubiquitous provision of the necessary equipment (and once the equipment was available there was, of course, no discouragement from using it), but the obstetricians' high hopes of its benefits were never realized and analysis of their accumulating results failed to show that its frequent use had contributed to the general decline in perinatal mortality or morbidity or indeed to any improvement in outcome for either mother or child (see pp. 177–9).

Senior obstetricians may have accepted, as their later writings show, the conclusions of impartial analysis of the results from their own data, but they do not seem to have passed on their revised conviction to their teacher colleagues in charge of training programmes; nor have they persuaded Courts of Law or Medical Insurance Societies that failure to use fetal monitoring cannot therefore constitute reliable evidence of professional negligence. Fear of this judgement in potential litigation has ensured that doctors and midwives continue to observe the practice.

When surveys are made of mothers' attitudes, it is found that, despite imposed discomfort, many claim to be reassured by continuous monitoring because it provides the information that care-givers say they need during pregnancy and labour. Mothers are not told that interpretation of electronic traces is totally unreliable; indeed that care-givers cannot be certain how to interpret the information of electronic traces so as to ensure that only beneficial treatment will be given thereafter. As in many other instances of obstetric management, mothers are not given unbiased evaluated information on which to make an informed choice. The history of electronic fetal monitoring is a clear example that mothers continue to be hoodwinked by false propaganda to acquiesce in treatment that can only benefit the advocates of obstetric management.

Obstetric management continues also to reflect obstetricians' unwavering faith in the value of ultrasound, a much used procedure whose safety for mother and baby has always been assumed, but never established by the results of a randomized controlled trial. Ultrasound scans provide a reliable technique for dating pregnancies, for confirming pathological conditions, such as breech and other malpresentations, multiple and ectopic pregnancies, the rare cases of persisting low placental site, and whether the fetus has survived an antepartum haemorrhage. Scans can identify lethal congenital malformations and provide baseline data useful in the monitoring of fetal development, using tests which have different significance at different gestational ages and can alert obstetricians to conditions which they believe their interventions can improve.

If conventional imaging scans are to detect retardation in fetal growth, they must necessarily be repeated at intervals during the later stages of pregnancy. Information on fetal growth retardation can be derived profitably by using Doppler ultrasound to monitor umbilical blood flow. By this means small fetuses which are healthy and will not benefit from intervention can be distinguished from small fetuses which are unhealthy and for which intervention to curtail the pregnancy may be life saving.

No record is kept of any baby's cumulative exposure to ultrasound – conventional or Doppler – and this will relate not only to the number of scans or assessments of feto–placental circulation, but also to the duration of each (and more is likely to be learned from a longer than a shorter exposure) and the power of the instruments used (later instruments probably being more powerful than earlier ones). Until such data is collected and accumulated and related to long-term outcomes, there can be no verdict on the ultimate safety or dangers of ultrasound.

Controlled trials have shown that routine ultrasound measurement of fetal size in late pregnancy results in an increased rate of antenatal hospital admission and possibly of induction of labour, with no evidence of substantive benefit to the baby, but the use of Doppler ultrasound in high-risk pregnancies does prompt interventions which do bring benefit to the baby.

The up-dated *Guide to Effective Care in Pregnancy and Childbirth*, evaluating all evidence by then available, concludes that 'trials provide no support for routine ultrasonography for fetal measurement ... its routine use in late pregnancy is unlikely to be beneficial'. The verdict on early ultrasound is that the evidence is equivocal – some good effects, some harmful. Likely to be beneficial is the selective use of ultrasound, imaging or Doppler, to answer specific questions about fetal size, structure or position, or assess amniotic fluid volume, and to estimate gestational age in first and early second trimesters.

Clearly, the essential findings of scientific analysis of the results of maternity care have not changed since the Winterton Committee and the Expert Maternity Group collected the evidence on which they based their conclusions and made their recommendations in 1992 and 1993. Just as clearly no committed attempt has been made since then to pass on this knowledge to pregnant women to enable them to exercise informed choice in their willingness to participate in obstetric treatment, nor to educate doctors and midwives to enable them to practise only evidence-based medicine.

Marjorie Tew
Nottingham
May 1998

Glossary

Alphafetoprotein A substance which, when present in abnormally high concentration in the maternal blood, may indicate gross malformation of the fetal skull (**anencephaly**) or spine (**spina bifida**) and when present in abnormally low concentration may indicate the chromosomal anomaly **Down's syndrome**

Amniotic sac Contains the fluid surrounding the fetus and may be punctured via the abdomen (**amniocentesis**) to yield a sample of fluid for test purposes or ruptured via the vagina (**amniotomy or Artificial Rupture of Membranes**) to induce labour

Anencephaly A defect in the development of the neural tube in which the uppermost part of the brain and skull of the fetus are either missing or incorrectly formed, with fatal consequences

Auscultation Listening directly to the fetal heart sounds via a trumpet-shaped tube, the **Pinard stethoscope**

Betamimetic A drug intended to produce relaxation of uterine muscle

Caesarean Section Extraction of the fetus from the uterus by means of a surgical incision in the abdominal and uterine walls

Cardiotocography A graphical correlation between fetal heart rate patterns and uterine contractions recorded by an **electronic monitor**

Cephalhaematoma An egg-shaped swelling on the head caused by a collection of bloody fluid between one of the skull bones and its covering membrane, most commonly seen in newborn infants after delivery by forceps or vacuum extraction

Cervical Cerclage A reinforcing suture intended to make an effective sphincter of an incompetent **Cervix** (neck of uterus)

Disproportion, cephalo-pelvic A fetal head unusually large or presenting by an unfavourable diameter in relation to a small or abnormally shaped maternal pelvis

Dystocia Difficult or abnormal labour

Eclampsia Dangerous maternal complication following **pre-eclampsia** which is signalled by raised blood pressure (**hypertension**), oedema, and protein in urine and was formerly called **toxaemia** (poisoned blood)

Ectopic Pregnancy The embedding of a fertilized ovum outside the uterus

Endocrinology The study of the endocrine glands and the hormones they manufacture and secrete directly into the bloodstream

Endorphins A group of chemicals manufactured within the brain, including beta-endorphin which, like opiates, relieves pain and has other regulatory effects on the mind, body and other hormones

Epidemiology The study of disease as it affects whole populations, its causes and distribution

Epidural Analgesia Injection of a local anaesthetic agent into the epidural space in order to block the spinal nerves and cause total numbness of the lower trunk and limbs

Ergometrine A synthetic oxytocic drug which reproduces the strong uterine contractions produced by the natural drug, **ergot**, without its most serious dangers

Fundal Relating to the top part of the uterus furthest from the cervix

Haemoglobin Pigment in red blood cells which contain iron. This combines with oxygen and carries it to body tissues. Deficiency of haemoglobin indicates anaemia

Hyperinsulinism The excessive secretion of the hormone, insulin, made by the pancreas

Hypoglycaemia The deficiency of glucose in the bloodstream causing muscular weakness and incoordination, mental confusion and sweating; if severe and not counteracted with glucose, it can lead to hypoglycaemic coma

Hypoxia, Anoxia, Asphyxia Increasing degrees of deprivation of oxygen suffered by the fetus before or during birth to the point of suffocation, resulting in transient or permanent morbidity (e.g. **neonatal fits, cerebral palsy**) or early death

Iatrogenic Treatment induced

Intubation Introduction by the birth attendant of a tube or catheter into the trachea of an asphyxiated infant, followed by insufflation with oxygen or air at a controlled pressure

Involution Gradual return of the uterus to normal size after labour

Lochia Discharge from the uterus of the residual products of pregnancy following childbirth or abortion

Oestrogen, Progesterone Hormones secreted by endocrine glands which orchestrate sexual development and the maintenance of pregnancy; secreted also by the placenta later in pregnancy

Oncology The study and practice of treating tumours, abnormal growths benign or malignant

Oxytocin The hormone secreted by the pituitary gland which stimulates uterine contractions and controls bleeding; now produced synthetically as **syntocinon** which, combined with **ergometrine** and called **syntometrine**, is used in the third stage of labour to hasten expulsion of the placenta and control postpartum haemorrhage.

Parity The number of viable children already borne: **primipara**, a woman bearing her first child; **multipara**, a woman bearing a later child

Partogram A graph of progressive cervical dilation in labour

Parturient Being in labour; relating to childbirth (**parturition**)

Perineum, Perineal Body The fibro-muscular pyramid from the lowest third of the vagina in front to the anal canal at the back and across the transverse diameter of the pelvic outlet

Placenta The organ formed for each pregnancy with the function of transmitting oxygen and nutrients from the maternal blood to the fetus, and carbon dioxide and other waste products excreted by the fetus to the mother; it also produces hormones. Serious problems arise if it is attached low on the uterine wall and obstructs delivery of the fetus (**placenta praevia**) or if there is undue delay in evacuating it after the birth of the baby (**retained placenta**)

Presentation That part of the fetus which first enters the pelvis, most often the head (**cephalic, vertex**), sometimes the buttocks (**breech**), occasionally the face, brow or shoulder

Prostaglandins Substances produced in human cells and having an oxytocic effect on the mechanical properties of cervical tissue

Psychoprophylaxis A method of physical and psychological preparation for childbirth to control mental and physical responses to the processes of labour and modify perception of painful stimuli

Puerperium The period following childbirth when the organs of reproduction revert to their pre-pregnancy state, raw tissues being especially vulnerable to infection (**puerperal sepsis, fever**)

Pulmonary Embolism The blocking of a pulmonary blood vessel by a solid, e.g., a floating clot detached from a leg vein thrombosis (**phlegmasia alba dolens**), or by a foreign substance which has entered the circulation, e.g. an **amniotic fluid embolism**, or by an air bubble – a cause of maternal death

Pyrexia Fever – rise in body temperature above normal usually caused by bacterial or viral infection

Rhesus Factor An antigen which may be present (+) or absent (−) in human blood. **Iso-immunization** occurs if Rh (+) blood cells from a fetus with an Rh (+) father pass into the circulation of an Rh (−) mother, causing her to produce antibodies (**anti-D**). If the antibodies pass into the circulation of a later fetus, they cause **Haemolytic Disease of the Newborn**, leading to anaemia, jaundice and often death. This condition can be treated with **Exchange Blood Transfusion** or prevented by giving the mother **anti-D gamma** globulin to prevent her from forming her own antibodies

Rubella German measles
Teratogenic Of drugs, like **thalidomide**, which produce as a side-effect congenital malformations
Uterine Inertia Inability of the uterine muscle to contract efficiently
Vacuum Extraction Method of assisting delivery by attaching a metal cup by suction to the fetal scalp and pulling gently in time with uterine contractions
Version A manoeuvre to turn the fetus to a more favourable presentation – **cephalic** to make the head present; **podalic** to make the breech present; **external** by manipulation through the abdominal wall before labour; **internal** by manipulation partly from inside, partly from outside the uterus
Vulva The fleshy folds surrounding the openings of the vagina and urethra and extending forward to the clitoris

The revolution in maternity care: the diverse strands of a complicated tapestry

THE SETTING OF A DOCTOR-DEPENDENT SOCIETY

In Britain, by the 1980s, society had come to accept that birth, the essential physiological event by which the human race has perpetuated itself, must now take place in a medical institution. The family home was the traditional birthing place right up to the start of the 20th century and for many years thereafter, yet by the early 1980s hardly 1% of British births took place there. For such a revolutionary concept to be accepted by a culture within such a short period of its history and with such unanimity must be a rare phenomenon. How did it come about?

Britain cannot claim to have been the pioneer of this revolution. It began rather earlier and progressed rather faster in many of the other economically developed countries, with the outstanding exception of Holland. The change was most rapid among the European immigrant populations of the New World, the United States of America (USA) and the then Dominions of the British Commonwealth, Australia, Canada, New Zealand and South Africa, where a vigorous medical profession was seeking to establish itself. The revolution in maternity care was even more complete in countries, as in Eastern Europe, where a political revolution had ordained that social and economic betterment was to be achieved through systems of planning and control by experts, and betterment in maternal and infant welfare through a system of childbirth care planned and controlled by medical experts. By the 1980s in all these countries birth at home was as rare as in Britain. The same underlying reasons for the change, through immensely complex, can be recognized in different places.

At first, the advantages of a medical institution of any kind were recommended as an alternative to the family home, but gradually the specialist consultant obstetric hospital, equipped with increasingly sophisticated technological instruments, has become favoured at the expense of the non-specialist hospital, not so equipped and used by general practitioners with the co-operation of midwives for delivering their patients. In England and Wales in 1990 only 1.6% of births took place in geographically separate general practitioner units (GPUs) compared with 12% in 1969.

Hospital care in several countries is organized on three levels of specialization. Level 1, the least specialized, corresponds approximately to the British GPU. The tertiary level 3 hospitals are the most specialized and provide care similar to that provided in the largest of the obstetric hospitals in Britain. British data are rarely published by size of unit, so it is not possible to identify separately the British equivalent of level 2 and 3 hospitals overseas.

But why should birth take place in any kind of hospital? One reason is because a hospital is the place where doctors can best deploy their technical skills and harness the instruments of developing technology to assist them. But why does birth need the technical skill of a doctor? Surely the success of human reproduction is demonstrated by the enormous expansion in the world's population and this has been achieved over the centuries without the mediation of obstetricians or hospitals for all but the tiniest proportion of people. Given favourable environments, other species reproduce successfully without medical or veterinary intervention. Given a favourable environment could not the human species do likewise?

The response to this question would seem to be that civilization has often not provided a sufficiently favourable environment and its price has been to submerge the human mother's natural instincts and deprive her reproductive system of its natural competence. Human reproduction has been numerically successful, but there have been many casualties on the way. This has brought great suffering to the individual families involved. In addition, it has created anxieties for communities and nations which see their survival as depending on constant replenishment with healthy babies ready to grow into productive citizens and sturdy warriors. Individuals and communities, therefore, share concern to find whatever assistance they believe will reduce the casualties of reproduction.

Every culture has its own medicine men to whom it looks to solve its problems of illness and death. Western cultures look to their academically trained doctors and their confidence in doing so has increased greatly over the last two centuries. Cures have no longer had to depend on mystery, magic and faith, or at least they are no longer perceived as doing so. The spirit of scientific enquiry, which became particularly lively in the 18th century, led to greater understanding of the physiology and anatomy of the human body and of its pathology. Understanding the causes of illnesses offered a first step along the path to surviving them by finding methods of prevention or cure. It was, however, still to be a long time before medical science developed effective treatments for the most frequent causes of death.

In England, as in other industrializing countries in the 19th century, populations were expanding rapidly, despite the very high death rates in all age groups which caused personal and social concern. One expression of the social concern was the introduction in 1837 of the legal obligation to register every death, with the sex and age of the deceased. Live births were also to be registered, but it was not until 1874 that it became compulsory to do so. The information collected was linked with that obtained from the decennial censuses of population, the first of which was carried out in 1841, so that patterns of mortality could be described and trends discerned. The statistics were presented, often with commentaries, in the *Annual Reports* of the Registrar General of England and Wales [1] until 1973 and thereafter in other official publications of the Office of Population Censuses and Surveys [2,3].

Great changes took place in the industrial and social environment in the 19th century. The expansion of industry led to increased pollution but also to increased employment and incomes. In general, the extra food and clothing people could buy compensated for the unhealthy conditions in which they had to work and live. Cheaper, more abundant and more varied food became available from the rising output of the farming industries, both at home and in the New World. Municipal authorities carried out impressive feats of sanitary engineering to supply pure water to town dwellers and safely remove domestic waste.

Death rates remained high until 1870, but thereafter they experienced a spectacular and sustained decline. The grateful public were disposed to give the medical profession the credit for this improvement and the medical profession was certainly not disposed to disclaim the honour. Instead it enjoyed the heightened prestige.

The honour was, however, misplaced as later epidemiological analysis, which evaluates the effects of the treatment of disease on patients as a whole, was to prove [4]. The great decline in mortality was brought about not by life-saving medical treatments, but by the life-saving consequences of non-medical developments. The most frequent causes of death had been infectious diseases, including cholera and tuberculosis. The chief reason for the decline in mortality was the decline in deaths from these causes. Through the discoveries of 19th century doctors and scientists, like Edward Jenner, Louis Pasteur, Robert Koch and others, much had been learned about the causes and modes of transmission of infections, but few effective medical treatments were developed for more than sixty years after the great decline in the death rate started. Certainly, vaccination against smallpox was available in the 19th century and antitoxin treatment for diphtheria from the early years of the 20th, but these diseases made up only a relatively small proportion of the killing infections. By the time that antibiotic drugs like sulphonamide, penicillin and streptomycin were available to treat specific infections and immunizations had been developed to prevent them, the diseases concerned had long since ceased to be frequent causes of death. Mortality rates from them had fallen dramatically and continuously since 1870 and would almost certainly have gone on falling without the added impetus of the new treatments, welcome bonus though these were.

The outcome in infectious illnesses depends on the balance between the prevalence and virulence of invading organisms on the one hand and the strength of the hosts' defences on the other. The work of the sanitary engineers greatly reduced the prevalence of harmful bacteria. Improvements in diet and living conditions helped strengthen the hosts' defences. The balance shifted in the hosts' favour so that gradually they won the contest. Their greater resistance to infectious diseases, including tuberculosis, was reflected in the rapidly declining mortality from these causes in all age groups. This change took place during the years before the advances in medical knowledge could make an appreciable contribution to the cure of the diseases or, except for smallpox, to their prevention. Analysis of the historic succession of events led the epidemiologist, Professor Tom McKeown [4], to conclude in 1965

> We owe the advance in health mainly, not to what happens when we are ill, but to the fact that we do not so often become ill. And we remain well, not because of specific preventive measures, such as vaccination and immunisation, but because we enjoy a higher standard of living and live in a healthier environment.

Earlier analysis of experience in Australia had led to the same conclusion – that improvements in provisions for public health, in nutrition and in other living standards had been more effective in combating infectious diseases and reducing infant mortality than the immunization and serum treatments which became available in the 1930s [5]. It is virtually certain that the reasons for the parallel decline in mortality which took place in other industrializing countries over the same period were the same.

The most frequent causes of death have changed during the 20th century. Effective, indeed spectacular, treatments have been developed for many diseases and death rates from them have been reduced. But it is still true that the general level of health depends much more on people not contracting diseases, by adopting a life-style which enables them to build up their own natural defences, than on medical cures for diseases contracted or medical preventive immunizations (Chapter 9, pages 381–2).

That this explanation for the decline in mortality, disclosed by epidemiological analysis in the 1950s and 1960s, was greeted with general surprise and scepticism, not least among the medical profession, revealed how deeply ingrained was the popular misconception about the powers of doctors. That it has remained a misconception is due to popular misinformation, fostered on the one hand by the medical profession which has, on the whole, more to gain by treating disease than preventing it, and on the other hand by the public. For it is perhaps essential as a reassurance to human vulnerability that people want to overrate the powers of those on whom they rely for the help they need when illness has not been prevented. While such ill-informed attitudes towards health and sickness in general prevail, it is understandable that society should believe that, although reproduction is not a disease, its problems are also better solved by medical intervention than by environmental improvement and healthy life-styles. And since the prosperity of doctors concerned with maternity care is vitally dependent on this belief, it is understandable that they should make great efforts to propagate it.

MATERNAL AND INFANT MORTALITY: EXCEPTIONAL CASES

The decline in mortality after 1870 was experienced by all subgroups in the population except for two. These were mothers in childbirth and infants in the first year of life. Surprisingly, these two groups did not seem to have benefited from the improved standards of living, at least according to the statistics. But the apparently high maternal and infant death rates towards the end of the 19th century may have been due, in part, to more complete recording. There are many problems involved in the certification of death to particular causes. Changes in the climate of public opinion may have made doctors more willing to attribute the death of mothers frankly to their maternity instead of to other contributory causes with less emotive connotations [6]. For whatever reason, the maternal mortality recorded for 1896–1900 was 5.5 per 1000 live births, having fluctuated around 5.0 throughout the 19th century.

The compulsory registration of births after 1874 probably led to the reporting of both the birth and early death of some infants, events which previously the parent had not considered it necessary to record officially. The average infant mortality rate, at 153 per 1000 live births, was as high between 1891 and 1900 as between 1841 and 1850, though rather higher than in the 1880s when it averaged 142. More complete recording was likely at most to have raised these death rates only marginally and was very unlikely to have obscured a real downward trend in the mortality of mothers or infants coincident and commensurate with the general experience.

The causes of infant death are different at different stages: those which occur within the first four weeks, the neonatal period, are most strongly related to conditions experienced during fetal development and birth – the sooner after birth the death occurs, the stronger is this relationship; deaths which occur in the next eleven months, the post-neonatal period, are most strongly related to conditions in the physical environment to which the infant is exposed. Soon after the turn of the century the persistently high infant mortality rate at last began to fall and when after 1906 the statistics showed separately the deaths at different stages, it was clear that all the improvement was happening in the post-neonatal period. The benefits of the improving environment were obviously now extending to these children also. Apparently only the deaths of mothers and infants associated with maternity were not so reduced.

England was a pioneer in the collection of demographic statistics. Records in other countries are not always as reliable or as readily available, but where they do exist they show the same experience as in England: from the later 19th century downward trends in mortality were experienced by most of the population but not by mothers and their new babies. The phenomenon was common to all the more economically developed countries.

These results caused much public disquiet. What was preventing maternity-related mortality from falling? How could this disturbing experience be reversed? When death threatens, societies in search of a remedy turn to their medicine men, to their doctors. And the doctors of Western medicine were very willing to accept the challenge (Chapters 7 and 8).

BIRTH ATTENDANTS AND THEIR CHANGING STATUS

There had, of course, been a long history of outstanding medical men who studied and tried to relieve the problems of childbirth. There was an even longer history of competent midwives who eased the problems of childbirth in practice and of a few midwives who were able to study the subject and write instructional books about it. But in the later 19th century many birth attendants were not competent. The great majority of them were then, as they had always been, women. They could be professional midwives, trained by apprenticeship with or without some formal, theoretical instruction; or self-trained handywomen who picked up their skills by observation and practical experience and who were cheaper to employ than the trained midwives; or the untrained, unskilled helpers, the relations, friends or neighbours, who were cheapest of all to employ for they only expected to be paid by some reciprocal service.

It is probable that some of the practices of the handywomen and untrained helpers actually added to the already considerable risks of the poor women they attended. Doctors might condemn these birth attendants, but they would not have considered replacing them for such low financial rewards. As their interest in childbirth extended, however, doctors soon recognized professional midwives as commercial rivals who undercut the market they wanted by charging lower fees. Doctors were, therefore, only too willing to attribute the high mortality in childbearing to the incompetence of midwives. They claimed, without any supporting evidence, to provide a safer service, albeit at a higher price. Attacks on their professional skills gave increased urgency to the aspirations of midwives to regulate their profession and improve their training, but ironically their success in doing so involved the sacrifice of their traditional supremacy as providers of maternity care.

As the 20th century progressed, the formally trained midwife ousted her informally trained colleague and the untrained handywoman, but her role became increasingly subordinate to that of the doctor. It was particularly so in hospital where she worked virtually as an obstetric nurse. She had more respect and greater independence of practice when she delivered mothers in their homes. The policy of the increasing hospitalization of birth advocated by doctors, allegedly to improve the welfare of mothers and babies, was in fact a very effective means of gaining competitive advantage by reducing the power and status of midwives and confirming the doctors' ascendancy over their professional rivals.

Professional rivalry was not limited to the contest between the male-dominated medical profession and the female midwifery profession. The medical profession was itself divided into generalists: those doctors who undertook maternity care as an integral part of general patient care – indeed it was the corner-stone around which general practices were built up – and specialists: those doctors whose whole time was devoted to the study and treatment of the illnesses associated with reproduction. Until the 1920s, the generalists predominated in numbers and influence. Most of their maternity patients, like their other patients, were attended in their homes, though a fashion was growing among their richer clientele for treatment in private nursing homes and small local hospitals. The trend towards delivery in such institutions continued in Britain after maternity care became free on the introduction of the National Health Service in 1948.

The territory of the specialist obstetrician was always the hospital, the workshop where cases of obstetric pathology could be assembled, their problems studied and treatments devised and monitored. But the speciality of obstetrics, or midwifery as it used to be called, did not yet have a separate status as an academic discipline. It received little esteem from the ancient faculties of medicine and surgery, to which it was related. In the 1920s, obstetricians campaigned successfully to assert their independence. The British (later Royal) College of Obstetricians and Gynaecologists was founded in 1929 and quickly became very influential in exalting the status of obstetricians and eventually ensuring their domination of maternity care.

To do this they had to discredit and constrain not only the independent midwives, but also the general practitioner obstetricians. The latter were gradually persuaded that they were competent to attend only restricted categories of women defined as being at low risk, while after 1970 in Britain administrative Health Authorities were gradually persuaded to close the small hospitals where obstetricians had little influence. Indeed, after the operation of the National Health Service had relieved general practitioners of the obligation to ensure their incomes by building up their practices by themselves, they no longer found complete maternity care to be so essential a corner-stone. A survey of practices before 1955 found that only 30% of the general practitioners interviewed were anxious to do midwifery [7]. Many, probably most, found that it suited them to be persuaded that they were not competent to provide any intranatal care, which made unpredictable and often inconvenient demands on time in exchange for the disproportionately small additional reward their terms of service provided. It turned out that the method which was adopted by the new National Health Service of remunerating general practitioners, mainly by capitation fee for patients registered on practice lists and only marginally by fee for specific service, was to have an unintended side-effect of great importance to the maternity service, that of discouraging their involvement in intranatal care (Chapter 2).

CHANGING PRACTICES IN INTRANATAL AND ANTENATAL CARE

The place of birth is related to the kind of care that different categories of birth attendant are qualified to give. But more fundamentally, the relationship is with the different kind of care which different birth attendants believe that it is biologically right to give. The traditional role of midwives was, as the medieval derivation of their name denotes, to be 'with woman' throughout her labour, giving her emotional support and encouragement. The midwife's skills lay in ensuring the necessary hygiene and in knowing how to help the labouring woman to use her own reproductive powers to bring forth her child naturally and without damage. Her skills were essentially non-interventive and the philosophy which underlay her practice was of the biological rightness and sufficiency of the natural process. As the influence of obstetricians on the midwifery training programmes increased, the philosophy became compromised and midwives were permitted and taught to perform certain interventions, but mostly at a low level of technology and capable of being practised in the home without fixed equipment. They were not allowed to acquire technical skills which would have made them effective substitutes for obstetricians.

But when the woman's pathological state raised obstacles to natural delivery too great for the woman's powers and the midwife's skill to overcome, the doctor had to be called in to complete the process with the use of instruments. Until the 20th century, this was done primarily to save the life of the mother; later motivation was more often to save the life of the baby and ease the distress of the mother. Doctors, whose predecessors invented obstetric forceps in the 17th century, retained the monopoly of their use thereafter. The manipulation of forceps requires the doctor to stand by the supine woman, the position which the Latin derivation of their name, obstetrician, describes.

To their monopoly of instrumental delivery, the doctors added in the 19th century another monopoly, the administration of general anaesthesia for the relief of pain. These extra services, despite their extra cost, increased the demand for doctors as birth attendants. The services could be performed in the home, but more conveniently for the doctor in a hospital where he encouraged his patients to come. In other respects the doctor's midwifery practices were similar in restraint to those of the midwife. Well into the 20th century, undergraduate medical schools were still preaching the doctrine of 'masterly inactivity', waiting for the birth process to complete itself naturally. When serious complications in labour called for operative delivery (and after advances in surgery had made obstetric operations less hazardous) or when they called for continuous intensive supervision, the appropriate place of delivery had to be the specialist obstetric hospital. When, after 1950, the range of interventions, surgical, pharmacological and electronic, proliferated and required the use of expensive technological equipment the only place they could be carried out was the obstetric hospital. As obstetricians became more confident to use the interventions at their disposal, they increasingly abandoned the philosophy of restraint. They redefined normality in pregnancy and labour to justify the widespread practice of antenatal, intranatal and postnatal interventions, so that the need, as they perceived it, for most births to take place in hospital became inevitable. And since obstetricians, despite their vaunted skills, could never predict with accuracy when a complication would arise, the sensible precaution was to take every step to ensure that all births should take place in their kind of hospital.

There was no possibility around this time of making birth in hospital a legal obligation, much as some obstetricians, then and later, might have wished it, for any proposal to do so would have incurred the immediate disapproval of public opinion as an assault on individual freedom. It would have aroused lively opposition from defenders of human rights. It was not until the 1980s, with near total hospitalization secured, that some obstetricians in the USA and Australia, noticing with apprehension the signs of renewed interest among women in giving birth at home, thought it necessary finally to assure their monopoly by advocating compulsory hospitalization (pages 26, 245). But before this recent panic, legal compulsion was judged to be superfluous as long as the objective could be attained by more subtle strategies designed to overcome every obstacle and close up every loop-hole by one means or another. The overriding need was to propagate the belief that birth was essentially dangerous and only under obstetric control could the danger be reduced. If parents wanted live, healthy babies, if communities wanted to replace themselves with vigorous stock, they had to be persuaded that this could only be achieved by entrusting the management of pregnancy and delivery to obstetricians working in obstetric hospitals.

And the earlier the indoctrination started, the more effective would it be. Antenatal care, a concept of the 20th century, was soon embraced as the perfect example of preventive medicine. Regular clinical examinations would detect deviations from normality in time to correct them or at least keep them from jeopardizing a safe birth. Although most diagnostic techniques and available therapies have in reality never been accurate or appropriate enough to meet the challenge, antenatal clinics have provided an excellent medium for replacing the mother's trust in the adequacy of her own physiology to achieve safe reproduction, by trust in the powers of obstetric management to achieve a superior outcome.

In most spheres of human activity, confidence is of great importance in leading to successful results. In no sphere is this more true than in childbirth where the physiological processes are so intimately dependent on psychological states. In the sphere of maternity care the obstetricians' objective was to make their profession the sole repository of confidence. To achieve this objective required an unremitting campaign of propaganda. This proved to be astoundingly successful in winning the approval, active or passive, of the vast majority of the population, through tactics which roused both positive and negative reactions. The propaganda won the approval, or certainly numbed the critical faculties, of the wider medical profession, as well as of legislators and administrators whose responsibility it is to formulate and execute policies for the organization of the maternity service. It inspired the confidence of the lay public, but most critically, it destroyed the confidence of mothers in their own reproductive efficiency and it destroyed the confidence of the alternative birth attendants, midwives and general practitioners who believed in restraint and practised accordingly (Chapters 3 and 4).

TARGETS FOR PROPAGANDA

The medical profession

The message propagated received a positive welcome, or at least it was accepted with little hesitation, from the wider medical profession. All branches of medicine were becoming more scientific in outlook. Advances in the understanding of all aspects of human biology led to the development of effective, scientifically based treatments for illnesses, both curative and preventive. It seemed a reasonable analogy that greater understanding of the physiology of childbirth should lead to the development of effective treatments, both curative and preventive, for its pathology. It was accepted as an inevitable corollary that preventive treatments would involve interference in the natural process of apparently healthy pregnancies. There is a long history in all fields of medicine of failure to evaluate new treatments before approval of their adoption as standard practice. There seemed no reason to have a different attitude to obstetric innovations.

After 1950, academic departments of obstetrics burgeoned, but their activities in the fields of biochemical and biophysical research far outstripped their activities in psycho-social or in epidemiological research. They did not investigate and so did not come to understand the fundamental interrelationships between emotional and physical processes, underestimating the importance of the former and overestimating the independence of the latter. When the results came to be reported of evaluative research which did not support accepted doctrine, doctrine and practice have been modified reluctantly or not at all in accordance with the findings.

For many years, despite the increased input of medical resources into maternity care, the mortality rates remained stubbornly high. But now at last obstetricians were propounding a new doctrine and now at last mortality rates had fallen and were continuing to do so. It was all too easy to believe that the decline in mortality was the result of the new obstetric methods.

Separate departments within university medical faculties show great mutual tolerance. They do not criticize each other's research nor the principles which underlie what they teach to students. Thus developments in obstetrics were taken on trust as worthy of scientific respect. The logical pitfall of assuming a causal relationship between coincidental trends was ignored, without consideration, by obstetricians. It was likewise ignored by the wider medical profession, which had often been lured into the same pit by the prospect of promoting their interests, directly or indirectly, by such illogical assumptions, for example in encouraging the public's belief that its health depends chiefly on medical care. The obstetricians' position was greatly strengthened by having at least the tacit, and more often the explicit, approval of the leaders of medical thought (Chapter 9).

Official advisory committees and administrators

The logical pitfall of spurious correlation and the lack of analysis of results were more culpably ignored by official committees which were appointed in Britain, ostensibly to give sound and impartial advice to the Minister of Health on what provisions should be made for the maternity service. Naturally, the members of the committees or their advisors included medical experts and the influence of obstetricians was particularly strong. So-called 'evidence' was taken from interested parties, but their submissions amounted to no more than statements of their sectional opinions, which they seem never to have been asked to support with factual evidence, and the material they submitted was never critically scrutinized for validity. The recommendations made in the reports of these committees were not at all impartial but largely endorsed the fallacious submissions of the most eloquent witnesses, the obstetricians' representatives, and gave the sanction of official authority to the obstetricians' ambitions.

An abrupt and radical break with this traditional approach to assembling and assessing information was made by the House of Commons Health Committee under its chairman, Nicholas Winterton, when in the session 1991–2 it conducted a further inquiry into the maternity services. It took evidence from a wide range of individuals and groups, users and providers of the services, as well as impartial researchers who had evaluated relevant outcomes (the first edition of this book, *Safer Childbirth?*, being included). In sharp contrast to its predecessors, the committee considered the evidence with open minds and came to the conclusion that the arguments put forward by the critics of the service, with supporting evaluated data, were far more convincing than the unsupported assertions of obstetricians. Therefore in 1992 it produced its Report which recommended a fundamental change in the philosophy which underlies the service which should henceforward be organized in the interests of the users, the mothers and babies, and no longer in the interests of the providers unless there was clearly no conflict between these [8].

Such recommendations implied radical changes in practical provisions. To ensure that the Winterton Committee had properly understood the issues involved and judged impartially, the Department of Health appointed an Expert Maternity Group to carry out a further review of policy. The title, *Changing Childbirth* [9], of the report in 1993 of this independent committee announces that it too was convinced that reorganization was necessary and that 'women and their families should be at the centre of maternity services which should be planned and provided with their interests and those of their babies in mind'. Not surprisingly, organized obstetricians disapproved of future changes to their disadvantage and did what they could to obstruct them.

The lay administrative and executive officers should also have been impartial on clinical issues. Management control, however, is probably simpler when deliveries are concentrated in institutions, preferably large institutions, than when they are dispersed throughout the community. The officers had no professional interest in disputing the policy of their medical colleagues whose views they are accustomed to respect. They were apparently quickly persuaded of its rightness and willingly played their part in its implementation by extending facilities for delivery in obstetric hospitals and curtailing facilities for delivery anywhere else, if necessary colluding with other health personnel to do so (page 17 and Chapter 5). Their reactions to changes called for by the Winterton and Changing Childbirth Reports cannot yet be known in 1993.

General practitioners of the 'old school'

The lack of validating evidence was not, however, seized upon by opponents of hospitalization and obstetric management. Most of the doctors who believed in non-intervention reluctantly came to concede that the propaganda must be true since everyone else believed it. They found themselves swimming against the ever-rising tide of pressure from their professional colleagues. Certainly, they increasingly conformed to the restrictive booking rules that were being imposed on them and participated less and less in intranatal care.

A few of those who were most sceptical about the new obstetric dogma and who had kept their own careful records were able to write up their results. They produced evidence of perinatal mortality rates very much lower under their care than in hospital and showed that this was not achieved by booking for or transferring to hospital all the potentially difficult cases. (Perinatal mortality comprises stillbirths and deaths in the first week of life.) In the 1950s and 1960s in areas where hospital beds were scarce or considered to be too far away, most bookings were for general practitioner care. Inevitably, they included some at high predicted risk and some which developed complications whatever their predicted risk, but the general practitioners were accustomed to managing abnormal deliveries and did so while maintaining a perinatal mortality rate below, often far below, the national average. For example, a general practitioner reported that in a rural practice in Kent, between 1946 and 1970, there was

a low rate of booking and delivery in hospital, a relatively large proportion of high risk cases under sole practitioner care, a low rate of transfer from GP to consultant care at all stages, a majority of complicated cases managed by GPs

and a perinatal mortality rate, including transfers, about two-thirds of the national average [10]. Other general practitioners in Scotland and Essex were able to estimate from their results that they could have cared safely for 95% and 80–85% of cases in their respective practices [11,12]. Yet such carefully documented analyses carried no weight with obstetricians and those responsible for policy in the maternity service:

Obstetric indications for booking . . . appear to be based on the assumption that general practitioners should never be placed in the position that they should have to exercise their judgement on an obstetric matter [12].

A few of the diminishing number of general practitioners who have continued to offer intranatal care since 1970 have reported their results [13–19]. They are allowed to deal with fewer complicated cases, but the outcome for the low-risk women they do attend is very good indeed. Obstetricians are adamant, however, that these good results are only achieved by the transfer to hospital at some stage of all cases with the slightest risk of an unfavourable outcome and that they do not constitute a satisfactory reason for opposing total hospitalization. The validity of this counter-claim will be examined in Chapter 8.

This minority of 'old school' doctors found themselves increasingly at odds with the majority of their colleagues. These included an older group, who found it more convenient to hand over intranatal care to hospital obstetricians, and a younger group of post-1950 graduates.

General practitioners of the 'new school'

For recently trained doctors the convenience argument could be rationalized by positive conviction of the rightness of the new practices and by negative fear, for their teachers impressed on them that they were not competent to conduct a delivery without specialist supervision (pages 17, 68).

By referring patients, and if necessary directing the less willing of them, to hospital, these converts became the most effective instrument through which the obstetricians' monopoly of childbirth was secured. In many cases, the tactics they used to persuade or direct were unethical and reprehensible. They frightened women by exaggerating the dangers of confinement at home or in a GPU, while they omitted to mention the dangers of confinement in hospital. They rebuked unwilling women for selfishness and irresponsibility in preferring their personal comfort to the safety of their babies' lives. They raised every conceivable objection, real and imagined, practical, medical and legal, to home delivery. If all else failed, they withdrew their medical service, not only to the woman for conditions connected with her pregnancy, but also to the rest of her family for any illness.

Journals and newsletters, such as the organs of the National Childbirth Trust and the Association for Improvements in the Maternity Services (pages 234–9) in which consumers can report their personal experience of maternity care, have over the years printed many testimonies of women from all parts of Britain of the deliberately unkind and unjust treatment they have received from their family doctors and obstetric consultants when they dared to ask to give birth at home. Doctors who behave in this way disregard the prejudicial effect on outcome of the stress they cause to the pregnant woman. Their behaviour flouts the founding rule of the profession, first do no harm, yet organized medical bodies have taken no action to prevent it. Apparently they accept the doctors' defence that their behaviour is necessary to protect the true interests of stubborn, unreasonable and misguided women and those of their babies or, alternatively, to protect themselves from any liability should the predicted disaster occur and be the subject of litigation.

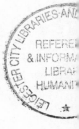

The experience of British women has not been unique. It has been repeated many times over in countries like the USA, Canada and Australia, where medical policy is antagonistic to home birth and medical tactics serve the same purpose.

Midwives

Throughout the 20th century, the thinking of leaders of the midwifery profession has been much influenced by the opinions of obstetricians and they have been steadily weaned from adherence to the philosophy of non-intervention to acceptance of the advantages claimed for intervention. Moreover, like the doctors, they have found practical compensations for the erosion of their independence and responsibility. To set against the loss of the job satisfaction of providing total, continuous midwifery care is the attraction of predictable hours of work in hospital, albeit with the impaired satisfaction of providing fragmented care. In hospital they are likely to work only in the antenatal clinic or in the labour ward or in the postnatal wards. Even in the labour ward their responsibility finishes at the end of their shift, whatever the stage of delivery the mother has reached.

For many years, the official voice of the Royal College of Midwives was in harmony with that of the Royal College of Obstetricians and Gynaecologists. Though dissent among midwives started to be organized from the mid-1970s, many midwives in senior administrative posts remained converted to the policy of hospitalization and made their contribution to frustrating the aspirations of non-conforming mothers.

To protect mothers from treatment by incompetent midwives, a system of supervision of midwives was introduced as one of the reforms following the *Midwives Act, 1902* (pages 242–3). The office of Supervisor of Midwives continues to be carried out with commendable attention to the duty of ensuring that high standards of practice are maintained. The standards set, however, tend to be those that would be acceptable to obstetricians. Practice that is more in accordance with the principles of non-interventive midwifery or with the acknowledgement that the mother's wishes, even if not conforming with current orthodoxy, should be respected is liable to provoke stern disapproval and suspension for the offending midwife, without pay and sometimes for a long period. Deregistration is the ultimate penalty. With the risk of such threats to their careers and livelihoods, midwives are effectively deterred from offering mothers a service deviating from officially accepted standards, even when in their judgement these are not in the best interest of the mother concerned.

The rising generation of birth attendants

Whatever problems there had been in converting established birth attendants to the new orthodoxy, obstetricians took effective steps to ensure that they were not repeated with their successors. Once the dogma had been proclaimed and accepted by staff in the obstetric departments of Universities, Teaching Hospitals and Schools of Midwifery, the students were soon indoctrinated and the favoured attitudes firmly implanted. They were required to believe unquestioningly what they were taught on their teachers' authority alone and without supporting evidence. Students found that, to be sure of passing examinations, it was safer to conform, whatever their original attitudes had been.

Instruction in theory and clinical practice was appropriately revised, so that new medical graduates and, to a lesser degree, certified midwives, found themselves qualified to carry out intranatal care only with reliance on interventions which they were conditioned to believe were usually necessary and certainly beneficial. They were deprived of experience of physiological childbirth, of delivery achieved by the natural process throughout. They were deprived of confidence in their ability to supervise the event without the immediate availability of technical aids of lesser or greater sophistication, which means in any place other than the obstetric hospital.

In consequence, it came to pass that local health authorities in Britain were able to argue that, although a woman had a legal right to demand a home birth and they had a legal obligation to supply a midwife, the law was unrealistic and could not be complied with, for they had no midwives in their employment with the experience, confidence and competence to conduct a home delivery and could not count on finding a general practitioner willing to provide medical cover for the birth. Hence they adopted a variety of stratagems to absolve themselves from their legal obligation: they tried to persuade the woman to withdraw her demand in the face of the concerted contrary advice of medical officers, midwives and health visitors. If that was insufficient persuasion, they could convince her to withdraw by supplying an attendant who was disposed quickly to diagnose an impending complication for which care in hospital was mandatory. Thus did local health authorities interact with educators to add their contribution to the obstacle race any mother must run if she sought to avoid a hospital confinement.

For one reason or another, it was hardly surprising that so few women finished up by giving birth at home, whatever their original preferences might have been (Chapter 2).

Mothers

Obstetricians, contemplating the fait accompli, like to say that women showed their approval of the obstetric management of childbirth by opting for hospital delivery 'with their feet'. The strength of forces propelling them in that direction left women with little alternative. In addition to the advice of their doctor, they were bombarded from all sides with admonitions that to give birth anywhere else was to endanger their own and their baby's life. They heard the message on television and radio programmes; they read it in the daily press and women's magazines. The media, for all their vaunted mission to expose injustice and discuss both sides of an issue, devoted far more time and space to relaying obstetric orthodoxy than to questioning its soundness. Irrespective of political persuasion, they appeared to be curiously timid about conducting any sustained campaign opposing the medical establishment. Any temporary episodes of interest stirred up by enterprising journalists were soon extinguished. In this behaviour, the lay media reflected the attitude of their medical counterparts, who seemed equally unwilling to press criticisms of obstetric orthodoxy.

Women's self-confidence was under continuous attack and was often not improved by their experience of antenatal care, which obstetricians had come increasingly to dominate. Monitoring the health of a woman during pregnancy was a 20th century innovation (Chapter 3). At first in Britain it was mainly organized by local health authorities and carried out by their own medical officers and midwives. When the National Health Service enabled all mothers to have free antenatal care from their family doctor, most of them did so and general practitioners then found themselves the usual provider of this part of the maternity service. But at the same time, more antenatal clinics were being set up or extended in hospital to cater for the increasing number of women booking for hospital delivery.

The objective of antenatal care had at first been to build up the mother's general health. Under the influence of obstetricians the emphasis changed to detecting, and if possible correcting, any condition in pregnancy which could endanger a safe outcome. Some of the diagnostic tests require only modest equipment and can be carried out satisfactorily in the woman's home or her doctor's surgery. Recent scientific advances have made possible more sophisticated diagnostic procedures, like ultrasound scanning, amniocentesis, cardiotocography (Chapter 3) and others, which require expensive technological equipment and specialized technical staff to operate it. These facilities can only be provided in an obstetric hospital where most women must now expect to have at least some of their antenatal care. Women whose pregnancies are found to deviate in any way from accepted normality are almost certainly referred to hospital for care. Diagnostic tests never give results which are 100% accurate, so they tend to be interpreted over-cautiously to avoid the risk of missing real danger signals. Apprehension is increased among mothers suspected, whether rightly or wrongly, of some abnormality and so, in turn, is their willingness to accept the need for specialist care.

The treatment prescribed for certain conditions in pregnancy requires antenatal inpatient care in hospital. It has been found that women of comparable health status are more likely to be admitted for such care if they have their antenatal care at hospital clinics than elsewhere [20]. The criterion of need seems to depend, not simply on the maternal condition, but also on the accessibility of hospital beds. Unless financial restrictions apply, there are medico-political incentives to fill vacant beds and patients can most easily be recruited from among women attending the hospital's outpatient antenatal clinic. Women are thus conditioned to regarding hospital as the appropriate haven for the care of the ills, real or suspected, of pregnancy and in due course labour. The increase in antenatal admissions to hospital from 15% of deliveries in 1973 to 34% in 1985 suggests a much more generous interpretation of maternal morbidity [21].

It is the inherent disadvantage of any system for the detection of prognostic signs of abnormality that it may implant in the subject some fear that the abnormal condition already exists or is likely to develop. Unless certain cure or prevention can be offered to give complete reassurance, the anxiety created may bring its own dangers which have to be set alongside the dangers of the undisturbed, although possibly false, confidence of ignorance.

It would, however, be quite wrong to imply that all women, or even a majority of them, complied against their wills with a system imposed on them. Most came to acquiesce with greater or lesser enthusiasm in the new arrangements. They certainly did want to produce live healthy babies and they were willing to concede that 'doctor knows best' and accept the new advice he was giving. In Britain and other Western countries, but not apparently Holland where the influence of midwives has remained considerable, mothers had learned to fear labour as an ordeal at best unpleasant, at worst unbearable. The prospect of handing over responsibility for its conduct to a doctor versed in technical skills for assisting the process was not unattractive, especially with the added inducement of effective pain relief. At all events it seemed a reasonable and brief sacrifice for that promised long-term advantage, declared to be otherwise unattainable.

But in any case many women did not regard hospitalization as a sacrifice. Since the 19th century women in the upper and middle classes had been choosing doctors rather than midwives as their birth attendant and gradually some kind of hospital rather than home as the place of delivery (Chapter 2). The practical attraction of a hospital confinement increased as standards of comfort there were raised and the environment made less austere. Some mothers were glad to be relieved briefly of their domestic responsibilities and to avoid disorganization in their own homes. Problems of later readjustment could be faced if and when they arose.

In time, hospital confinement became the model to which women of the lower classes aspired. It was desired as an assertion of social equality. So the co-operative attitude of women of all social classes was another potent factor in facilitating the transition to total hospitalization.

As with the poorer classes in a relatively rich country, so with all classes in a relatively poorer country, the demand for hospital maternity care represents escape from the stigma of poverty and social inferiority. Though misguided, this may prove to be as powerful a motive as the desire to reduce the risks of childbirth in influencing the organization of maternity care in less economically developed countries. The organized medical profession will always be glad to encourage such aspirations.

When given the opportunity to choose between birth attendants, the woman's preference for doctors (once always male) may have been based on more than the promised superiority of their clinical skills. Psychologists have hypothesized that the changed attitude arose from deep psycho-sexual causes – the female fantasy of the weak woman being rescued from distress and danger by the strong male. The doctor's motives for becoming involved in maternity care may arise from similar deep causes – the male fantasy of the strong man rescuing the weak woman from distress and danger. After his essential contribution to initiating the process, the male takes no further part, biologically, in reproduction. The mystery and power of creation is vested in the female. The male is said to resent, at least subconsciously, this exclusion and the implication of inferiority.

Anthropologists detect different ways in which this resentment is manifested in different cultures. In Western medicine, the male obstetrician reasserts his superiority over the female when he finds her body unable to carry out its function of reproduction competently by itself and he can take over her prerogative by intervening to assist and complete the process. He reasserts his superiority most emphatically when he cuts open the womb and extracts the baby without any cooperation from the mother, an intervention apparently so deeply satisfying to the operator that, now that its danger to life is relatively small, is imposed on ever slighter pretexts (Chapter 4).

At a personal and superficial level, the socially approved obstetrician/patient relationship legitimates a limited and non-committal physical intimacy which gives pleasure to some men and some women. For women at the other extreme, the physical intimacy from which they can only escape by forgoing professional care is a constant source of disgust, distress and tension.

At a general and deeper level, a more cynical theory is that the male acquisition of the domination of childbirth and society's acceptance of this situation represent a fundamental counter-attack on the female's strivings and achievements along the road towards political and economic equality. Cynics see this as a salutary demonstration that inroads into man's territory have been accompanied by the surrender of her own, woman's territory – a universal acknowledgement of her essential subservience.

Many male obstetricians would resent having their choice of career attributed to any of these psycho-sexual or socio-sexual motives. A more prosaic explanation is that their choice was unemotional and quite pragmatic: their first ambition was to be a specialist doctor and obstetrics, combined with surgical gynaecology, was the speciality with the most promising career appointment vacant when they made their choice.

THE POWER STRUGGLE

Hospitalization of childbirth is the medium through which the philosophy of interventive obstetrics is carried into practice. That philosophy, now held by most obstetricians, is opposed to the philosophy of non-interventive midwifery, once held by all and still held by many midwives. One philosophy cannot take precedence over the other unless its practitioners likewise take precedence. For the realization of total hospitalization of birth, a necessary condition was the resolution of a power struggle between the rival providers of maternity care, a struggle in which career obstetricians gained victory over career midwives. However, the original reason for the struggle was, not the idealistic aim of asserting the superiority of a philosophy, but the self-centred aim of securing better career opportunities for male obstetricians in a hitherto female occupation. They won the interprofessional contest partly because of the poor fighting qualities of the midwives and the weakness of their occupational organization, inherent female characteristics (Chapter 2).

Unlike men, women in all occupations seem to have a basic disinclination to grasp the material advantages to be gained for themselves through organizing in a trade union in order to pursue their group interests at the expense of competitors. Midwives in earlier centuries never succeeded in doing so. They were never persuaded to try to emulate the success of male trade guilds and professional colleges. When in the late 19th century their thinking changed and they got around to setting up their own professional organization, they were heavily dependent on advice and support from sympathetic doctors. In any case, the regulation of midwives was, from 1902 to 1983, in the hands of the Central Midwives Board (CMB), the body which was appointed to implement the provisions of the 1902 *Midwives Act* but which for most its life included only a minority of midwives among its members. The College (later Royal) of Midwives was prevented from exercising the same authority over its members as the medical Colleges did over theirs and the authority was further weakened by the considerable influence on it of obstetrician colleagues. This has been a sort of 'Trojan horse', which discouraged organized midwives from perceiving their professional interests as opposed to those of obstetricians and so from organizing effective self-defence. Obstetricians' influence at this level was greatly assisted by their influence, through the CMB, over midwives' training, which progressively undermined new midwives' faith in an old, and opposing, creed.

But in fact, many individual midwives did not see obstetricians, on whose interventions they relied in cases of complicated delivery, as opponents. Exemplifying the 'inferior sex' stereotype, midwives (weak and female like their clients) recognized the limitations of their skills and waited to be rescued by obstetricians (strong and male). Whether or not the intervention called for would also rescue the mother or the baby, the midwife had let someone with different skills take over responsibility for the outcome. She deferred to a superior profession and her defence was enshrined as a legal obligation under the regulations of the *Midwives Act*, 1902.

Organized midwives, from inclination and legal necessity, shared this attitude of ultimate inferiority and were disposed to bow to the superior wisdom of organized obstetricians with whom they would have preferred to co-operate than dispute. While they were agreeably co-operating, the interests of midwives as midwives with a philosophy of their own were steadily being eroded and their occupational subordination confirmed. But the significance of the struggle was wider than its direct effect on the professional groups concerned. The obstetricians' victory for their occupation implied also victory for their philosophy, victory for the medical management of procreation, which directly affects everyone.

As obstetric management came increasingly to dominate intranatal care in the 1970s, some midwives became urgently aware of the threat to their survival as a profession and as practitioners of a fundamental philosophy. A group of them organized a movement, which they called the Association of Radical Midwives [22], within the Royal College of Midwives to reassert their role as the guardians of normal childbirth, which, in the absence of obstetric interference, would be completed without complication in around 80% of cases. Their thinking, backed by impartial analyses of the results of maternity care which had been published since 1977 and investigations by the World Health Organization, influenced the Royal College of Midwives to adopt a more independent stance and introduce their own proposals for reform (Chapter 2).

BIRTH ATTENDANTS ABROAD

In the course of the 20th century, the British midwife has undoubtedly sacrificed much of her independence of practice and public esteem for her profession as midwife, in favour of her role as obstetric nurse, increasingly competent to operate sophisticated technological instruments but less competent to empathize with the mother and facilitate the physiological process of labour and delivery. But she has not sacrificed all her independence, all her status, all her traditional skills. This is in marked contrast to experience in some other countries, notably the USA, Canada and Australia, where the midwife has been all but annihilated through the actions and propaganda of a politically powerful obstetric profession.

Since professional midwives in so many countries are weak, it is not surprising that their International Confederation, formed again in 1951 after its wartime disbandment, has been unable to give its members effective support in re-asserting the philosophy of non-interventive midwifery and winning political recognition for its practice. But if it can do little to protect the professional status of midwives, its triennial conferences generate great enthusiasm and mutual comfort among the members who participate, so that hopes are kept alive that future reforms are worth fighting for (Chapter 2).

In this regard also, obstetricians have been much more effective. In the 1930s, the young British College of Obstetricians and Gynaecologists was quick to extend its influence to the then Dominions of the British Commonwealth. The American College of Obstetricians and Gynecologists was founded in 1951. International co-operation and consultation flourished and was soon formalized in 1954 in the International Federation of Gynaecologists and Obstetricians, an organization with considerable influence and success in propagating widely the beliefs and practices of interventive obstetrics.

OTHER ALLIES FOR OBSTETRICIANS

Anaesthetists

Obstetricians have been joined in recent decades by powerful allies who profit from the operation of obstetric management. As new anaesthetic agents and techniques for their administration have been developed, the discipline has become too complicated to be left under the control of anyone other than a specialist anaesthetist. The service of an anaesthetist is required whenever general anaesthesia has to be administered, as when delivery is by caesarean section – an increasingly favoured procedure in many obstetric hospitals – or when the mother asks for epidural anaesthesia to relieve her pains while she remains conscious, a plea encouraged increasingly by her birth attendants.

Anaesthetists have acquired a vested interest in the kind of obstetric management that creates jobs for them by making them essential members of the obstetric team. A very small number of maternal deaths are caused by the tragic side-effects of anaesthesia. If these are to be prevented, specialist anaesthetists claim that they must be involved. If their availability is essential for a safe delivery, and if all mothers are to be given the option of comprehensive pain relief, as anaesthetists advocate, then birth must take place in their workplace, the hospital. Adequate, or indeed any, anaesthetic cover cannot be provided in GPUs or the family home and this makes them, in the opinion of organized anaesthetists, totally unsuitable places for birth, whatever other advantages may be claimed for them (pages 175, 212).

Neonatologists

Many babies, born after operative or instrumental deliveries or to an anaesthetized or drugged mother, are in such a poor condition to start independent life that they have to be resuscitated and removed to a special or intensive care unit where their progress can be monitored through a battery of highly sophisticated electronic instruments. A complex science of neonatology has been built up to save the lives of sick and underdeveloped infants, and doctors have become specialists in this fascinating, often distressing, often rewarding, branch of paediatrics. It is plausible that the sooner special care starts, the sooner will the child recover. For this reason neonatologists can advocate that birth should take place close to the facilities for special or intensive baby care, which exist in the larger obstetric hospitals. This is to ignore the evidence that a much smaller proportion of the babies born outside obstetric hospitals, like the babies born in hospital who escape the invasive interventions, arrive in such poor condition that they need special care at all. The careers of neonatologists depend largely on a regular throughput of sick and immature babies, the victims or perhaps the successes of interventive obstetrics (Chapters 4, 5 and 8).

Manufacturers of drugs and equipment

The advances in interventive obstetrics, anaesthesia and neonatology are dependent on the technological instruments and pharmaceutical products by means of which the interventions are carried out. The manufacturers of these have a strong commercial interest in promoting their use. The sale of drugs has to comply with legally imposed safety regulations, which take account of known dangers, but some dangers do not become known until after, sometimes long after, a drug has been used. Until their products are proved harmful, the drug companies have every incentive to encourage obstetric practices which will maximize their sales.

There is no corresponding restriction on the sale and use of equipment. Instruments of one kind and another have been developed with admirable ingenuity, so that hitherto inscrutable processes or states can be observed or deduced. They have certainly helped to increase knowledge. Whether they have helped to increase wisdom is very doubtful. They are sold on the merits of their fascinating appeal to technologically minded doctors. They are bought and put into routine service without having to show that they result in a net improvement, short-term or long-term, in the welfare of mothers and babies. The sale of medical equipment is a commercial enterprise, pursued with all the techniques of aggressive marketing to achieve immediate gain. The techniques go as far as the financial sponsorship of obstetricians to attend prestigious international conferences at which the sponsor's equipment is displayed and promoted. Such conferences can be educative, but it is difficult for the recipients of gifts to maintain an impartial attitude to the donors and their wares.

The interests of the manufacturers of medical equipment and drugs coincide exactly with the interests of those who preach and practise obstetric management and conflict directly with the interests of those who preach and want to practise natural childbirth. Only the former group of clients has access to the valuable financial support, liberally provided from commercial sources, in the dissemination of propaganda. Also sharing a commercial interest in hospitalization are the manufacturers of baby products, particularly substitutes for breast milk, for they have found the concentration of births there a most convenient environment for sales promotion, though the goods they advertise and later sell are often not in the baby's best interest.

Bringing in the law

More ironic is the obstetricians' success in winning the support of their brother professionals, the lawyers (Chapter 5). The essence of the legal system is that it should probe and sift evidence impartially before a judgement is made. Judges acknowledge their ignorance of medical matters. Their criteria are that treatment given should be in the best interest of the patient and administered by the most effective methods currently known, so that they turn to the reputed experts in the discipline concerned. The experts on childbirth to whom they refer are obstetricians, not midwives.

The experts' integrity is taken for granted. The possibility of a conflict of interest between the providers and receivers of treatment is not addressed. The obstetricians' assertions are accepted without ascertaining that they are based on an unbiased evaluation of clinical and statistical evidence. In particular, lawyers have accepted expert submissions that caesarean section offers the safest solution in cases of obstetric complication and that a record of the fetal heart rate by an electronic monitor is an indispensable indicator of the correctness of further treatment, both opinions for which there is discrediting evidence (Chapters 4 and 8).

Pursuit through litigation of grievances arising in maternity care has become more popular in recent decades. Fear of litigation is quoted as one of the chief reasons for the impressive rise in the incidence of caesarean section and the continued use of electronic monitors. Obstetricians have got themselves into the ridiculous position of having to perform an operation, or carry out a diagnostic procedure, in order to forestall successful litigation on the grounds that they did not do everything possible to secure a safe outcome, when in fact their action is much more likely to prejudice a safe outcome in most cases.

In the USA, hysteria has gone even further. Courts have been persuaded to grant orders forcing women to be detained in hospital and undergo obstetrical procedures, in particular caesarean section, against their will. A body of legal thought is growing that, once it has reached the stage of viability, the fetus has rights distinct from the mother and these rights are to be safeguarded according to the obstetrician's, not the mother's, judgement. The mother is to forfeit her right to be protected from physical assault, which is what a surgical treatment for which she withholds her consent actually is.

Obstetricians would clearly like a legal embargo on any alternative to hospital intranatal care if this were politically and practically feasible. In Britain, the Royal College of Obstetricians and Gynaecologists has suggested to successive Government Committees reviewing the maternity service that recommendations in this direction would be welcome, but the recommendations have not been made, nor have politicians acted on the suggestion. In 1987, a prominent Australian Professor of Obstetrics, who claimed to have widespread support among the medical profession, certainly among obstetricians, called for laws banning home deliveries on the unsustainable grounds that they are much less safe [23].

Despite their almost total monopoly of childbirth care, the anxiety of obstetricians the world over to prevent the slightest competition, by any means however offensive to human rights, surely betrays an uneasy lack of confidence that their style of management is indeed as superior as their propaganda proclaims.

And it was the effectiveness of their propaganda which ensured the obstetricians' ultimate success. Their universally appealing argument in favour of hospitalization was that birth would thereby be made safer for mother and child. Obstetric management would reduce, not only the dangers of complications which had occurred, but also the dangers of complications ever occurring. The natural process, the immensely complex and wonderfully co-ordinated sequence of interdependent events and relationships, the product of aeons of evolution, would be made safer by the interventions devised by 20th century obstetric scientists.

STATISTICAL EVIDENCE

What evidence did obstetricians have to justify their ambitious claim? They constantly drew attention to the coincidental trends of rising hospitalization and falling mortality and implied, indeed asserted, a causal relationship between them (Chapters 6–8). Neither they nor anyone else thought it necessary to test statistically whether this conclusion was valid. When the simple test was eventually carried out by the present author, the claim was found to be unsustainable. The correlation between the annual proportional increases in the rate of hospitalization and the annual proportional decreases in the rate of perinatal mortality was strongly negative. This implies that, if births in obstetric hospitals had not increased, perinatal mortality would have fallen by more than it actually did (pages 344–8 and Figure 8.1).

For the statistical test to be carried out, however, the necessary data had to be available and progress towards total hospitalization was well advanced before this happened. Nevertheless, other statistics were available by the mid-1960s from which highly relevant inferences in the same sense could have been drawn by impartial analysts.

If obstetricians were to be able to show that mortality rates were lower when births took place under their management than when they took place under the supervision of midwives or of general practitioners, they needed to measure the results of care under each system. Measuring results means collecting and collating appropriate statistics and making them available for impartial analysis, so that fair and informative comparisons can be made and valid conclusions drawn.

Collecting and processing statistics is an expensive undertaking. It requires a considerable degree of skill and judgement from those who have to decide what statistics it will be appropriate to collect and how they can be most informatively collated and presented. It requires accuracy and honesty on the part of those who actually collect the original information and compile the necessary data forms. It requires even more skill, judgement and honesty on the part of those who carry out the analysis if their interpretation is to be accurate and impartial. These attributes are just as necessary in the days of computers as they were before.

Specific statistics may be collected prospectively for the research purpose of testing some hypothesis and the cost will be met by whomsoever finances the research topic. No one in any country ever set out to test the hypothesis that hospitalizing birth made it safer. So precisely appropriate statistics for this purpose were never collected. Analysts have to make the best use they can of existing statistics, whether these are derived from official or unofficial sources, provided they are reliable. Most of the official statistics come as the by-product of some administrative requirement, such as the compulsory registration of births and deaths and the management of health services at central and local levels. The collection is financed more or less generously from the public purse.

As stocks of data go, Britain is relatively well endowed, but even so routinely published official statistics before the 1960s were rarely classified by place of birth and the sparse stock of statistical results for earlier years comes mainly from specific investigations. Not many more were so classified after 1960. Nevertheless, they make a useful contribution towards evaluating outcome at each place during the period before the 1980s when hospitalization became virtually complete and effectively put an end to the possibility of making informative and valid comparisons.

SOURCES OF BRITISH STATISTICS

Because total hospitalization came later in England than in most other comparable countries, while at the same time her collection of medical statistics was relatively advanced, she is in a unique position to supply material referring to large national populations and relevant to the evaluation of different systems of care.

Since 1952, the Ministry of Health and its successors, the Department of Health and Social Security and later the Department of Health, have commissioned a continuous review of the causes of the maternal deaths which occur each year. By 1952, the number of these had fallen low enough to make individual enquiries a feasible exercise. The results of these confidential enquiries have been published triennially, but it was only between 1964 and 1975 that they were classified by place of delivery and mortality rates shown relative to the number of births booked, though not necessarily delivered, at each place. The data given did not make it possible to control for differences in the predicted risk status of the mothers booking at each place, beyond their age and parity (the number of children they had previously borne), but mortality rates, in total and at specific ages and parities, were highest for births booked for hospital (page 321). After 1975, maternal deaths were too few to support meaningful analysis by place of confinement (Chapter 7).

In the field of perinatal mortality the endowment is richer. Because infants of low birthweight are at such high risk of dying and because their perinatal deaths make up such a large proportion of the total, the Ministry of Health routinely collected information about them, along with their place of birth. Between 1954 and 1964, the Chief Medical Officer published his analysis of the results in his annual reports. They showed that the rate for stillbirths plus neonatal deaths was very significantly higher if delivery was in a hospital, a category which then included GPUs. He continued to collect the data after 1964 but ceased publishing the results. The unpublished returns for the years 1967 to 1973 were later supplied to the present author in response to her private request. They confirmed the significant excess mortality in hospital (Table 8.3).

Annual records derived from registration data of births and stillbirths, which were published by the Registrar General from 1965 to 1968, also showed that stillbirth rates were much higher in hospital than at home. From 1969 to 1981, the figures were given separately for obstetric hospitals and GPUs and made it clear that it was in the former that the excess mortality occurred. In the course of the 1970s, a drastic reduction was enforced in the number of births at home. This affected principally women who would otherwise have had planned midwifery care and low mortality. Without them, the stillbirth rate for the remaining home births was left increasingly to reflect the high mortality of the small core of women who, though at high risk on account of biological or social factors, made their own choice to reject professional care of any kind. Nevertheless, by 1981 the stillbirth rate in hospital was still significantly higher than in GPUs and home combined (Table 8.7).

The meagre store of official statistics can be supplemented with data obtained from two nationwide sample surveys of births and associated deaths (Chapter 8). These were conducted in 1958 and 1970 under the auspices of the Royal College of Obstetricians and Gynaecologists and were financed by a charity, the National Birthday Trust Fund. They had in fact been preceded in 1946 by a survey of maternity in Great Britain (Chapters 3 and 4), but the statistics published in the report contribute hardly at all to the evaluation of outcome at each place of birth. In 1946 the importance of this issue was not apparently realized.

In the later surveys an immense amount of detailed information was collected about every birth, live and still, that occurred in Britain in one single week of each year, 1958 and 1970, providing representative samples of experience around these periods. The 1958 survey went on to collect information about every stillbirth and neonatal death which occurred in the following three months. The characteristics of these larger numbers of deaths could then be related proportionally to the characteristics of all births to reveal instructive associations. In 1970 information collected on deaths was limited to those occurring in the survey week and so the smaller numbers gave less scope for cross-classifications and subanalyses.

The published results of the surveys (Chapter 8), particularly the one in 1958, provided an invaluable store of information on many aspects of childbirth and quantified many significant associations between predicting risk characteristics and outcomes. The terms of reference for the Steering Committee of the 1958 survey included the gathering of information about the possible effects of the place of confinement. But the published reports, for no explained reason, presented only a few cross-classifications relevant to this issue. To the impartial observer the statistics which were published in whatever detail they were categorized and whatever the predicted risk status of the births concerned, showed consistently and unmistakably an excess of mortality among the births in hospital (Table 8.1). Yet, amazingly, they were interpreted as showing precisely the opposite – an excess of danger for births outside hospital and especially for births at home.

If cross-classifications with other risk factors for which there were survey data would have satisfactorily explained the apparent excess of mortality in hospital it is incredible that they were not published. The distortion of fact was quite out of keeping with the scholarly quality of the rest of the report, which commanded wide respect and probably served to gain credence for the distortion. The other findings did not conflict with professional interests. The finding of excess mortality in obstetric hospitals was in total contradiction of them and proved to be too great a challenge to impartiality.

The biased interpretation or deliberate misinterpretation, reiterated many times in the report, was accepted not only by those who had a professional interest in believing it, but also by a much wider public who mistakenly trusted the experts to be impartial. If anyone, disinterested statistician or other, protested at the time about this blatant misrepresentation, there seems to be no record of such protest in medical annals. On the contrary, frequent references can be found in the literature to the 'conclusive' finding of this survey that the family home is the most dangerous place for birth and this view certainly informed the thinking of those in a position to influence official policy for the maternity service. Its influence in propagating this belief was not limited to Britain. The welcome message was repeated uncritically by obstetricians around the world.

In 1970, about one-third of British births were still taking place outside the obstetric hospitals, but the number of associated perinatal deaths there in the survey week was very small, both absolutely and relatively to births. This was used as the reason for not publishing detailed comparisons with the much larger number of deaths, both absolutely and relatively, associated with births in hospital. Careful scrutiny and re-assembly of the published data, however, enabled mortality rates in specific subgroups of births to be closely estimated. Comparison between results for births in hospital and outside repeated the true findings of the 1958 survey, a consistent excess of deaths in hospital. Explicit data, which would have confirmed this unequivocally, could be derived from the collected material, but they were not published by those in charge of the survey. It was not until 1983, after a persistent campaign carried on for two and a half years by the present author, that the data were finally released. The results were devastating to obstetricians' claims, for they showed that at every level of predicted risk measured, high and moderate as well as low, perinatal mortality was highest by far for births in obstetric hospitals and lowest for births at home (Table 8.6).

But by 1983 revelation of the facts came far too late to influence the course of events. Whether or not by deliberate intention, the results of the 1970 survey, which confirmed the true findings of the 1958 survey and of every other relevant source of data and thus should have changed policy if policy is to benefit the users and not the providers of the maternity service, were obscured and withheld until it was too late to matter. Total hospitalization had already been achieved.

THE EFFECT OF INTERVENTIONS

Was there reason to doubt that these results, which reflected the outcome of obstetric care as a whole, were giving a less than fair picture of the promised benefits of hospitalization? If hospitalization and obstetric management were going to reduce mortality overall, this could only be achieved if mortality was lower in cases when particular interventions were practised than when they were not.

After 1950, maternal mortality from all causes was already falling quickly, related to certain medical treatments but only marginally related to obstetric interventions. Intervention was not often called for in order to save the life of the mother. Even in morbid conditions like severe toxaemia or pre-eclampsia, where the mother's life is in danger until the pregnancy is ended, there is no evidence that the downward trend in mortality was hastened, markedly or indeed at all, by the rising incidence of the induction of labour or elective caesarean section (Chapter 7). By 1991 some leading obstetricians were voicing misgivings about the benefits of interventions. In a memorandum to the Winterton Committee, one Professor wrote, 'It must be recognised that diagnostic and therapeutic interventions have their own intrinsic risk. On some occasions an intervention may cause the harm one is trying to prevent.

An intervention without proven benefit cannot be justified on the basis that it will "do no harm"' [24, p. 800].

Most specific interventions are undertaken ostensibly in the interests of the infant. But in fact they were all introduced and adopted as routine practice without any trials having been conducted to confirm that they did reduce perinatal mortality in the circumstances in which they were being used. Retrospective results showed consistently that mortality was higher in the subgroups subjected to intervention. The conventional defence is that the interventions were only used to avert a greater danger, but this defence cannot be sustained. Induction, for example, was carried out in nearly as many births at low predicted risk as at high and often not as a response to medical indications (page 156). If mortality is higher after individual interventions, irrespective of the predicted risk of the birth, it must follow that overall mortality will be higher under the system of obstetric management which incorporates all the interventions and practises them liberally, even in low-risk subgroups which would otherwise have experienced low mortality rates.

Interventions which need the equipment and expert staff of a specialist hospital are very probably life-saving in certain, but infrequent, obstetric emergencies and when such emergencies occur some distance from a hospital, delay in performing the intervention may well increase the danger to the point of death. Avoiding this potential risk for the few is widely held to be the conclusive argument justifying the total hospitalization of all births.

But obviously, avoiding this danger must be to court others. There is absolutely no evidence that the routine use of interventions prevents the occurrence of emergencies. There is positive evidence that the routine use of interventions increases the dangers of death. In each case this increase may be small, but it affects a lot of cases. In aggregate these 'routine' dangers, added to by the dangers of unnecessary interventions which often follow mistaken diagnoses, far outweigh the 'emergency' dangers. This is what mainly causes the mortality rate for births in specialist hospitals, where such 'routine' dangers are prevalent, to be higher than that for births at home or in non-specialist hospitals, where both 'routine' and 'emergency' dangers are rare.

But the intention of obstetric interventions, devised by experts drawing on a wealth of scientific knowledge, is to improve the ease and safety of childbirth. Are there scientific reasons why they should fail in their purpose? Great discoveries have certainly been made about the physiological processes involved in childbirth, but a great deal about the essential interactions is as yet imperfectly understood. What has been demonstrated is that any artificial interruption at any stage of the naturally ordered processes upsets the co-ordination of the subsequent elements of the integrated sequence and so reduces the safety and efficiency of the whole. In the words of an eminent Dutch Professor of Obstetrics [25]

> . . . Spontaneous labour in a normal woman is an event marked by a number of processes so complicated and so perfectly attuned to each other that any interference with them will only detract from their optimal character . . . the danger will arise that the physiological part of obstetrics will be threatened by doctors who all too often will change true physiological aspects of reproduction into pathology.

Indeed the purpose of many interventions has to be to compensate for and if possible put right the harmful consequences of the damage created by an earlier intervention. Thus is generated the aptly described 'cascade of intervention' [26].

Induction may initiate labour, but it initiates many other problems as well. For the mother there are, inter alia, the physical problems of increased pain, increased need for analgesia or anaesthesia, increased restriction of mobility through having to have a fetal monitor applied, increased need for instrumental or operative delivery, increased risk of postpartum haemorrhage, increased risk of postpartum infection; she is also liable to experience the emotional problems of a sense of her own incompetence and failure and of delayed bonding with her baby. For the baby there are, inter alia, the physical problems of a lesser or greater degree of immaturity, of a reduced oxygen supply and increased distress, of respiratory depression through the absorption of sedative drugs given to the mother, of injury from instrumental or operative delivery. There are no means of knowing whether the baby suffers emotional problems, and how serious they are, from losing its control of the timing of its delivery, from the greater violence of induced contractions and of instruments, physical forces it has not evolved to cope with, or from its greater risk of being separated from its mother for special or intensive neonatal care. The interventions and their consequences will be described more fully in Chapters 4 and 8.

There are, therefore, sound biological reasons why obstetric interventions, however well intentioned, should have failed to make most births safer and sound biological explanations for results which show an excess of mortality among births in hospital under the management of obstetricians.

THE REASONS FOR FALLING MORTALITY

The facts are, however, that by the 1990s for some reason both maternal and perinatal mortality rates had fallen to a small fraction of what they had been fifty years before. The decline had taken place continuously after a long period when these mortality rates, unlike others, had remained persistently high. The English experience was shared by other developed countries and everywhere it happened over the period when the influence of obstetric thinking and practice was increasing rapidly.

The hypothesis that the decrease in mortality was caused by the obstetricians' increased domination of maternity care is seductive but, sadly for its proponents, it does not stand up to impartial investigation. It is opposed on the one hand by statistical results and on the other by biological expectations, factors which are mutually consistent. There must, therefore, be some other hypothesis to explain the decline in mortality and its timing. The obvious alternative is that the declining mortality was brought about by the improving fitness of the procreating population, principally of childbearing women but also of their mates.

In all living species healthy offspring are most likely to come from healthy parents. Declining death rates and increasing expectation of life are reliable indices of a population's improving health status resulting from rising standards of living, especially from better nutrition. But a woman's fitness to reproduce depends only partly on the standard of living and of nutrition she currently enjoys. It depends also on the nutrition she has received since her conception, throughout her fetal, infant and childhood life, when the structure of her body and her reproductive organs were developing.

The trend in death rates indicates that, although the current standards of nutrition enjoyed by women of childbearing age were improving in the late 19th century, their physical development had been inherited from more deprived times. Only after 1900 did the infant environment improve. Smaller family sizes meant more food for each child. Better nutrition not only increased an infant's resistance to infectious diseases, but also to diseases of malnutrition like rickets which impair skeletal development and, in particular, cause malformation of the female pelvis. For women, malformed pelves certainly cause problems at delivery which seriously threaten the survival of both mother and child and malformed pelves were very prevalent among the childbearing women of the 19th century.

As the prevalence of infant malnutrition diminished, so did the incidence of pelvic malformation and other maldevelopment affecting the reproductive system among future mothers. But it was not until the 1930s, two generations after the first decline in the general death rate, that the effect of this improvement began to show and the first signs appeared of a decline in maternal mortality.

It so happened by chance that these first signs were immediately followed by powerful life-saving innovations in medical treatment.

Popular opinion, medical and lay, was quick to give all the credit for the welcome improvements in maternal mortality to the new medical treatments and overlooked the possible contribution of improved maternal health and physique. The earliest and most striking of the medical innovations, the discovery and introduction of antibiotic drugs, was followed by a speedy and steep reduction in maternal deaths from puerperal sepsis. The less dramatic effect of increased resistance to infection by healthier hosts was overshadowed, though discerning observers did recognize that the use of antibiotics did not provide the full explanation of the reduced mortality and morbidity from what had hitherto been a most intractable, and the greatest single, cause of maternal death (Chapters 4 and 7).

The perinatal mortality rate was less quick to fall. Although from the 1940s it did so continuously, the pace of decline was not constant. It was particularly rapid in war-time Britain, but this pace was not achieved again until the 1970s. Most of the mothers in the 1940s had themselves been babies twenty or thirty years earlier when special programmes for maternal and infant welfare were adding to the benefits of generally improving standards of nutrition, or at least giving special protection to these groups from the privations imposed during the world war of 1914–18.

The effect on infants of the economic depression and widespread unemployment of the 1930s, although partially ameliorated by welfare programmes, was reflected in the sluggish decline in perinatal mortality in the 1950s. The high level of employment and the management of the economy during the war years of the 1940s, plus more intensive welfare provisions, led to higher standards of nutrition, particularly for mothers and babies. These were in due course reflected in the accelerated decline in perinatal mortality in the 1970s. Continued post-war economic prosperity and welfare programmes ensured a cohort of mothers sufficiently healthy to withstand the effects of the high level of unemployment in the 1980s and early 1990s, so that perinatal mortality continued to fall (Chapter 8).

Maternal and perinatal mortality are critically dependent on standards of maternal nutrition both during the gestation period and, no less importantly, during the mother's life since her own conception. The process is cumulative over generations. The health and physique of one generation of mothers depends on the health and physique of their mothers and, in turn, of their grandmothers and great grandmothers. The improvement in health of the general population, which manifested itself in lower death rates from 1870, took two generations to manifest itself in lower death rates for mothers and even longer for their babies. Just as improved health caused death rates in general to fall in the absence of effective medical treatments, so would maternal and perinatal death rates have fallen, after the appropriate time lag, in the absence of effective obstetric treatments.

Improving maternal health over the generations has led to a declining perinatal mortality rate to which the greatest contribution has always been made by births of low weight (those under 2500 grams or $5\frac{1}{2}$ pounds). Low-weight births are themselves also strongly correlated with poor maternal health. It might have been expected that the proportion such births make of the total would also decrease as maternal health improved. Surprisingly this has not happened. This may be because the expected decrease has been offset, to a greater or lesser extent, by some of the most frequent obstetric interventions which are designed to forestall the diagnosed impending dangers of continued uterine life, but which inevitably cut short the baby's gestation and may in the end bring dangers more life-threatening than those they avoid.

In the course of the 20th century many treatments have been developed to cure certain types of pathology and prevent others. Where they are effective, they reduce mortality and add to the beneficial consequences of the population's good health. Particularly in the second half of this century, treatments have been developed to cure or prevent certain types of pathology associated with pregnancy and childbirth. Where they are effective, for example, in the prevention of rubella, with its consequent congenital malformations, and of neonatal haemolytic disease caused by maternal rhesus iso-immunization, they reduce mortality of mothers and infants and add to the beneficial consequences of the mother's good health and physique. But they are not always effective and can do more harm than good. This is highly likely if treatments, which may be appropriate for specific pathological conditions which occur in the small minority of cases, are used in healthy pregnancies and labours, which make up the large majority.

FOLLOWING THE WRONG CLUES TO THE WRONG SOLUTION

The coincidence of the improving health status of mothers (and fathers) and of the increasing practice of obstetric interventions in maternity care has had the disastrous consequence of perverting the scientific understanding of what essentially makes birth safe. The professional bias of obstetricians and their medical colleagues, not surprisingly, is to attribute the decline in associated mortality which has already taken place mainly to the results of their treatments. This has suppressed any lingering doubts about the rightness of their philosophy, that nature unassisted is a poor midwife, that the natural process is always fraught with dangers which obstetric interventions can in most cases reduce and in no case increase. It has inspired in them a misplaced confidence that their research should be directed towards creating ever more sophisticated clinical procedures. In fact it has produced a vast amount of information, of value in the study of fetal development and its pathology but of little relevance to the long-term objective of making human reproduction safer.

Research to unlock nature's secrets has been directed down channels at the end of which the Holy Grail does not lie. For obstetricians' interventions concentrate on the physical and biochemical processes of birth and neglect the no less essential emotional processes, the function and effect of which they undervalue. Obstetricians are motivated to undervalue them because emotional processes fall outside their sphere of expertise and acknowledgement of them would impede rather than facilitate implementation of their theories.

From their unsound reading of history they go on to recommend that future improvement can be achieved only by the continuation and intensification of their efforts. Conviction that their diagnosis and prescription are correct blinds them to the overwhelming evidence that supports the alternative philosophy so eloquently summarized by Professor Kloosterman [27]:

> ... giving birth is mostly a normal physiological event which does not require any form of medical intervention ... a natural phenomenon that only requires medical interference in pathological and rather exceptional situations.
>
> ... we cannot improve labour in a healthy woman. We can change the process, we can shorten it, we can speed it up, we can try to take away pain, but at best we will do this without doing any harm. This leads to the conclusion, that the ideal obstetrical organization brings aid to women and children who need help (the pathological group) and protects the healthy ones against unnecessary interference and human meddlesomeness.

HOW OBSTETRICIANS REACHED THEIR GOAL

The later stages of the process which culminated in the obstetricians gaining pre-eminence as providers of maternity care have been completed quickly in the last twenty years. But the foundations for change had been well laid in the development of the contributory and interacting factors over earlier decades and even centuries. Understanding the present situation requires more detailed knowledge of the changing earlier states which led up to it: of the changing roles and changing training of the rival birth attendants; of the changing practices in maternity care, antenatal as well as intranatal and postnatal; of the changing attitudes and expectations of childbearing women; of the changing involvement of society; of the results of maternity care at different periods and how they were misinterpreted, misrepresented and ignored in the determination of policy. This unsatisfactory state should be brought to an end if the reforming recommendations of the recent reports of the Winterton Committee and the Expert Maternity Group are implemented.

The following chapters will outline the historical sequence and inter-action of the events which led up to the revolution in maternity care and make it clear that the chief beneficiaries of the revolution are not, as we are led to believe, mothers and babies, but the dominant provi-ders of care and the supporting professions who share the same interest. The diverse strands of the complicated tapestry will be brought together and the implications for the future will be indicated in the epilogue.

REFERENCES

1. General Register Office/Registrar General. *Reports/Statistical Reviews, Annual 1838–1973*, HMSO, London.
2. Office of Population Censuses and Surveys (1974–92) *Mortality Statistics, Annual. Series DH 1, DH 2, DH 3*, HMSO, London.
3. Office of Population Censuses and Surveys (1974–92) *Birth Statistics, Annual. Series FM 1*, HMSO, London.
4. McKeown, T. (1965) *Medicine in Modern Society*, George Allen and Unwin, London.
5. Lancaster, H.O. (1956) Infant mortality in Australia. *Med. J. Aust.*, **2**, 100–8.
6. Macfarlane, A. and Mugford, M. (1984) *Birth Counts: Statistics of Pregnancy and Childbirth*, National Perinatal Epidemiology Unit, Oxford, in collabora-tion with Office of Population Censuses and Surveys, HMSO, London, Chapter 10.
7. Gillie, A. (1956) in *Proceedings of a Conference on General Practitioner Obste-trics*. College of General Practitioners, London, pp. 2–3.
8. House of Commons Health Committee (1992) *Maternity Services*, vol. I (the Winterton Report), HMSO, London.
9. Department of Health (1993) *Changing Childbirth*, Report of the Expert Maternity Group, Part 1, HMSO, London.
10. Wood, L.A.C. (1981) Obstetric retrospect. *J. R. Coll. Gen. Pract.*, **31**, 80–90.
11. McGregor, R. and Martin, L. (1961) Obstetrics in a general practice. *J. Coll. Gen. Pract.*, **4**, 542–51.
12. Bury, J.D. and Garson, J.Z. (1963) Home or hospital confinement? *J. Coll. Gen. Pract.*, **5**, 590–605.
13. Taylor, G., Edgar, W. *et al.* (1980) How safe is general practitioner obstetrics? *Lancet*, **ii**, 1287–9.

14. Cavenagh, A., Phillips, K. *et al.* (1984) Contribution of isolated general practitioner maternity units. *Br. Med. J.*, **288**, 1438–40.
15. Shearer, J. (1985) Five year prospective survey of risk of booking for a home birth in Essex. *Br. Med. J.*, **291**, 1478–80.
16. Young, G. (1987) Are isolated maternity units run by general practitioners dangerous? *Br. Med. J.*, **294**, 744–6.
17. Lowe, S., House, W. and Garrett, T. (1987) Comparison of outcome of low-risk labour in an isolated general practice maternity unit and a specialist maternity hospital. *J. R. Coll. Gen. Pract.*, **37**, 484–7.
18. Garrett, T., House, W. and Lowe, S. (1987) Outcome of women booked into an isolated general practitioner maternity unit over eight years. *J. R. Coll. Gen. Pract.*, **37**, 488–90.
19. Marsh, G.N. and Channing, D.M. (1989) Audit of 26 years of obstetric practice. *Br. Med. J.*, **298**, 1077–80.
20. Flint, C. and Poulengeris, P. (1987) *The 'Know-Your-Midwife' Report*, 34 Elm Quay Court, London SW8 5DE.
21. Department of Health and Social Security/Office of Population Censuses and Surveys. *Hospital Inpatient Enquiry Maternity Tables*, Series MB4 No. 8 (1973–76) (Table 4) and No. 28 (1982–85) (Table 2.2), HMSO, London.
22. *Midwifery Matters – The Association of Radical Midwives Magazine.* Regular statement on inside cover page.
23. *Sydney Morning Herald* (7 November 1987) quoting Warren Jones, Professor of Obstetrics and Gynaecology, Flinders Medical Centre, Adelaide, Australia.
24. House of Commons Health Committee (1992) *Maternity Services*, vol. III, Appendices to the Minutes of Evidence, pp. 654–922.
25. Kloosterman, G.J. (1982) The universal aspects of childbirth: human birth as a socio-psychosomatic paradigm. *J. Psychosom. Obstet. Gynaecol.*, **1**, 35–41.
26. Inch, S. (1981) *Birthrights.* Hutchinson, London, Appendix 5.
27. Kloosterman, G.J. (1978) Organization of obstetric care in the Netherlands. *Ned. Tijdschr. Genieskd.*, 1161–71.

2

Birth attendants and their places of practice

THE FIRST BIRTH ATTENDANTS

For most of human history procreation has been managed by the individuals concerned, as it is with other animals in the wild which, as the close observations of modern zoologists confirm, give birth unaided and without apparent pain or distress. Likewise in different times and places, there have been many records of women, unattended, giving birth simply and safely. For example, the American squaw, living in her tribal culture, carried on her normal activities throughout pregnancy. Then,

> When she realises that her hour of delivery is at hand, she enters her cabin or betakes herself to some stream or spring, gives birth, washes the young 'injun' in the cold water, straps it on her back, and before she has been scarcely missed, has returned a full-fledged mother, and resumes her labours. [1, p. 113]

Dr Grantly Dick-Read, who inspired the Natural Birth Movement of the 20th century, was first drawn to this philosophy 'by witnessing a woman in the battlefields of Flanders calmly delivering her own child and walking off laughing with the child at the breast. The woman followed her natural instinct and tradition' [2]. The American anthropologist, Margaret Mead, recorded 'I have never heard primitive women describe the pain of childbirth' [3].

But civilization seems to have robbed women of the certainty of a safe, pain-free, uncomplicated delivery, just as intensive stock rearing has done with farm animals. Certainly, by Biblical times some difficulty in labour must have been a common experience, explained in the Book of Genesis as God's punishment of woman for Eve's disobedience in eating the forbidden fruit: 'in sorrow thou shalt bring forth children' [4].

Nature's objective is to perpetuate the species, so she is concerned primarily with numerical success and can tolerate many failures on the way, especially since failure is most likely when the parents or their offspring are in some way unfit. Nature is not concerned with the distress felt by individuals when failure occurs or the process is too painful.

Although their bodies are biologically programmed to give birth unaided, women in many societies have felt the need for a helper and companion to support them throughout labour, so that some system of birth attendants has become an integral part of their cultures. The word 'midwife' literally describes this function of being 'with woman'. Pregnancy and childbirth were traditionally recognized as 'women's business', from which men, including husbands, were firmly barred. The dominance of female birth attendants has continued in societies where religious rules require the social segregation of women or where women are the possessions of their husbands and must be protected from contact, especially intimate physical contact, with other men. But in Western, Christian cultures opposition to male involvement was already being broken down by the 17th century.

The first birth attendants were probably the labouring woman's female relations or friends, women who learned their skill from their own experience of childbearing and from watching other birth attendants performing their office. The more births they attended, the more skilful they became and the more their services were sought. Those with most experience came to be recognized as having a distinct occupational status in the community. They had to cope, not only with uncomplicated deliveries, as they could with confidence, but also with deliveries complicated at any stage. Complications such as abnormal presentations, haemorrhages, obstructions, retained placentas and eclamptic convulsions have been recorded.

Often the midwife's skills were equal to the challenge of the complication and mother and infant survived. But in cases of extreme difficulty, when it seemed that only by surgery could the process be ended, she had to call for male assistance. The men to whom the mediaeval English midwife turned were barber-surgeons. They were organized in trade guilds which ensured that their members first learned their skills in the use of instruments in an apprenticeship system and thereafter had the exclusive right to practise this function. They rarely admitted women who were thus prevented from adding instrumental delivery to their midwifery skills, an embargo that has remained ever since [5, p. 2].

At first, the instruments were used to remove dead fetuses to save the mother's life, but early in the 17th century the Chamberlen family, which included eminent barber-surgeons over three generations, invented obstetric forceps by means of which the fetus could be delivered alive [6, pp. 77–81]. Such a weapon gave a much prized advantage to those who could use it. With it men were encouraged to offer their services as midwives.

THE ACQUISITION OF THEORETICAL KNOWLEDGE

At that time men were much more likely than women to have received some general education. The barber-surgeons had more chance of reinforcing their technical dexterity with theoretical study of the relevant anatomy, physiology and pathology and so equip themselves to practise as man-midwives. Not only did the female midwife lack theoretical knowledge, she was unlikely to be able to acquire it because of her inability even to read and write.

Her handicap kept her from profiting from the books on midwifery which appeared in English from the 15th century onwards [6]. Some of the advice in them merely described standard practice which had changed little over preceding centuries. Some advice, however, incorporated new knowledge or new fashions and some of it was obviously to warn against the danger of certain interventive techniques which had become prevalent (Chapter 4).

The very existence of books, sources of knowledge, which were open to her male rivals but were closed to her because of her illiteracy, probably served to increase the frustration the female midwife felt at her ignorance of the biology of childbirth. Her sense of inferiority was exacerbated by her realization that her richer customers were coming to rate the new technical qualifications of the man-midwives so much more highly than her own traditional competence, based on accurate observation of the inherent efficiency of the natural process, and her continuous moral support, that they were not only prepared to pay the men higher fees, but also to overcome their inbred female modesty in such an intimate context.

Midwives' suspicion and jealousy of their potential rivals led them to reject the Chamberlen proposal that a Corporation of Midwives be established where they would be taught by the man-midwives. Nor was their petition granted to form their own society which might have advanced its members' interests [6, pp. 78–9], as the College of Physicians and the Guild of Barber-surgeons had done for theirs. Women seem always to have been less naturally inclined than men to form organizations for the benefit of their occupation. Midwives did not do so until the later 19th century, and then less effectively than their medical rivals (pages 82, 383).

The pioneer man-midwives of the 17th century had in the 18th century a number of distinguished successors who sought to improve their understanding of the birth process and to develop methods of dealing with complications which were beyond the practical skills of the uneducated midwives who lacked such understanding. The humanity which prompted their endeavours should not be questioned, but it was not unnaturally combined with self-interest [6, pp. 101–27].

In an age of quickening scientific enquiry, discoveries in a little-explored field brought intellectual rewards of their own. But the man-midwives had correctly identified a deficiency in maternity care; ability to overcome it would bring great prestige and with that increased financial rewards. Moreover, it would subtly but effectively assert the superiority and dominance of the male sex in the power of creation, of which they had been deprived by nature. The prospect of such rewards has inspired obstetricians ever since and their successful pursuit of them has increasingly determined the organization of maternity care.

COMPETENT ENGLISH MIDWIVES OF THE 18TH CENTURY

Man-midwives were forced to concentrate on abnormalities because female midwives, no less self-interested, were concerned to protect their own market and excluded men as far as possible from participating in normal births, or even in births with the quite considerable complications they felt able to manage. Thus, deprived of the opportunity to witness how simple and safe childbirth could be, the men's experience was biased towards its complexity and problems, a bias which has continued to dominate obstetricians' thinking and practice despite vastly changing social conditions.

Many more books were written by the man-midwives, but some educated female midwives also made their contributions to the literature [6, pp. 104–25]. The experiences they describe illustrate their competence, for example, in dealing with unorthodox presentations. Sarah Stone, who practised in the West of England in the 18th century, recounted being called to a difficult birth and 'When I got there I found the child's arm out of the birth, I immediately searched for the feet which I soon found, and in a little time completed the delivery' [7]. She had obviously mastered the technique of podalic version, the ancient art of delivering the fetus feet first, rediscovered by the French obstetrician Ambroise Paré in the 16th century and recommended as the solution to obstetric problems in the 17th century by the English barber-surgeon/man-midwife, Percival Willoughby.

Towards the end of the century, Margaret Stephen described how the 'passage of the aftercoming head in a breech presentation should be facilitated by the technique of jaw flexion and shoulder traction' [8, p. 124]. She had been taught by a male pupil of William Smellie, the distinguished Scottish doctor of the period of whom it is said that he 'created the Obstetrician, elevated midwifery as a speciality for doctors and in so doing earned for himself in perpetuity the title "Master of British Midwifery"' [6, p. 103]. Mrs Stephen appreciated her tutor's instruction, but she was far from conceding to men the major role in intranatal care. She recognized the value of the discriminate use of forceps in saving babies' lives but, believing that 'the vast majority of pregnancies would have a successful natural outcome', she therefore deplored the fact that 'an increasing number of men were regarding childbirth as an unnatural event which required their instrumental assistance' [8, p. 123]. If forceps and other obstetric instruments were needed, then it should be the midwives, after training, who should use them – a proposal that was never to be implemented.

Although the intranatal interventions of the best of man-midwives had almost certainly saved the lives of many women and babies, Mrs Stephen wrote that 'so general a use of men in the business of a midwife has introduced a far greater number of deaths among society than it has prevented [8, p. 124], an observation for which there was to be repeated evidence in the course of the next two hundred years (Chapters 7 and 8). But attention was distracted from the dangers of their obstetric techniques by the men's political strategies, by their deliberate misrepresentations, by casting aspersions on the characters of the female midwives and impugning their professional reputations, and by their insinuations which taught mothers to believe they endangered their own lives and the lives of their children, by employing women [8, p. 124]. Such unsupported propaganda has a familiar ring, so similar is it to that with which mothers ever since have been misled. It has been constantly used to great effect to influence the choice of birth attendant.

Mrs Stephen recognized that training, theoretical and practical, was a great advantage, and indeed a necessity, for midwives if they were to compete with men. Being female implied being ignorant and so to be little respected; being male implied being educated and so to be much respected. She deplored, as she might have done in the succeeding centuries [9], that '. . . midwives with ability (but less theoretical knowledge), and even less prestige, were encouraged to consult men who were without practical experience and sometimes little relevant theoretical knowledge, but greater prestige by virtue of their profession and gender' [8, p. 125].

Nevertheless, her insight into human nature and human reactions, as typical today as then, led her to advocate sending for a doctor in cases of obstructed labour 'because, should any misfortune happen, which perhaps is unavoidable, people are more readily reconciled to the event, because there is no appeal from what a doctor does, being granted he did all he could on the occasion' [8, p. 124].

Mrs Stephen's astute observations were not sufficiently persuasive to counteract the propaganda and halt the increasing involvement of men in maternity care. Man-midwives, whatever their actual qualifications and these varied greatly, had the reputation of coming from the more educated classes and were on that account more acceptable to women of these classes. Education was, then as now, an esteemed virtue, assumed in itself to guarantee better service.

CLIENT PREFERENCE

It was a mark of a man's economic success that the female members of his family did not have to be economically useful. Society encouraged them to be ornamental, delicate and physically modest. Persuaded that they were indeed delicate, they were ready to believe that for them childbirth needed the stronger management of male doctors and that this need transcended their innate physical modesty. It was as though doctors were saying 'Let us of the stronger sex overcome your difficulties for you', while the midwives were saying 'Let us of the same sex support you while you overcome your own difficulties, which most of you are well able to do'. The leisured ladies preferred the doctors' option.

As the upper and middle classes increased in numbers, so did the demand of their womenfolk for man-midwives, whose intrusive touch, if not sight, they permitted. Ability to pay their higher fees was in itself a public demonstration of their economic advance. They set a standard to which other women would aspire once they could afford it.

By no means all the men who practised midwifery did possess the qualifications which the upper class women admired. Many had not studied in medical schools or served recognized apprenticeships which would have fitted them for this employment. Indeed, except in Edinburgh, medical schools did not offer formal teaching in midwifery before the 19th century (pages 47, 49–50). Like their female counterparts, they could act as midwives without passing any test of ability and the ready use of instruments gave them the potential to do great damage. Presumably the charlatans concealed their incompetence behind masculine charm. At all events, their existence did not prevent the increasing acceptability of men as midwives.

As their confidence grew, they considered the title 'man-midwife' unsuitable. By the early 19th century, those who specialized in midwifery preferred to be known as obstetricians, the word derived from Latin and describing those who 'stand before the woman as she delivers her child'. The description 'accoucheur', derived from the French verb meaning to bring to bed, was used by general practitioners whose work included midwifery. These titles not only describe new occupations, but also indicate a change in the favoured position for the woman giving birth (Chapter 4).

The demand for medical attendants, before 1900 almost exclusively male, was further increased after the introduction in the mid-19th century of chloroform, which midwives were not allowed to administer. Women could then be spared, not only from the pains of normal labour, but from the excruciating agonies of instrumental deliveries. The use of chloroform, like the services of doctors, was available only to those who could afford to pay for it.

THE LYING-IN HOSPITAL: A LANDMARK IN MATERNITY CARE

A development which was to have critical significance for the future direction of maternity care was the establishment in the course of the 18th and 19th centuries of lying-in hospitals in major cities and towns. The primary purpose of these was charitable, to provide shelter and care for poor, homeless parturient women. In addition, they fulfilled a quite different purpose which was to be of great lasting significance. This was to provide centres for obstetric teaching and research, the linch-pin for the future spread of education for birth attendants. In the long term, the development of maternity hospitals was to benefit obstetricians more than mothers and babies or midwives. It was ultimately to confirm the ascendancy of the male doctor as birth attendant, to establish his dominance in the management of childbirth and to change the concept of reproduction from being a natural condition, appropriately completed in a domestic setting, to a pathological condition, appropriately completed in a medical institution.

The mother as patient

For the charity patient, the lying-in hospital brought advantages and disadvantages. In exchange for receiving free treatment, food and rest, the women were used by obstetricians as material for extending their own knowledge of the physiology and pathology of parturition, for experimenting with interventions and treatments and for teaching medical students and midwives. These facilities were possible, and were considered ethical, because the women concerned were assumed not to share the physical modesty and sensibilities of the obstetricians' higher class clients, which would have precluded using them as objects for study. Poor women who lived near teaching hospitals were likewise offered attention in their homes in exchange for the clinical experience they provided for medical students. As in other fields of medicine, scientific advances from which all classes have benefited owe much to the generous, if involuntary, co-operation of the poor.

The midwife

For midwives also the lying-in hospital brought advantages and disadvantages. Little progress had been made in meeting the midwife's need, recognized by Mrs Stephen and others, for theoretical training in anatomy and pathology. In this respect, the English midwife had lagged far behind her colleagues in France and Germany, for whom some such training had been available since the Middle Ages. In Scotland training flourished in the 18th century and the University of Edinburgh appointed a Professor of Midwifery whose function was initially to teach female midwives but was extended when he opened a voluntary class for medical students and a small maternity ward in the Royal Infirmary [10].

Even if the facilities had existed in England, most midwives could not have taken advantage of them because of their illiteracy and their inability to afford the cost. Very few could have paid, as Mrs Stephen had done, for private tuition from a more qualified man. Most had to learn their craft, as they had always done, in the unofficial apprenticeship system. The quality of their training depended on the quality of the midwife they followed and that could range from the very good to the very bad, from the wise and well-informed to the foolish and ignorant. The better the midwife, the more she could charge her pupils; pupils who could not afford to pay had perforce to copy their incompetent mistress.

The lying-in hospital created the first opportunity in England for combining training in theory as well as in practice in an institutional setting, but the benefit was available only to the minority of midwives who could live in the larger towns where the hospitals were located. Moreover, the training given must have been limited to have been completed in the period of about three months, which seems then to have been standard. Since it was the doctors who provided it, the theoretical instruction must inevitably have reflected something of the masculine and medical approach to midwifery, which in the circumstances would impress the trainee midwife as superior. To be offset against the gain in theoretical learning was her loss of status, for the midwife who continued to work in the hospital had, like her continental counterpart, to accept a role subservient to the obstetrician and sacrifice some of the traditional independence of the domiciliary midwife who lacked formal training.

A further disadvantage was that the hospitals provided the medium through which the midwife was faced with a new rival, the 'monthly nurse'. Whether the birth was to take place in hospital or, like most, in the mother's home, obstetricians or accoucheurs wanted to manage the actual birth, the exciting and financially rewarding culmination, but begrudged the tedious time being 'with woman', waiting for the preparatory processes to take their course. Doctors have consistently undervalued the psychological and biological importance of this part of labour and have never claimed expertise in its exercise. It was in their economic interest to delegate this time-consuming duty to some lowly paid assistant who would be incapable of rivalling them by conducting the actual delivery. They therefore encouraged the lying-in hospitals to give a simpler training to nurses who, for a small part of the doctor's fee, would do the waiting for them, judge when to summon them and look after mother and baby for the first month after birth. In fact, the hospitals trained more monthly nurses than midwives [6, p. 146].

The obstetrician

The advantages for the doctors, in terms of status, power and opportunities for extending their knowledge, were obvious. Hospitals are the workshop of the obstetricians where they feel most confident and in charge and where a useful number of cases are conveniently assembled for study. Less obvious was the disadvantage to obstetricians, who probably did not realize its importance, and to their patients that concentration on the cases treated in the early lying-in hospitals meant that their experience was increasingly biased towards the pathological. It came from the two extremes of the social scale, neither representative of the majority of births.

Though society expected that the low-class patient for whom the hospitals were specifically intended should give birth with the ease of an uncivilized animal, her impoverished background was likely to have left her with impaired strength and skeletal malformations and so likely to develop obstetric complications.

At the other end of the scale, obstetricians were able to persuade a few of their richer clients that their needs would be better met if they had their confinements as private patients in hospital. So started the process of making hospitals respectable and more desirable places for giving birth than the family home, however comfortable that might be. The high-class patient was prone to believe herself too delicate to give birth without medical intervention and her expectation easily became self-fulfilling.

The obstetricians' opportunities for observing normal birth were increasingly restricted and they were ceasing to believe that it could ever be uncomplicated. Their bias towards pathology and the weight of their influence in policy making and in the direction of education and research were growing hand in hand. 'The overriding considerations were that midwifery could be learnt only in a lying-in hospital, and that human reproduction was not a natural process but was associated with a high rate of dangerous complications in pregnancy and labour' [10].

Centres for training medical students

An early benefit of lying-in hospitals to obstetricians was in the facility they provided for teaching medical students, from whose fees the obstetrician could earn a considerable part of his income. Because of the cost, the first apprentices were more likely to be medical graduates, who intended to make their careers in midwifery, than undergraduates, for it was not until well into the 19th century that midwifery became one of the subjects in the undergraduate degree syllabus of the British University Medical Schools. It was added to medicine and surgery as a compulsory part of the final examination first in the Scottish Universities in 1840 and later in other Universities of Ireland and England and there was no uniformity in course requirements. Candidates for membership of the Royal College of Surgeons of England or the Licentiate of the Royal College of Physicians of London, which were qualifications for medical practice, did not have to pass an examination in midwifery until 1886, following an Act of Parliament [11]. That examination, however, was governed entirely by physicians and surgeons.

The General Medical Council had been set up by the 1886 Act and, although rarely including an obstetrician among its members, had constantly concerned itself with the state of midwifery education. By 1888 it was still dissatisfied that its proposals for improvement, in particular increasing the students' practical experience, had not been implemented. This dissatisfaction was shared by a body of 337 general practitioners who, in a petition to the Council, deplored

> . . . the very inadequate teaching of midwifery, and the bad results to the women of the country resulting therefrom; so inadequate an amount of training in this most important part of medical practice is averse to the public good and the highest interests of the profession. [11, p. 710]

The number of cases of labour the various licensing and teaching bodies required their candidates to attend was found to vary between six and thirty. Proof of attendance was haphazardly applied and attendance at labour did not mean its actual conduct by the student [11]. The state of affairs had not been remedied by 1900.

Possibilities for greater theoretical instruction in midwifery were restricted by the demands of other subjects in their crowded curriculum which then lasted for four years. Possibilities for greater practical experience were restricted by the relatively small number of beds in lying-in hospitals to which the Medical Schools had access and which were needed also for the training of the rival midwives. The priority given to the training of midwives was dictated, not by any recognition that childbearing women would be better served by competent midwives than by competent doctors, but for financial considerations, for pupil midwives served the dual purpose of providing cheap nursing care in hospital while they were learning to manage deliveries. This bonus would be sacrificed if deliveries were reserved for medical students and any alternative nursing care would be too costly. The short-term gains of preference given to midwives were, however, largely squandered in the longer term, for a substantial proportion of successful trainees did not pursue careers as midwives [11, p. 737], a source of wastage that has been repeated ever since.

But, however great their lack of practical experience in both quantity and range, compared with that of midwives, doctors managed to maintain the reputation of being the superior authority on childbirth.

THE CHANGING STATUS OF MIDWIVES

The lowering of the midwife's professional status in hospital intensified the loss of both social and professional status which she had already suffered when her richer clients preferred her male rival. But this image of the profession was more seriously tarnished by the adverse publicity given to the shortcomings of its ignorant, incompetent members. Many criticisms were no doubt deserved, but midwives' rivals found it to their interest to exaggerate. Reputable midwives were made to feel disgraced by the disreputable claimants to the title. This embarrassing association, together with the puritanical prudery which was increasingly expected of their class, deterred educated women from becoming midwives. The 19th century saw a deterioration in the quality of the average English midwife.

There were, however, a few leaders who, motivated by the desire to improve the lot of their sex as childbearers and as political members of society, sought to preserve the career of the midwife and elevate its professional and social status by improving the quality of its practitioners. They urged increased training to higher standards, both practical and theoretical, and the awarding of certificates to those who were found, by examination, to have completed the courses successfully [6, pp. 135–76]. Ambitions were not restricted to achieving competence in normal deliveries. Florence Nightingale, whose reforms had achieved great improvements in the standards and status of the nursing profession, proposed that a midwife should receive

> . . . such a training, scientific and practical, as that she can undertake all cases of parturition, normal and abnormal, subject only to consultation, like any other accoucheur. Such a training could not be given in less than two years . . . no training of six months could enable a woman to be more than a Midwifery Nurse. [12, p. 158]

Midwives, however, depended for their scientific training on their rivals, the doctors. Even the more sympathetic of these had always co-operated with some reservation and were not so magnanimous as to agree to their trainees encroaching on the preserve they had marked out for themselves. By 1880 the London Obstetrical Society, an early organization of obstetricians, was offering written and oral examinations to women who met their entry requirements and followed their exacting syllabus, but the diploma awarded guaranteed only that its possessor was a skilled midwife competent to attend natural labours [6, p. 164].

Entry for this qualification was restricted to women aged between 20 and 29 years. Indeed, older women with their schooldays, if they ever had any, further behind them would have found it more difficult to adapt to the required theoretical study. But women in their twenties, who were free to study for a career, were likely to be those who had not themselves borne children and so were prevented, like men, from empathizing with the labouring women through personal experience. Thus the reforming midwives' quest for a scientific grounding for their work and the higher value placed on this than on experience was to lead to a change in the character of the typical midwife; the traditional matron who had learned much, or little, wisdom from life was to give way to the intelligent spinster who would first learn from academic teaching and then from the other women's experience (page 77).

The aim of the reforming midwives was not that appropriate education and certification should be made available for the elite few, but that it should be made available for all midwives and that only certified midwives should be allowed to practise. By 1886, the medical profession had dealt with the problem of charlatan practitioners by securing legislation by which only persons who had obtained a recognized qualification in medicine, surgery and midwifery could be registered as doctors. Campaigns were launched to obtain similar legal sanction for the restriction of midwives, but they met much opposition from the rival practitioners bent on preserving their own markets, on the one hand from the very articulate and politically influential doctors who feared qualified competitors and on the other hand from illiterate midwives who would be unlikely to pass a written examination. It was only after many years of intense political activity and bitter controversy between groups with rival professional interests that the British Parliament passed the *Midwives Act* in 1902 to enforce the registration of English midwives [5]. The interests of the mother and baby, though nominally paramount, were in reality subordinated to the interests of the birth attendants.

THE CHOICE OF BIRTH ATTENDANT AROUND 1900

In England a woman's birth attendant depended mainly on her income, her social or civil status and where she lived. If she belonged to the upper or middle classes, she was likely to engage a doctor, a specialist obstetrician or a general practitioner accoucheur, whose fee she could afford and who would in most cases attend her at her home or in a few cases in a maternity hospital, if she lived in a town where there was one suitable. She would also be looked after by a monthly nurse.

If her family was less affluent or if she belonged to the working class or lived in the country, she was likely to engage a midwife; the more she could afford to pay, the more likely was her midwife to be well trained. If she could afford to pay very little, she risked being at the mercy of the ignorant, incompetent midwives who brought disgrace to the profession. If she could not afford to pay anything at all, her attendants, if any, would be relations or friends, performing a neighbourly act, probably on a reciprocal basis. If she was unmarried or homeless, she might be delivered in a public or workhouse hospital, under the care of obstetricians, including teachers of obstetrics.

Regular statistical records were not kept of the number of births attended by each type of attendant. A survey of infant mortality, carried out in 1869 by the Registrar General's office on behalf of the London Obstetrical Society, produced rough estimates that, overall, medical men attended 10–30% of births, but in London's West End they attended nearly all of them; midwives were estimated to attend 30–90% of births in large provincial and manufacturing towns and in agricultural villages, but only 30–50% in London's East End; all of which left 'a considerable number' without any professional attendant [6, p. 160].

BIRTH ATTENDANTS IN THE USA

By the end of the 19th century in most societies the birth attendant was still predominantly a female midwife with at least practical training or experience. However, in North America her 18th century pre-eminence was already being seriously eroded [13]. The young American doctor, whether college trained or not, was eager to establish a practice for himself and willingness to attend births was a good recommendation for a family doctor. He shared with his patients an outlook that was progressive rather than conservative. Both had great faith in the promise of science and were disposed to believe that interventions would improve on the natural process.

Far earlier than in Britain, doctors in this branch of medicine had organized a professional association to advance their interests. In 1877, the President of the newly formed American Gynecological Society, ignoring established evidence on how intervention spread infection (Chapter 4, pages 111–12), was shifting the blame for the high incidence of puerperal fever in public lying-in hospitals to the demoralized state of the unmarried women who used them and suggesting 'that doctors consider using the forceps to expedite delivery rather than standing by the anguished, labouring woman and crooning to themselves that meddlesome midwifery was bad' [13, p. 118].

More thoroughly than in the Old World, the culture, which had expected women to share their menfolk's toil as they struggled after economic prosperity, changed to glorifying their idleness as prosperity was achieved, so women from the successful classes were less interested in becoming midwives, while at the same time were more readily convinced of the advantages of obstetric interventions. Thus in a society becoming rapidly more prosperous, both the supply of and demand for midwives diminished. They were still found among poorer, more isolated communities, white and non-white, and among newer immigrants. They included some who were ill-trained and incompetent and who, however unfairly, earned disapproval for midwives in general. There was no effective movement to defend their reputation by improving their competence through better training. The doctors' increasing domination of obstetric management was largely uncontested and set a pattern which maternity care the world over was to follow in the 20th century.

Other English-speaking countries of the New World, Australia, Canada, New Zealand and South Africa, shared many of the characteristics of the USA, the social and economic ambitions of their growing populations and the professional ambitions of their doctors. These were as eager and as determined as their fellow migrants to their adopted countries to stake their claims to future prosperity. The promising gateway to assuring their social importance was somehow to persuade their young compatriots that their medical assistance at childbirth was indispensable and far superior to what a midwife could offer. Their market proved to be rewardingly amenable to their persuasion.

REGISTERED MIDWIVES

The purpose of the English *Midwives Act* of 1902 was to secure better education for midwives and to regulate their practice, so that in due course all of them would have formal training and on its successful completion they would gain a qualifying certificate, without which they could not practise. The Central Midwives Board was appointed to implement these objectives and control registration. But until the training courses were set up and functioning, the register had to admit not only midwives who already had a formal qualification, but also so-called bona fide midwives, women of good character who had practised for at least one year [6, pp. 177–246].

The first roll of 22 308 names, published in 1905, was made up of 44% of the former group and 56% of the latter. Progress towards the goal was gradual but certain: by 1916 only 25% of the registered midwives were untrained, by 1933 only 3%. It was not until 1947, however, that no bona fide midwife was admitted to the roll.

The number of bona fide midwives was reduced because some of them failed to comply with the ever more stringent rules laid down by the Central Midwives Board. These affected not only the personal habits and behaviour of the enrolled midwives, but also their professional responsibilities. The latter were widened from time to time, making it increasingly difficult for illiterate or barely literate women, which many were, to carry them out. Requiring midwives to record the mother's pulse and temperature at each visit was a simple device for weeding out the least literate.

The campaign to eradicate the untrained midwife and handywoman was to some extent frustrated for over twenty years by the collusion of some doctors who got around the regulation which after 1910 prevented an uncertified midwife from attending women in childbirth 'habitually and for gain' except under the direction of a medical practitioner. They did this by agreeing, for part of her fee, to represent that she was only acting as their temporary substitute. Collusion was more frequent in rural areas where births were too few for full-time certified midwives to make an adequate income and the occasional need was met by uncertified women. Collusion persisted until 1936 when local authorities were made responsible for the payment of midwives (pages 60, 198). The doctors' willingness to collude implies a fair degree of confidence in the untrained midwives' skills and that, despite all the propaganda to the contrary, the chance of an adverse outcome, which would have exposed the illegal practice, was small. Moreover, the unqualified midwife, unlike her certificated counterpart, was hardly a serious competitor among the richer clientele that the general practitioner wished to reserve for himself.

Training registered midwives

The increase in the proportion of trained midwives on the roll testifies to the efficiency of the Central Midwives Board in organizing training courses and instituting its own examinations which, from 1905, superseded those of the London Obstetrical Society. By 1910 it had already recognized 103 institutions for training in the UK, in some cases in hospitals, in others through District Nursing Associations and approved independent midwives [6, p. 194], and from 1911 a pupil had to attend a course of lectures given by an approved lecturer [14]. More exacting courses were progressively introduced and the necessary training provisions progressively extended. After 1938, approval was only given to schools which could offer a sufficient number of cases to give pupils experience of complicated, as well as uncomplicated, deliveries [6, p. 229]. This usually meant hospitals where specialist obstetricians were in control and excluded the smaller general practitioner hospitals [15].

From 1924 courses for the training of midwifery teachers were organized in several centres, leading first to a Teacher's Certificate in 1926 and then to a Diploma in 1936. In 1950 a Midwife Teachers' Training College was opened and functioned until 1986 when it was superseded by more ambitious educational arrangements (pages 75–8). All midwives were required to attend a seven (later reduced to five) day residential course every five years [6, p. 227].

The long-standing training period of three months was increased by stages and by 1938 was twelve months for qualified nurses, which most entrants then were, with an extra year for those who had still to learn basic nursing skills. To reduce the deterrent of a longer training period, which inevitably required a greater investment of time and money by the pupil midwives, financial allowances were made available by the State. Although their higher standard of training should have made the midwives' services more valuable, there was no assurance that most of their future clients would be able to pay them higher fees and so reward the investment.

The content of midwifery courses

In her three months' training in 1903, the pupil midwife had to prepare for oral, practical and written examinations covering the elementary anatomy of the female reproductive organs; pregnancy and its principal complications including abortion; the symptoms, mechanism, course and antiseptic management of natural labour; and the management, including feeding, of the mother and baby during the ten day lying-in period. She had to recognize abnormalities at any stage for which she should call in a doctor. These included haemorrhage, malpresentation of the fetus, suspected cephalic-pelvic disproportion, fits and convulsions, offensive discharge, retained placenta, malformation or morbidity of the child and the death of the mother. She had to learn to cope with obstetric emergencies until the doctor's arrival and how to manage puerperal fever according to the current state of knowledge. She had personally to conduct twenty deliveries, making the appropriate abdominal and vaginal examinations, and follow up these mothers and babies for ten days [6, pp. 181–3].

In fact, she had to learn a very great deal in a very short time and the desirability of a longer period in which to study these and additional subjects in greater detail was undoubted. Teaching of elementary physiology was introduced in 1916 and some instruction in antenatal investigations was added to the syllabus in the 1920s and 1930s.

Domiciliary delivery was the dominant model for intranatal care right up until the 1940s. Only about one-quarter of the seventy-one schools surveyed by the Ministry of Health in 1923 provided hospital experience, although this was increasingly considered to be valuable and even essential [6, p. 205].

Midwives were allowed to administer several drugs, but did so infrequently. For the relief of pain in labour they were restricted to the use of mild sedatives. Chloroform was considered too dangerous for midwives to use and 'gas (nitrous oxide) and air' was only permitted after the invention of a portable apparatus had made its administration safe enough for the British College of Obstetricians (page 58) to recommend its use by midwives who had received the necessary training, for which special courses were provided from 1936. Midwives' training and examination in the use of inhalational analgesia did not, however, become mandatory until 1947 [16]. It was not until 1950 that midwives won permission to use the drug pethidine, which obstetricians had used since 1939 to relieve pain in labour [6, pp. 222, 237, 241–2].

The longer training period after 1938 was divided into two parts. Part I covered the theory of normal and abnormal midwifery and neonatal paediatrics, with some relevant sociology and psychology; it required the conduct of ten deliveries and was completed with a written and oral examination. In Part II, theory was applied to practice, followed by clinical and oral examinations.

> The clinical examination included history taking, general and abdominal examination/palpation, urine testing, blood pressure estimation, examination of the placenta and membranes, and the use of inhalational analgesia. . . . The oral part related to the candidate's written case studies, twelve of which were submitted at this time. [6, pp. 228–9]

THE LACK OF PROGRESS IN THE EDUCATION OF DOCTORS

In England, doctors and their representative bodies had strongly opposed the training and registration of midwives, wishing to preserve the market for themselves. Although many midwives were incompetent and without training, many doctors with a training of sorts were no less incompetent. Improvement in their undergraduate education in midwifery continued to be slow. Proposals to this end by the General Medical Council and others were constantly opposed and defeated by physicians and surgeons, for reasons not understood by obstetricians.

> It is a curious thing that those medical practitioners who turn their attention more particularly to medicine and surgery, should for all these years have belittled the necessity of students being adequately trained in midwifery. The reason for such an attitude is difficult to understand, but it must charitably be attributed, in part at any rate, to ignorance of the immense importance of this subject to the community. [11, p. 718]

Recommendations that every medical student should personally deliver thirty or twenty or even fewer cases were frustrated by the continued limited access to childbearing women. Student doctors still had to compete with student midwives for training material and Medical Schools had to adjust the regulations accordingly. They also condoned the frequent attitude of students that 'this part of their training was a nuisance to be completed in the shortest possible time. ... They allowed cases to be rushed through and not uncommonly one case was counted to a number of observing students' [17, p. 12].

In 1922 the Council made fresh recommendations, similar to those eventually adopted in 1947. These stipulated that the syllabus should include systematic instruction in the principles and practice of midwifery and gynaecology, including the anatomy, physiology and pathology of pregnancy and labour, with six months' instruction and practical experience in a maternity ward and out-patient clinic of antenatal and postnatal care and the care of the neonate. For two of these six months the student should be resident in the maternity hospital, concentrating on midwifery and infant hygiene, and should attend at least twelve cases of labour under proper supervision.

These precepts were not promptly fulfilled in all medical schools. A wide diversity of standards regarding practical experience continued to prevail. Attendance at far less than twelve deliveries was common. Little instruction was given in antenatal conditions. By 1928, the training period in three-quarters of teaching centres was less than six months and of this the larger part was devoted to gynaecology, and its more serious cases, knowledge of far less practical value to a general practitioner than knowledge of midwifery [11, pp. 728-9].

While the recommendations were being digested, serious disquiet persisted over the obstetric competence of medical graduates, for 'as soon as the student was qualified, the public trusted him to perform the most difficult obstetric operations which he had rarely seen and almost certainly never performed' [17, p. 12]. Some post-graduate training and experience was clearly necessary and the machinery for arranging it needed to be organized.

ORGANIZING OBSTETRICIANS

Since the *Medical Act* of 1886, candidates for admission to the medical register had to be trained and examined in medicine, surgery and midwifery, but midwifery was the neglected Cinderella of the family. For centuries, physicians and surgeons had had their own Colleges to regulate their affairs, to set and maintain the professional standards of their disciplines. Neither College showed much interest in promoting the professional standards of the newly elevated discipline, midwifery. Towards the end of the 19th century, the leading obstetricians had been Fellows of the Royal College of Physicians. In the early 20th century it was becoming more usual for them to be Fellows of the Royal College of Surgeons. Neither of these qualifications required the candidates to demonstrate proficiency in the theory and practice of midwifery. There was in fact no recognized route leading to the status of consultant obstetrician.

Leading obstetricians of the 1920s believed that 'there ought to be a portal through which all must pass who wished to be consultants in this branch of medicine, that portal to consist of equal parts of training and examination' [17, p. 8]. To form this portal was the first reason for proposing the foundation of their own separate College. Other stated reasons were to prevent the divorce of obstetrics from gynaecology and to speak as the representative body of all obstetricians and gynaecologists, but it was also concerned to bind the teachers of obstetrics and gynaecology together, so that they could demand adequate facilities for the teaching and examining of students. It saw as urgent the need to supplement the scanty undergraduate curriculum with post-graduate training [17, p. 18].

The foundation of the College met with much opposition, in particular from the Royal Colleges of Physicians and Surgeons, which required a great deal of argument and negotiation to be overcome before it was finally registered in 1929 as the British College of Obstetricians and Gynaecologists. More problems had to be surmounted before the College was able to establish, in 1931, its examination for the Diploma in Obstetrics and Gynaecology, intended as a post-graduate qualification for general practitioners. This required candidates to have completed six months in a resident or non-resident medical or surgical post; six months in a resident obstetrical post; six months in a resident or non-resident gynaecological post; six months in an antenatal clinic; and finally pass written, clinical and viva-voce examinations. The title was changed in 1945 to Diploma in Obstetrics, with the abbreviation D.Obst.RCOG [17, p. 89].

Medical support for midwives

The lack of interest shown by many medical undergraduates was followed by the same lack of interest from many doctors after they had qualified and were registered. Yet it was for registered doctors that registered midwives were obliged to send whenever they detected signs of abnormality before, during or after birth. The complaint of the midwife, Margaret Stephen, in the 18th century (page 44) was no less apposite in the 20th.

The midwives' first rule book of 1903 specified the warning signals to be looked for at each stage (pages 55–6). The respective duties of midwife and doctor were reiterated in 1928 by a government committee commissioned to review the working of the *Midwives Act* from 1902 to 1926.

> The midwife as the person responsible in the majority of cases for the care of the mother throughout pregnancy, confinement and the puerperal period is the one on whom the main burden would rest. In all such cases there should be available the services of a doctor, with certain well defined duties towards the mother, to whom the midwife should be able at all times to look for assistance when she is faced with difficulties beyond her ordinary competence and skill, and an obstetric specialist would be called in by the doctor to deal with exceptional emergencies. [6, p. 211]

The registered midwives were more punctilious in this duty of seeking medical aid than their independent predecessors. The proportion of cases in which they sent for the doctor rose steadily after 1902 [5, p. 185]. The doctors, however, were not always so punctilious in responding to the midwives' calls, which they were not legally obliged to do. Lack of interest and of self-confidence may sometimes have been their reasons. In some cases at first their reluctance arose because they hoped, by non-co-operation, to force their rivals out of business. Frequently it arose because of uncertainty about being paid for their trouble. If the patient could not afford their fee, either the midwife paid it out of her own pocket or the doctor went without. This grievance was settled by the *Midwives Act* of 1918 under which the local authority had to reimburse the doctor if necessary [5, p. 185].

By then, however, general practitioners were not so keen to be involved in onerous, time-consuming midwifery care, because they could be guaranteed a certain income in payment for attending insured patients after the *National Insurance Act* of 1911 [5, p. 185]. They became even less involved after the *Midwives Act* of 1936 which required all Local Authorities to provide an adequate, salaried domiciliary service, although this reform brought to an end the need for commercial rivalry between the two professions [6, p. 226].

The doctors' reduced involvement in normal midwifery led to further reduction in their competence to deal with complications. Fewer of them were willing to try. It was estimated that in London only one in twenty answered midwives' calls for help [6, p. 226]. But among those who did maintain their interest were many who became highly skilled in combining the gentle patience of midwifery with the technical dexterity of obstetrics.

It was obviously unrealistic to expect all doctors to answer midwives' aid calls. When the National Health Service was launched in 1948, a subgroup who would do so were to be listed in every area. These so-called general practitioner obstetricians were required to have shown an interest in midwifery by having held a resident appointment in a maternity ward and dealt with a certain number of midwifery cases in their own practice for several years. The D.Obst.RCOG qualification was accepted as providing a convincing testimonial of their fitness for the responsibility of undertaking midwifery care on their own account or acting as back-ups for midwives in cases of complication.

Qualifications for specialist obstetricians

The first objective of their College was to define specific qualifications for the specialist obstetricians, its future Members and Fellows, and prescribe how they were to be attained by training and examination [17, p. 82]. It took seven years of debate and development before practical problems and professional opposition, particularly from the rival Royal Colleges of Physicians and Surgeons, were surmounted, so that the Membership qualification, intended for consultants, could be finally separated from the Diploma, intended for general practitioners.

A serious difficulty lay in the shortage of facilities for residential appointments in teaching or affiliated hospitals, so that compromises had at first to be made. But insistent pressure led to increased provision of hospital beds and suitable inducements to women ensured that the beds were soon utilized. Increased hospitalization was thus primarily to satisfy the training requirements set by obstetricians to implement their theories of good maternity care. More hospital patients made it possible to demand residential posts of six months in both general medicine and general surgery, with one year each in obstetric and gynaecological departments. Thus candidates for Membership of the College (after 1947 Royal) of Obstetricians and Gynaecologists had to have completed three years of resident posts in hospital.

The candidate had to submit notes on twenty obstetrical and ten gynaecological cases which he had treated, thus redressing the bias in favour of gynaecology deplored in undergraduate education (page 57), and also a short commentary on one obstetrical and one gynaecological case, with a review of the relevant literature. He had to take part in an oral discussion of his written submission and, from 1935, pass a clinical examination also. From 1936, a written examination covering anatomy, physiology and general medicine and surgery as related to obstetrics and gynaecology was added.

These more exacting requirements improved the quality of successful candidates, with the incidental benefits of raising the general standard of note-taking and ability to make use of a library. Membership of the College soon became a necessary qualification for senior registrarships and after 1947 the standard requirement for applicants for the increasing number of consultant posts to be filled in the National Health Service. The expansion of the discipline was illustrated by the expansion of the College. In its first three years, 1929–32, it had 120 Fellows and 108 Members. By 1949–52, these numbers had multiplied to 364 Fellows and 1027 Members [17, pp. 177–9]. At the same time, the College's supervision of the non-teaching hospitals where the post-graduate students could train served to improve standards there.

The founders of the College were well pleased with their achievements. The measures it had taken ensured that

> . . . the best trained men have had at least five or six years of post-graduate training. In this way a sound clinical training in hospitals visited and recognised by the College is insisted upon, and a test has been developed, by a system of trial and error, which has a profound effect on the training of the candidate, and yet which is as fair as can be devised. [17, pp. 86–7]

Establishing an entry portal for consultant obstetricians and gynaecologists was not the only one of its objectives which the College had reached by 1950. Its Council was reputed to represent the best of thought and practice, so that it was normally consulted about questions relating to obstetrics and gynaecology and spoke with authority on behalf of the profession. The roots of the great influence it was later to exert were already well established.

The influence of gynaecology on obstetrics

The foundation of the College had received valuable support from the small but influential Gynaecological Visiting Society which had existed since 1911. Over the years, the union between obstetrics and gynaecology had been firmly cemented and the attitude of obstetricians was much influenced by their interest in gynaecology.

Gynaecology is concerned with pathological conditions of the female reproductive organs. As a branch of surgery, its natural home is the hospital. Obstetrics is concerned with abnormalities of pregnancy and childbirth and, because their daily work did not bring them into contact with normal pregnancy and labour, obstetricians were increasingly confirmed in their belief that most pregnancies were abnormal. Abnormalities, they were sure, were best treated in hospital. Students, undergraduate and post-graduate, as well as midwives, learned more, they believed, from hospital experience. To meet the training needs the number of births in hospital had to be increased.

Hospitals are the places for the treatment of illness. If mothers are to give birth in hospital, they are susceptible to the suggestion that childbirth is an illness. The suggestion can predispose to the reality and so confirm the obstetricians' beliefs. For this reason, the hospital is an inappropriate setting in which students at any level can gain experience of normal delivery.

A very successful establishment

One of the founders of the Royal College of Obstetricians and Gynaecologists, its first honorary treasurer and its first historian, William Fletcher Shaw, summarized its past achievement and its future prospect:

> The movement which culminated in the foundation of the College became a crusade to put obstetrics and gynaecology, the third subdivision of medicine, into its rightful place. The initial driving force came from the teachers, who had nothing to gain for themselves, and who, without thought of reward, gave freely of their time and energy to raise the status of the subject to which they had devoted their lives. . . .

The time for crusading is past and to later recruits the College represents a portal through which they must of necessity pass. But their personal admission, admonition and public acceptance of the declaration, together with their representation on the Council, bring home to them a sense of personal responsibility. This is as it should rightly be, for the College still needs the full support of each Fellow and Member, the realisation that he is part of a College whose reputation is the sum total of the reputation of all its Fellows and Members. It still needs their proper pride in membership and their determination to retain all that has been won. [17, p. 175]

Undoubtedly, the College has been immensely successful in promoting the interests of this branch of the medical profession. Amidst his history of the educational improvements obtained for its members and the public honours bestowed on its leaders, Shaw makes only one claim, unfortunately unjustifiable (page 291), that the College has promoted the interests of mothers and babies, which was, after all, not one of the declared objectives of its founders.

Undoubtedly the College was immensely important in setting the pattern for the future development of the maternity service, a pattern propitious for obstetricians. It was immensely important in transforming the concept of childbirth from being a physiological process which could occasionally go wrong into a medical condition which could never be trusted to go right, a transformation unpropitious for mothers and babies. The change in direction initiated by the establishment of the lying-in hospitals in the 18th and 19th centuries was now greatly accelerated. The domination of birth by the medical attendants, not only over their rivals, the midwives, but also over the object of their attentions and their *raison d'être*, the labouring mother, was emphatically asserted.

Organized obstetricians abroad

The influence of the College was not limited to Britain [17]. Close links, with increasing autonomy, were established with countries which were then British Dominions, Australia, Canada, New Zealand and South Africa, and with India. As in the USA, the hospitalization of childbirth had become more prevalent in the cities and towns of the young countries than in Britain itself. Hope and faith in interventive obstetrics were more eager and more widely shared, so the professional reforms of the College's policies were welcomed as vindicating existing biases.

In the USA, hope and faith persisted despite the lack of practical confirmation that childbirth was less traumatic when doctors, rather than midwives, were in control. Though midwives were condemned for their ignorance and incompetence, and many probably deserved the condemnation, the charges were recognized as applying equally to doctors, for their midwifery education and training in the early 20th century were, as in Britain, woefully inadequate.

J.W. Williams, Professor of Obstetrics at Johns Hopkins Medical School, the best in the country at that time, wrote of his own students in 1911, 'I would unhesitatingly state that they are unfit on graduation to practice obstetrics in its broad sense, and are scarcely prepared to handle normal cases' [18]. His enquiries found that a graduate from one of the best medical schools might have attended thirty births, but from most schools he had attended one or none. 'They could not handle difficult labours, even if they could recognise them; they had no training that related obstetrics to gynecology or surgery; they attended home deliveries without supervision. . . . general practitioners lost as many women to infection as did midwives and their ill-judged and improperly performed operations killed as many women as died from infection' [18]. (In fact he greatly overstated the incidence of infection in midwives' cases.) Williams recommended that 'medicine should educate the laity that most doctors were dangerous in birth and that most of the ills in women resulted from poor obstetrics' (page 303). He believed that future improvement would come through maternity hospitals and urged doctors to tell women, rich and poor, that they were likely to receive better care there than at home. At the same time, the hospitals would provide much better training of doctors.

His recommendations bore fruit in that in due course hospital delivery became standard practice. Whereas in 1900 less than 5% of births were in hospital, by the early 1930s in various cities between 60% and 75% of them were there. But since the ill-qualified practitioners often accompanied the mothers to hospital and sought, incompetently, to emulate the interventive techniques of their specialist colleagues, the mothers did not in fact receive the better care promised. The specialists wished to eliminate untrained practitioners and raise the standards of care. Towards this end the American Board of Obstetrics and Gynecology was established in 1930.

Of greater influence, however, was the study by the New York Academy of Medicine which investigated the recorded births and maternal deaths in New York city between 1930 and 1932. Two-thirds of the births were attended by physicians in hospital and 8% by midwives at home. Two-thirds of the deaths were considered to have been avoidable, had it not been for the incompetence or carelessness of the attendant, whether obstetrician, general practitioner or surgeon [19].

Embarrassment at this revelation of the shortcomings of doctors and hospitals prompted the introduction of regulations designed to remedy them, particularly to promote an aseptic environment and to prevent operations by unskilled doctors. But faith was not shaken that hospitals were the best place for birth and that interventions correctly performed by qualified obstetricians were beneficial. In this study, the maternal mortality rate per 1000 births was found to be 4.4 if doctors attended but only 2.9 if midwives attended and this low figure included births with complications where a doctor had been called, whatever the outcome [19]. (Nationally the rate was nearer 7 per 1000.) The study commented favourably on the work of midwives, who more often attended poor and immigrant women, and on the advisability of home delivery, but this praise was not enough to prevent these options being withdrawn with the agreement of both doctors and clients. Doctors 'sensed that they had received a mandate from families and from society to perfect the medical management of birth, that patients shared their view that doctors knew what was best for birth and should manipulate as fully as possible.' [13, p. 167]

By 1946, when 54% of births in England and Wales were in medical institutions of some kind, the percentage in America had passed 80 overall, nearer 95 in urban and 70 in rural areas, a tempting example for British obstetricians and one already being followed in Australia. There births in public institutions had increased from 3% in 1907 to 7% in 1920, but then leapt ahead to 55% in 1929. The trend was never reversed [20].

The last steps to supremacy

British obstetricians after 1950 saw no reason to resist this temptation. Their conviction had grown ever deeper that the most important factor governing the safety of childbirth was the competence of obstetricians. They had taken effective steps to improve their competence through a rigorous programme of post-graduate education, so by the time the National Health Service (NHS) was instituted, they had achieved, deservedly in their own view, wide recognition as masters of the maternity service. Their training concentrated on improving their technical efficiency in actively managing a sequence of physical events. No more than lip-service was apparently paid to the importance of the mother's emotional reactions and to comprehending how these are integral to initiating and regulating the reproductive process.

Obstetricians' power and influence were consolidated with the setting up in 1954 of an international federation of gynaecologists and obstetricians, FIGO, to promote co-operation in the direction of science and assistance in scientific research through triennial congresses.

They clinched their ascendancy through the expansion of the university departments, one of whose functions was to press on with research, applying advances in the physical sciences to develop techniques intended to improve the conduct of pregnancy and delivery. This function they carried out with impressive enthusiasm and industry. The parallel function of evaluating their scientific innovations was carried out with much less thoroughness or timeliness. This omission adversely biased their third function, that of regulating the training of doctors, generalists and specialists, in the light of the new knowledge which from the 1970s was expanding at a rate which challenged the adequacy of training provisions.

A SUCCESSFUL BUT UNEASY PROFESSION

Yet having secured its pre-eminence over midwives and childbearing women in the delivery of maternity care, the obstetric speciality was disappointed to find itself in later decades the most frequent subject of litigation (page 244) and failing to attract as many of the young medical graduates choosing careers as it once did. It became anxious to find the reasons for its diminished popularity, but assumed ruefully that increased litigation, with consequent increased insurance premiums for medical defence, was an important cause [21, p. 146]. Another cause might lie in the training process.

Training undergraduates in the late 20th century

The undergraduate curriculum in medical schools in the United Kingdom and Eire, as in North America and Australasia, had become even more crowded. In 1989 the time allowed for training in obstetrics and gynaecology varied but averaged eleven to twelve weeks; the number of vaginal deliveries the students were required to have conducted varied but averaged eight to ten, greater numbers being reserved, as in the past, for midwives. Also as in the past, conduct of delivery did not require constant attendance throughout the stages of labour and hence understanding of its progress. The theoretical syllabus was biased towards the physical sciences; though some time was now given to teaching counselling in psychosexual and social matters, little was left for family planning, and even less for epidemiology or the importance of nutrition in pregnancy [22]. This last lack was probably because obstetricians themselves were still not agreed on what constitutes the ideal diet [23, 24].

However significant the contribution of social factors, current and historic, to the pregnant woman's present condition, it is rarely within the power of the individual doctor to change these; the doctor has to be trained to deal with the situation in front of him as best as he or she can. So the most that could be hoped for was that the doctor on qualification should have a basic knowledge of human reproduction, the principles and practice of normal obstetrics, including antenatal and postnatal care, and 'enough practical experience to be able to deliver a baby in an emergency and apply simple resuscitation to the newborn' [25].

But as the decades passed and many obstetric interventions became routine practice, 'normal' obstetrics in the hospital setting came to be understood as describing, not physiological delivery after a physiological pregnancy and labour, but just delivery without instrumental assistance, irrespective of previous and subsequent interventions. Medical students had even fewer opportunities of witnessing and participating in the practice of natural birth. They were shielded from believing that a satisfactory outcome from such a process was possible. They were firmly imbued with the doctrine that the process of reproduction was a medical condition, with the only safe place for birth a consultant hospital under the management of obstetric specialists, and they were firmly discouraged from questioning this authority. Few among succeeding generations of new doctors would have felt qualified to take responsibility for a birth outside hospital, away from the equipment for intervention, or support a mother who wished to make such an arrangement which they had learned to regard as culpably irresponsible.

Training general practitioners

From 1948, general practitioners who intended to undertake maternity care had to be on the Obstetric List, for inclusion on which the recommended criterion was six months' post-registration experience in a consultant obstetric unit, so confirming their acceptance of childbirth as a pathological event. For the increasing number of aspiring general practitioners who, in the following decades, wished to provide antenatal and postnatal care only, the recommended post-graduate qualifications covered a thorough understanding of the complications of pregnancy and the puerperium and of normal and abnormal neonatal conditions, as well as the ability readily to recognize the need for referral to a consultant. Doctors were also 'to be aware of the emotional aspects of childbirth' [25, Apps II and III], but in practice emotional aspects were much subordinate to physical aspects. The decreasing number of doctors who wished to provide intranatal care as well were required to master the same interventive techniques as the obstetric specialist. They had also to 'be able to communicate with women in labour so that they [the women] understand the procedures proposed for their own safety and that of their babies' [25, pp. 5–11]. Thus the general practitioners were to make their own authoritative contribution to the propaganda medicalizing and mystifying childbirth.

Vocational training programmes were introduced for all intending general practitioners and training in obstetrics and gynaecology had to be incorporated. The two Royal Colleges (RCOG and RCGP) recommended in 1981 that experience be acquired partly in consultant hospitals through residential appointments for six or three months (for full and part maternity care respectively) and partly as trainee practitioners in approved general practice. All requirements would be met by practitioners who qualified for the Diploma of the RCOG. Refresher courses should keep their skills up to date.

The results of these arrangements may have proved satisfactory to the RCOG but the most potent effect of their senior house officer experience in obstetrics, far from improving their competence and confidence, was to frighten most of the general practitioner trainees out of intranatal care [21, p. 223, 26, p. 858]. They were driven to share the obstetricians' view that birth is always too dangerous to be conducted away from institutions with the facilities for technological intervention. But this training is an inappropriate preparation for doctors whose place of work is in the community where most commonly the need is not to deal with serious pathology. The trainees' inculcated attitude was only likely to be modified if the principals in the general practice in which they received their vocational training actually gave or were interested in giving intranatal care and these constituted a minority of trainers. As long as the RCOG dominated the obstetric education of general practitioners, it had little to fear from their potential rivalry.

Such criticisms seem to have made the RCOG and RCGP slightly uncomfortable, for in 1992 they modified their recommendations for general practitioner vocational training, requiring that it should give sufficient opportunity for learning about normal labours, as well as instrumental deliveries, and now official blessing was to be given to the contribution to the training programme by hospital midwives. The training should serve to build up the confidence of trainees and their willingness to undertake intrapartum care, for which an extra six months' experience of obstetric management on maternity wards would be necessary, compared with trainees intending to offer antenatal and postnatal care only [27].

The changes recommended appeared to be minimal. Trainees' attitudes might be very different if their vocational training were dominated rather by community midwives supervising deliveries in the mother's home or in a small maternity unit and showing that most problems could be competently managed without high technology. Such a reform, however, might risk accentuating the ancient rivalry between the doctors and midwives.

Towards breaking down these barriers, the Association for Community-Based Maternity Care (AC-BMC) was formed in 1989 with the objective of fostering primary obstetrics and supporting consumer choice, in particular, of place of birth. By 1992 its members comprised roughly two-thirds general practitioners and one-third midwives, with a small number of sympathetic obstetricians and links with consumer organizations. The Association opposed the scientifically unjustifiable monopolization of maternity care by hospital-based obstetricians (pages 2, 204) and the denial of services which some women would prefer. It emphasized the common interests of all care-givers and care-receivers involved in community care, but conceded that the primary carer at birth should be the midwife and advocated the sharing of much midwife and GP training [26, pp. 598–606].

The general practitioners who founded the AC-BMC were among the few of the younger ones who, despite their training and professional pressure, were convinced by the experience of some older colleagues that most births needed little or no intervention to achieve a healthy outcome and they continued to provide gentle supervision to the satisfaction of their clients. In the 1950s and 1960s, deliveries for which they accepted responsibility were taking place less frequently in the mother's home and more frequently in unattached GPUs. But their independent conduct became more difficult to sustain, as after 1970 these were progressively closed and replaced with allocated beds in, or units attached to, consultant hospitals, staffed by midwives whose practice conformed to consultant standards.

The road to consultant status

Inevitably, it takes more time to master the ever expanding body of knowledge. In the 1950s five or six years of post-graduate training and experience had been considered sufficient to achieve the status of consultant obstetrician (page 61), but by the 1980s this learning period had stretched to about eleven years. The process involved first working excessively long hours as house officers in hospital, and then as registrars in short-term posts in different parts of the country, conditions disruptive of family and social life and especially disadvantageous for women doctors to combine with childrearing. Their goal once reached, some consultants took a belated reward for their gruelling apprenticeship in a more distant and leisurely performance of their duties and were criticized for not being readily available to advise and supervise their juniors, particularly on the labour ward [28, 29].

The consultants' post-graduate education, despite the comprehensive regulations laid down by the RCOG, including permission to argue controversial issues [30], was judged to give them 'little formal assessment of skills, no curriculum, few trained teachers, no critical forum for debate and challenge' [31]. This last lack, reinforcing their undergraduate indoctrination, helps to explain the persistence of the profession's biased beliefs and attitudes. The exacting examination for Membership of the RCOG was held to be merely a permit for further training; approved training and experience would be required for a further three or more years before an obstetrician or gynaecologist could be accredited to practise as an independent specialist.

The need for further in-service education in labour ward practices was recognized by the RCOG [21, p. 145]. Other proposals for reform were being made within the profession in the 1980s and early 1990s – making the course more structured, so that candidates would be prepared in fewer years for the Membership examination (a minimum of 3.5 years after registration) and Fellowship qualification, while conforming with the requirements for accreditation within the European Union [32]. On the other hand, arrangements should be made for the course to be followed part-time over a longer period to accommodate the needs of young women doctors with small children, in the hope of redressing the serious shortage of women consultants, much deplored by women patients [26, p. 870].

A more condensed course could not, of course, cover all the new knowledge but it could perhaps be split into subspecialities – reproductive medicine, perinatal medicine, and gynaecological oncology and urology – and young consultants would have, after accreditation, to continue their study to specialize in one or more of these. To relieve the pressure on their juniors and to increase their presence on the wards, more consultants would have to be appointed and more suitable candidates for promotion would have to be lured into the specialty. That there was a relative shortage of consultants was not, however, a finding of the 1983 Enquiry into Facilities Available at the Place of Birth, for they outnumbered registrars (all grades) by two to one and equalled the number of senior house officers [33].

Making the specialty more attractive to intending entrants might be achieved by a more structured and less protracted training course, at least as long as the accruing advantages were not offset by similar changes in rival specialities, and also by reducing the threat of litigation through always undertaking an internal enquiry into obstetric accidents which involve injury to a mother or baby, followed with disciplinary action if appropriate [21, p. 146]. The possibility that yet other factors deter young doctors from entering the obstetrics speciality was not explored.

FROM HOME TO HOSPITAL: THE CONSEQUENCES FOR MIDWIVES

Obstetricians in post-war Britain were indeed impatient to move towards hospitalizing birth, so that they might put into practice their developing theories about the advantages of their style of management. The most serious challenge to their plans lay in the rival profession, the midwives conducting deliveries in the mothers' homes, so domiciliary midwifery had to be discredited. Ammunition to do so came readily from the youthful experience of many leading obstetricians who, as medical students, had learned midwifery by delivering poor and often unhealthy women in slum dwellings around the teaching hospitals. Their encounters with complications, particularly postpartum haemorrhage, left lastingly unfavourable impressions. They were disposed to attribute the dangers less to the health status of the women than to the inconvenience of the setting, from which they proceeded to the unjustifiable conclusion (Chapters 7 and 8) that domiciliary delivery as such was dangerous.

Their propaganda was effective and, despite counter-claims by the midwifery profession, the administrative organization secured that the percentage of births at home was inexorably forced down to reach 36 by 1958, 13 by 1970, 3 by 1975 and around 1 throughout the 1980s and early 1990s. Once domiciliary delivery was being virtually eradicated, attention could be focused on eliminating the non-specialist hospital, which, not being equipped to deal with emergencies, was declared, in defiance of actual results, to be both unsafe (page 220) and uneconomic (page 232). In 1958 and in 1970 the percentage of births in unattached GPUs was 12, but by 1975 this was reduced to 7, by 1986 to 2.2 and by 1990 to 1.6 [34–37].

Obstetricians took over the care of more and more women, antenatally as well as intranatally. Obviously they needed assistants, but not from a rival profession which subscribed to a conflicting philosophy and claimed independent status. So a different role for midwives had to be engineered.

New roles

The shift of antenatal care away from the municipal clinics to the hospital and general practitioner clinics (page 102) left midwives with much reduced opportunities to practise the supervisory and diagnostic skills they had been taught. In the hospital antenatal clinic they were welcomed as clerks and chaperones; they were allowed to carry out routine checks sometimes, but abdominal examinations and palpations less often, and usually their authority was undermined by having these repeated by the obstetrician. How much responsibility they were allowed in GP clinics to which they were attached depended on the attitude of the doctor. In partial compensation for the attenuation of their antenatal role, their training was extended in mothercraft, nutrition, family planning, psychology, breast feeding and the importance of mother and baby bonding [6, pp. 250, 256]. Since most of the midwives in training were not yet themselves mothers, they could not reinforce the theoretical instruction in these subjects with the learning of personal experience.

But the greatest changes in their training were in the field of intranatal care. As new obstetric interventions were introduced and became routine (Chapter 4), midwives had to learn the techniques required to carry out their part in them, on their own, although more often on the obstetricians', initiative: to induce and accelerate labour surgically by the artificial rupture of the membranes and pharmacologically by setting up intravenous infusions for the administration of syntocinon; to record the progress of cervical dilatation on a partogram (page 161); to set up and operate the electronic cardiotocograph for monitoring the uterine contractions and the baby's heart rate, interpret the traces and if necessary initiate interventive action; to assist in taking specimens of capillary blood from the fetal scalp so that blood gas levels could be measured; to administer the stronger pain relief now required, including 'topping-up' the agent in epidural anaesthesia; to carry out and suture an episiotomy (page 165); to resuscitate and intubate distressed neonates; in short to become competent obstetric nurses [6].

All this attention to impersonal instruments left the midwife less time for personal interaction with the labouring woman, less time to sustain her with moral support. Instead of her traditional role of easing and comforting, she had at least temporarily to augment distress. Obstetricians' willingness to interfere with physiological labour meant that in practice 'few labours in hospital were allowed to follow their natural course, and so intrapartum care and delivery undertaken solely by midwives was rare' [6, p. 278]. The interventions increased the need for instrumental and operative deliveries, in which case the midwife was deprived of her reward of facilitating spontaneous birth. Interventions were far fewer in the GPUs and midwives working there enjoyed greater freedom and responsibility.

Yet even in hospital, midwives working in labour wards were the ones least robbed of their traditional function. Hospital organization usually separated antenatal, intranatal and postnatal work and as obstetricians wished to retain experienced and technically competent midwives in the labour ward [38], rotation between aspects of care was discouraged. Some midwives rarely had the chance to deliver a baby and virtually none was able to follow a pregnancy right through to its completion. Midwives delivering in GPUs carried out antenatal work rarely and postnatal care only until the mother's early discharge.

The role of most midwives working in the community was likewise restricted, for their main function became the postnatal care of mothers discharged early from hospital or GPU. The satisfaction of giving continuous care was enjoyed by only a few midwives booked for a home delivery or for a 'domino' (DOMiciliary IN and Out) delivery, when the midwife looks after the woman at home until labour starts, accompanies her to hospital and conducts the delivery there, and after a few hours brings the mother and baby back home.

From 1971, midwives' training in postpartum supervision was extended for the first time to 28 days [6, p. 263], a requirement which emphasized possible overlaps with the responsibilities of Health Visitors or general practitioners. The conflicts of professional specialization, in the hospital or community setting, were supposed to be overcome by all involved working as a team, the team leader being in practice a doctor, never a midwife.

For midwives had ceased to be leaders. They had proved very much less successful in organizing a powerful professional body than had obstetricians. The Midwives Institute, founded in 1881, was turned into the College of Midwives in 1941 and received its Royal Charter in 1947 [6, p. 244], but it was the Central Midwives Board, on which organized midwives had only minority representation, which regulated the profession, an indignity which organized doctors would not have tolerated. Although the objects of the new Royal College were to promote and advance the art and science of midwifery and to raise the efficiency of midwives, the profession was by then so far under the domination of obstetricians that it had to follow their interpretation of how the object should be approached and science was accorded preference over art. There was no record for over thirty years of any effective opposition by organized midwives to the relentless rejection of their philosophy and the erosion of their traditional service.

Responses to changes

In its silence the College was reflecting the views of many of its members, for not all midwives deplored the changes taking place. An investigation conducted in 1970 for the Central Midwives Board into the views of student midwifery teachers found that some, with regret, saw midwives as 'losing status, becoming handmaidens to obstetricians, . . . no longer practitioners in their own right and enjoying less job satisfaction', while others, with enthusiasm, saw them as 'mini-obstetricians needing greater expertise in advanced technical matters, . . . [and] in management' [6, p. 264]. Midwives who hold the latter view have been appointed to many senior managerial posts and use (or abuse) their authority to enforce obstetricians' policies (pages 242–3).

In disbanding in 1974 the Domiciliary Midwives Council and the withdrawal in 1977 of the requirement for training in domiciliary delivery, the Royal College of Midwives (RCM) signalled its acceptance of obstetricians' claims about the greater safety of their methods as uncritically as did everyone else and it was slow to modify its official view in the light of new contradicting evidence being published from 1977 onwards [39–50]. As late as 1985, when a conclusive analysis establishing the greater safety of midwifery methods (Table 8.6) was given wide coverage in the lay press, the spokeswoman for the RCM could only echo the invalid bluffing offered in self-defence by the spokesman for the RCOG [51], insinuating, without any supporting evidence, that the balance of safety had by then been reversed.

Certainly obstetricians had succeeded in weaning many leading midwives and midwife teachers away from their belief in the rightness of physiological birth, an attitude they passed on to some of their pupils. But all were not so convinced and in 1976 a protest group organized what they later called the Association of Radical Midwives (ARM), 'radical' signifying the need to return to the original philosophy and fundamental skills of midwifery. The strength of prejudice these rebels had to face is illustrated by the fact that 'the minutes of early meetings give only first names of those attending for fear of victimisation' [52]. Nevertheless, the movement continued to grow and gradually wore down some of the prejudice. By 1991 its members numbered 1500 and included many distinguished midwives, the leaders of thought in the profession. It came to be regarded more sympathetically by the RCM who were influenced to realize that the future of their profession was at stake and that the ARM was pointing the way to safeguard its survival.

CONTROL OF MIDWIVES' EDUCATION

Whereas the regulation of the midwifery profession had been embodied in a series of *Midwives Acts* in earlier years, in 1979 these were superseded by the *Nurses, Midwives and Health Visitors Act* which set up the United Kingdom Central Council (UKCC) and ended the reign of the Central Midwives Board. This Act followed the recommendations in 1972 of an independent commission (Chairman Professor Asa Briggs), which accepted official policy that all births were henceforth to be in hospital under obstetricians' control and therefore that midwives were no longer to be distinguished as a separate, distinct profession. They were to be treated rather as a small branch of the much larger nursing profession, with consequently limited representation for their specific interests on the new national governing Boards which were first elected in 1983. The views of the midwifery committee of the English National Board (ENB) were often disregarded, but they were often not even elicited.

One issue of anxious concern was midwifery education. In 1989 it was ruled that the Education Officer responsible for a Midwifery School need no longer be a midwife. Protests by the midwifery committee were outvoted in 1990. The dismay and anger felt by midwives was expressed by the President of the RCM in her address to their Annual General Meeting in 1990, 'If we lose control of our education, we lose control of our profession'.

The prospect of lost control was enhanced by the recommendation in a review of the work of the National Boards and the UKCC carried out in 1990 by government-commissioned researchers, Peat Marwick McLintock. Though they were aware of counter-arguments, their view was that for organizational reasons the responsibility of approving clinical areas where student midwives learn should be in the hands of nurse education officers or the Principals of Institutions of Higher Education. As a result, some 'inappropriate decisions concerning the clinical learning experiences necessary for student midwives to develop the skills of a midwife' have been taken [27, pp. 906–8, 52, 53, p. 400].

Regional Health Authorities, in responding to the aspirations of professional care-givers for higher academic standards, have required schools of midwifery to amalgamate with schools of nursing into colleges of nursing and midwifery or health care studies, so as to gain the educational and economic benefits, for students and teachers, of shared learning in a wider range of courses. The bait of a higher career ladder for midwife teachers was not realistic, for top posts needed experience specific to nurse teachers [54].

The RCM was more successful in persuading the House of Commons Health Committee of the separateness of its profession and its education needs. It was gratified that the Committee recommended in 1992

that midwives should be afforded the same rights as other professions over the control of their education. Whether in NHS or other institutions, midwifery studies should be afforded independent faculty status. Selection of candidates, curriculum planning, assessment processes and course validation must remain under the control of the midwifery profession. We would expect these principles to be upheld not only in the training establishments but also by the statutory bodies that set overall national standards for training and approve and monitor the courses. [55, para 417]

Many midwives cling to their hope for a new *Midwives Act* to give effect to the proposals which the Radical Midwives and their parent college had made in 1986 and 1987, and repeated in 1990 [21, p. 115, 56, 57]. Under these, most midwives (60–70%) would work in the community in new, small, locally convenient antenatal clinics, displacing the general practitioner as the pregnant woman's first contact with the maternity service, providing full care, including delivery either in hospital wards under midwives' control, probably on the 'domino' principle, or at home. The remaining midwives would work in hospital, in teams small enough for each mother to know each midwife, and co-operate with consultant obstetricians to care for women with complications. The same team would follow the individual woman from her first antenatal contact to her final postnatal discharge.

Visions are not always easily converted into reality. A survey in 1992 of all midwifery units in England and Wales [58] found that by then some form of team midwifery had been successfully organized in fewer than 40% of localities; in the others problems of persuading doctors or some midwives to co-operate willingly had not been surmounted and some schemes set up had been discontinued. Although it was hardly doubted that team midwifery resulted in greater satisfaction for mothers who received less intervention, less analgesia and shorter labours, and greater job satisfaction for midwives, systems for impartial evaluation and comparison with alternative methods of care were lacking, so that it could not be claimed unequivocally that the theoretical advantages, including even ensuring continuity of carer, were in most schemes actually achieved.

Problems were created, for example, by midwifery managers not allowing midwives to give continuity of care if that involved working outside prescribed shift hours, by general practitioners unwilling to cede their role as first contact, and by obstetricians unwilling to agree to most care taking place in the community (page 106) [27, pp. 906–9]. A leading obstetrician counselled dismissively that midwives would improve their status better by aiming to take a greater share in all aspects of care within the existing obstetrician-dominated team structure [59]. An apparent upsurge in the later 1980s in the harrying of outspoken midwives may have reflected defensive attitudes by those in authority. The harrying became less evident in the early 1990s, perhaps reflecting the ineffectiveness of this tactic (pages 243–4).

Other routes to midwifery qualifications

Other important changes were taking midwifery education further from the domain of nursing. To emphasize that childbirth is not an illness, the reforming midwives agitated for their profession to be opened more generously to women without a nursing qualification, as it is in Holland and Denmark and as it once was in Britain. This plea apparently met with unaccustomed approval, for the number of schools enlisting 'direct entry' students was increased from one in the mid-1980s to seventeen in 1991 with plans for still more thereafter [60]. Reversing the implicit policy when their training was first introduced (page 51), the midwives' explicit aim was now to attract women who had themselves borne children and would be able more easily to empathize with their clients. The authorities' prompt compliance was probably motivated less by midwives' arguments than by demographic forecasts of an impending shortfall in the population of school-leavers. The mature students, however, complained that their teachers did not modify their methods and attitudes appropriately, but were too inclined to treat the new entrants like schoolchildren and give them insufficient scope for directing their own learning [61].

The revised direct entry education schedule of theory and practice could lead after three years to the midwife's registration qualification, or students could in due course go further to a Diploma in Higher Education or later to a BA or BSc Honours degree. More midwives were to be encouraged to undertake research and evaluate practices in maternity care. The first Professors of Midwifery were appointed and courses leading ultimately to a Master's degree started. There were certainly arguments in favour of raising the academic status of the midwifery profession to the same level as that of the medical profession. But it would be a mistake to imagine that a successful academic, an expert in theory, is necessarily a successful midwife, for midwifery 'will always be a practice-based profession' [54]. It must not let itself be educated out of its appreciation of the overriding importance of positive emotions and basic good health in the mother by teachers whose untested scientific theories may fail to fit the facts. The midwife's formal education, while teaching technical competence, must also provide a fertile medium for developing common sense, kindliness, empathy, patience, and the ability to inspire confidence, which are the most valuable qualities in a midwife.

The outstanding midwife in charge of the outstandingly successful Farm Midwifery Center in rural Tennessee firmly believes that the most important contribution to her midwifery training came from women who gave birth within a women-designed context.

There are indispensable midwifery skills that cannot be learned from a textbook or inside of a lecture hall. I am sure that there are some skills that cannot be learned within the context of hospital birth as we know it in the United States. [62]

Directives and guidelines have been set out by the European Community Council, the UKCC and the ENB to ensure that the training and education of midwives will produce safe, competent practitioners. Exceptionally, the Department of Health has commissioned an independent research project to evaluate the direct-entry (pre-registration) programme. Detailed interviews with student midwives, teaching staff and service-based managers are to be carried out and the vast amount of data collected, together with that generated by on-going, in-depth group inquiry of student midwives at selected sites, will be analysed and interpreted. However, proposals to involve participation in evaluation by the users of the midwifery services were not included in the published research programme [60].

MIDWIVES IN OTHER DEVELOPED COUNTRIES

However unsuccessful British midwives have been in maintaining the status they claim as 'the guardians of normal birth', midwives in the other developed countries, except the Netherlands, have failed as much or more. Once predominant everywhere as independent practitioners, they have been superseded as primary carers by doctors, though they can, of course, work in hospitals as obstetric nurses, assistants to obstetricians. Experience in the USA has been typical. There the suppression of independent midwifery started in the 19th century. By 1900 midwives were conducting only about half of all deliveries, by 1935 only about 12% and by the 1970s about 2%.

> The dramatic disappearance of a centuries-old profession, almost to extinction, was no accident. It was not due to objective scientifically based health care planning to improve the quality of maternity care. It came about by a conspiracy on a grand scale, spanning more than a century and continuing to the present day, on the part of medical doctors seeking to eliminate their economic competitors. Their tactics included two major forms: (1) the waging of a propaganda campaign to discredit the practices and reputations of midwives (to gain public support); and (2) the enactment of legislation and licensing regulations (which granted them a monopoly and gave them regulatory powers over midwives). [19, p. 112]

The conspiracy was all too effective. In some of the American States midwives are still forbidden by law to practise outside a hospital unless they obtain a licence, the granting of which can be beset with medically imposed obstructions and which commits them to work under the supervision of a doctor [63]. Regulations are relaxed only in areas with too few doctors.

Increasingly from the mid 1970s, campaigns were organized by movements opposed to the medicalization of childbirth. To provide maternity care for women judged to be at low risk of obstetric complication, some free-standing birth centres, with low intervention policies and facilities and staffed mostly by midwives, have been set up, but they were often not welcomed by the medical establishment and have had to overcome obstacles to obtain licences to practise [64]. There has been some official discouragement from using them.

Seemingly as a precaution against any further revivals of midwifery and non-hospital delivery threatened by these ominous murmurings, the later 1980s and early 1990s saw an epidemic of repressive action, in the USA, Canada and Australia, as well as in Britain, against competent midwives alleged to have transgressed the rules (pages 243–4). Despite this reaction, some liberalizing regulations have been secured, but success has not been uniform, for the relaxations in some American States have often been offset by stricter regulations in others. Overall, however, the number of deliveries in the USA conducted by midwives, mostly in birth centres or at home, has tripled between 1980 and 1989, when it made up 3.7% of the total [65].

Midwives – certified and lay

Most midwives in the United States are certified nurse-midwives with two years' recognized midwifery training after completing their nursing course. They work in obstetric hospitals and in free-standing birth centres, always with the support of a back-up obstetrician, and sometimes in joint practice with one. Lay midwives, the most likely targets of legal prohibition, are not trained nurses; as direct entrants to midwifery, they may have learned their craft in schools abroad or as apprentices to experienced midwives, sometimes in schools attached to birth centres [66].

The greatest moves towards legalization took place in the early 1990s in Canada and its Provinces: Ontario was quick to launch an official training course, based on the philosophy that birth is a normal, physiological process, for direct-entry midwives without prior nurse training; Alberta passed legislation in 1992 which designated midwifery as a profession [67], encouraging British Columbia to follow suit in 1993. The effect of legalization, however, while obviously of material benefit to licensed midwives, may be to formalize medically directed licensing systems to benefit the providers of care rather than protect the users.

The status of midwifery as a profession is unquestioned in the Netherlands, but midwives' independence is most assured when they deliver mothers in the family home or in small hospitals. In 1986, they gave sole care in 43% of deliveries, more than half of them at home [68], but they too are forbidden by law to attend women classified as 'at risk', on criteria laid down by obstetricians [69] (pages 348–54). When they work in obstetric hospitals, even the Dutch midwives tend to become doctors' assistants (70, p. 33]. The notable success of midwives' care in the Netherlands has been enhanced throughout the 20th century by the provision of maternity aid nurses who are specially trained, not only in hygiene and mother and child care, but also in all aspects of looking after the mother's family while she recuperates from the exertions of birth. The modern aid is also able to assist the midwife by relieving her of some of her more time-consuming functions and by keeping a detailed log of relevant events [71]. This is an institution which might with advantage be copied by other countries: it would certainly be appreciated by mothers and might well be a more profitable, though less glamorous, use of resources than investments in costly high technology, ante- and intrapartum.

Where independent midwifery is illegal, as until recently in Canada, there is no official provision for training midwives. A few unofficial midwifery schools provide training, often for students without a nursing qualification. Care by lay midwives, some self-taught, is usually good; irrespective of results, however, their treatment by doctors can vary from sympathetic co-operation in some places to extreme hostility in others. Mothers, who engage them because their methods are more acceptable and their fees lower, have more often than not to face considerable disapproval from official providers. Yet it has been these much harried lay midwives who have gone on carrying the flickering torch, at great personal risk of career and freedom, and so kept alive the prospect of non-medical maternity care.

BIRTH ATTENDANTS IN UNDERDEVELOPED COUNTRIES

There is not the same opposition to midwives in countries where the population is too poor or too dispersed to support a powerful medical profession, yet the phenomenon of the 'disappearing midwife' is becoming apparent there, to the detriment of the maternity services [72]. A basic problem is to find suitable midwifery tutors, qualified in both the theory and practice of midwifery and also in the demands of the local environment. Aspiring midwives may not have the prior educational qualifications to be accepted for training in midwifery schools in developed countries, but those who do may not find what they learn appropriate for their less developed homelands. Midwives trained in large maternity hospitals may find it difficult to practise without technological aids and in turn to teach student midwives to do so.

The shortage of midwives is only partly made good by training more of the traditional birth attendants (TBAs) – upgrading their skills so that they can perform deliveries and cord care hygienically and use techniques within their scope to prevent or control postpartum haemorrhage, as well as enabling them to give advice about nutrition, family planning, the sexual transmission of infections, breast feeding and healthy child-rearing. Thus they should help directly to reduce the two most frequent causes of maternal death (sepsis and haemorrhage) and indirectly many others (pages 305–6).

Despite these potential gains, there are some reservations that training TBAs is the most profitable investment towards achieving the immediate objective of reducing the high toll of maternal mortality, for there are many complications, including obstructed labour, which the trained TBA could not deal with, but which, it is thought, could be treated effectively in small, modestly equipped, local hospitals and health centres, and better rewards might result if money were spent on creating more of these. As well as the problems of recruiting trainers, TBA training programmes are not easy or cheap to organize. They usually last three months and the amount the trainees can learn in that time is limited, as it once was for the early midwife trainees in the developed countries (page 56). The area in which the TBA can practise is also limited, since she has other domestic responsibilities, which means that she is likely to attend fewer than twenty births in a year, a small number over which to spread the cost of her training [72, 73].

Midwives world wide

An international association of midwives, based in Belgium, was founded in 1922. It was disbanded during the 1939–45 war but formed again as the International Confederation of Midwives in 1951. Its purpose is to link national associations and promote standards of midwifery practice. To this end it holds triennial conferences. Politically, the organization has in the past been no more powerful than its member associations in reasserting its philosophy of non-interventive midwifery and the claimed status of midwives, but it may have been instrumental in ensuring that the recent spirit of protest, arising in some countries, has been spread to many others.

The spirit of protest has been fuelled by the realization that, wherever comparisons are possible, care by midwives using low technology is found to lead to better outcomes for mothers and babies than does care by obstetricians using high technology (Chapters 7 and 8). Such findings after painstaking research have led the World Health Organization to recommend that care during normal pregnancy, birth and following birth should be the duty of midwives, with doctors assisting only in cases of complication and that all interventions, whether of high technology or low, should be used sparingly and discriminately, for strictly medical indications only [74, 75].

The WHO reports have no force beyond recommendations. National governments are not bound to take notice of them. Neither are the professional organizations of obstetricians, for whose continued prosperity the implications are very damaging. Once again it is a question, not of factual evidence, but of relative political power. In maternity care, political power derives from legal monopoly and the obstetric profession has been much more adept than the midwifery profession at exploiting for its own advantage the legal protection granted to each of them. The greater restraint shown by midwives in pursuing their self-interest means less potential conflict with the disinterested aim of any birth attendant, which is to facilitate the delivery process and ensure that no impairment, immediate or later, is sustained by either the mother or her offspring.

REFERENCES

1. Wertz, R.W. and Wertz, D.C. (1977) *Lying-in: a History of Childbirth in America*, The Free Press, New York. (Quoting J.H. Dye (1884) *Painless Childbirth*, Buffalo, pp. 53–4.)
2. Briance, P. (1985) Childbirth with confidence do it yourself. *J. Psychosom. Obstet. Gynaecol.*, **4**, 67–70.
3. Mead, M. (1972) *Blackberry Winter: My Earlier Years*, Morrow, New York, p. 51.
4. Genesis 3:16.
5. Donnison, J. (1977) *Midwives and Medical Men*, Heinemann, London.
6. Towler, J. and Bramall, J. (1986) *Midwives in History and Society*, Croom Helm, London.
7. Towler and Bramall, *Midwives in History*, p. 118. (Quoting S. Stone, 1735, *A Complete Practice of Midwifery*, London.)
8. Towler and Bramall, *Midwives in History*, p. 123–5. (Quoting M. Stephen (1795) *The Domestic Midwife*, London.)
9. Drife, J.O. (1988) My grandchild's birth. *Br. Med. J.*, **297**, 1208.
10. Holland, E. (1954) The medical schools and the teaching of midwifery, in *Historical Review of British Obstetrics and Gynaecology, 1800–1950*, (eds J.M. Munro Kerr, R.W. Johnstone and M.H. Phillips), Churchill Livingstone, Edinburgh, Chapter XXX.
11. Berkeley, C. (1929) The teaching of midwifery. *J. Obstet. Gynaecol. Br. Emp.*, **37**(4), 701–55.
12. Towler and Bramall, *Midwives in History*, p. 158 (Quoting F. Nightingale (1872) *Notes on Lying-in Institutions and a Scheme for Training Midwives*.)

13. Wertz, R.W. and Wertz, D.C. (1977) *Lying-in: A History of Childbirth in America*, The Free Press, New York.

14. Walker, A. (1954) Midwife services, England and Wales, in *Historical Review of British Obstetrics 1800–1950* (eds J.M. Munro Kerr, R.V. Johnstone, and M.H. Phillips), Churchill Livingstone, Edinburgh, Chapter XXXIII.

15. Cookson, I. (1967) The past and future of the maternity service. *J. Coll. Gen. Pract.*, **13**, 143–62.

16. Claye, A.M. (1954) Obstetric anaesthesia and analgesia, in *Historical Review of British Obstetrics 1800–1950* (eds J.M. Munro Kerr, R.V. Johnstone, and M.H. Phillips), Churchill Livingstone, Edinburgh, Chapter XXVII.

17. Shaw, W.F. (1954) *Twenty-Five Years. The Story of the Royal College of Obstetricians and Gynaecologists 1929–1954*, Churchill, London.

18. Wertz and Wertz. *Lying-in*, pp. 145–7. (Quoting J.W. Williams (1912) Medical Education and the Midwife Problem in the United States. *J. Am. Med. Assoc.*, **58**.)

19. Stewart, D. (1981) *The Five Standards for Safe Childbearing*, Napsac Reproductions, Marble Hill. (Quoting New York Academy of Medicine (1933) *Maternal Mortality in New York, 1930–32*, The Commonwealth Fund.)

20. Commonwealth Bureau of Statistics (1907–70) *Demography*, Canberra.

21. House of Commons Health Committee (1991) *Maternity Services: Preconception*, vol II, Minutes of evidence pp. 1–291. HMSO, London.

22. Biggs, J., Harden, R. and Howie, P. (1991) Undergraduate obstetrics and gynaecology in the United Kingdom and the Republic of Ireland, 1989. *Br. J. Obstet, Gynaecol.*, **98**, 127–34.

23. Royal College of Obstetricians and Gynaecologists (1983) *Nutrition in Pregnancy*, RCOG, London.

24. Rush, D., Green, J., Mahomed, K. and Hytten, F. (1989) Dietary modification in pregnancy, in *A Guide to Effective Care in Pregnancy and Childbirth* (eds M Enkin, M. Keirse and I. Chalmers), Oxford University Press, Oxford.

25. Joint Working Party of the Royal College of Obstetricians and Gynaecologists and the Royal College of General Practitioners (1981) *Report on Training for Obstetrics and Gynaecology for General Practitioners*, RCOG, Appendix I.

26. House of Commons Health Committee (1992) *Maternity Services*, vol III, Appendices to the Minutes of Evidence, HMSO, London, pp. 651–922.

27. The Royal College of General Practitioners and the Royal College of Obstetricians (1993) *General Practitioner Vocational Training in Obstetrics and Gynaecology*, RCGP, London.

28. Department of Health, Welsh Office, Scottish Home and Health Department, Department of Health and Social Services, Northern Ireland (1991) *Report on Confidential Enquiries into Maternal Deaths in the United Kingdom 1985–87*, HMSO, London.

29. Ennis, M. and Vincent, C. (1990) Obstetric accidents: a review of 64 cases. *Br. Med. J.*, **300**, 1365–7.

30. Tindall, V., Martin, R. and Burslem, R. (1989) *Preparation and Advice for the MRCOG*, Churchill Livingstone, Edinburgh.

31. Bewley, S. (1991) The future obstetrician/gynaecologist. *Br. J. Obstet. Gynaecol.*, **98**, 237–40.

32. Department of Health (1993) *Hospital Doctors – Training for the Future* (The Calman Report), HMSO, London.

33. Chamberlain, G. and Gunn, P. (1987) *Birthplace: The Report of the Confidential Enquiry into Facilities Available at the Place of Birth*, John Wiley, Chichester, Table 5.5.

34. Butler, N.R. and Bonham, D.G. (1963) *Perinatal Mortality*, Churchill Livingstone, Edinburgh, Table No. 12.

35. Registrar General (1972) *Statistical Review of England and Wales for the Year 1970*, Part II, HMSO, London, Tables B1 and B2.

36. Office of Population Censuses and Surveys, *Birth Statistics* (Annual 1974–1991), HMSO, London, Tables 8.1–8.3.

37. Office of Population Censuses and Surveys (1985) *Mortality Statistics: Perinatal and Infant: Social and Biological Factors*, Series DH3, no. 18, HMSO, London, Table 23.

38. Royal College of Obstetricians and Gynaecologists (1982) *Report of the RCOG Working Party on Ante-natal and Intra-partum Care*, RCOG, London.

39. Tew, M. (1977) Where to be born? *New Society*, 27 January 120–1.

40. Tew, M. (1977) Obstetric hospitals and general practitioner units – the statistical record. *J. R. Coll. Gen. Pract.*, **27**, 689–94.

41. Tew, M. (1978) The case against hospital deliveries: the statistical evidence, in *The Place of Birth* (eds S. Kitzinger and J. Davis), Oxford University Press, Oxford, pp. 55–65.

42. Tew, M. (1979) The safest place of birth – further evidence. *Lancet*, **i**, 1388–90; **ii**, 523.

43. Tew, M. (1980) Facts not assertions of belief. *Health Soc. Serv. J.*, 12 September, 1194–7.

44. Tew, M. (1981) The effect of scientific obstetrics. *Health Soc. Serv. J.*, 17 April, 444–6.

45. Tew, M. (1982) Obstetrics versus midwifery – the verdict of the statistics, *J. Matern. Child Health*, May, 198–201.

46. Tew, M. (1984) Understanding intranatal care through mortality statistics, in *Pregnancy Care for the 1980s* (eds L. Zander and G. Chamberlain), Royal Society of Medicine and Macmillan, London, pp. 105–25.

47. Tew, M. (1985) Safety in intranatal care: the statistics, in *Modern Obstetrics in General Practice* (ed. G.N. Marsh), Oxford University Press, Oxford, pp. 203–223.

48. Tew, M. (1985) Place of birth and perinatal mortality. *J. R. Coll. Gen. Pract.*, **35**, 390–4.

49. Tew, M. (1986) Do obstetric intranatal interventions make birth safer? *Br. J. Obstet. Gynaecol.*, **93**, 659–74.

50. Campbell, R. and Macfarlane, A. (1987) *Where To Be Born? The Debate and the Evidence*, National Perinatal Epidemiology Unit, Oxford.

51. (1985) *The Times*, 13 and 21 August.

52. Cronk, M. (1992) How did we get into this mess in the first place? *MIDIRS Midwifery Digest*, **2**, 6–8.

53. House of Commons Health Committee (1992) *Maternity Services*, vol. II, Appendices to the Minutes of Evidence, HMSO, London, pp. 338–650.

54. Warwick, C. (1992) Reflections on the current management of midwifery education. *MIDIRS Midwifery Digest*, **2**, 251–4.
55. House of Commons Health Committee (1992) *Maternity Service*, vol. I, Report together with Appendices and the Proceedings of the Committee, (The Winterton Report), HMSO, London, paras 1–452, pp. i–xciii.
56. Association of Radical Midwives (1986) *The Vision. Proposals for the Future of the Maternity Service*, ARM, Ormskirk, Lancashire.
57. Royal College of Midwives (1987) *The Role and Education of the Future Midwife in the United Kingdom*, RCM, London.
58. Wraight, A., Ball, J., Secombe, I. *et al.* (1993) *Mapping Team Midwifery*, Institute of Manpower Studies, University of Sussex.
59. Macdonald, R.R. (1987, 1988) In defence of obstetricians, *Br. J. Obstet. Gynaecol.*, **94, 95**, 88, 205.
60. Kent, J. and Maggs, C. (1992) *An Evaluation of Pre-registration Midwifery Education in England: Working Paper 1, Research Design*. Maggs Research Associates, Bath.
61. Hindley, J. (1991) Pre-registration midwifery education: a student's view. *MIDIRS Midwifery Digest*, **1**, 382–3.
62. Gaskin, I.M. (1992) Non-medical midwifery training. *Napsac News*, **17** (1), 19–21.
63. Midwifery and the Law (1983) *Mothering*, special education, (ed. P.O. McMahon), Mothering Publications, Albuquerque, USA.
64. Rooks, J., Weatherby, N., Ernst, E. *et al.* (1989) Outcomes of care in birth centres. *N. Engl. J. Med.*, **321**, 1804–11.
65. (1992) News item. *Birth*, **19** (2), 107.
66. Korte, D. and Scaer, R. (1992) *A Good Birth, A Safe Birth*, 3rd edn. The Harvard Common Press, Boston, Massachusetts.
67. Relyea, M. (1992) The rebirth of midwifery in Canada: an historical perspective. *Midwifery*, **8** (4), 159–69.
68. Tew, M. and Damstra-Wijmenga, S. (1991) Safest birth attendants: recent Dutch evidence. *Midwifery*, **7**, 55–63.
69. Teijlingen, E. and McCaffery, P. (1987) The profession of midwife in the Netherlands. *Midwifery*, **3**, 178–86.
70. Houd, S. and Oakley, A. (1986) Alternative perinatal services: report on a pilot survey, in *Perinatal Health Services in Europe* (ed. J. Phaff), World Health Organization, Croom Helm, Kent, p. 33.
71. Teijlingen, E. (1990) The profession of maternity home care assistant and its significance for the Dutch midwifery profession. *Int. J. Nurs. Stud.*, **27**, 355–46.
72. World Health Organization (1992) *Traditional Birth Attendants: a Joint WHO/UNFPA/UNICEF Statement*, WHO, Geneva.
73. Kwast, B. and Bentley, J. (1991) Introducing confident midwives: midwifery education – action for safe motherhood. *Midwifery*, **7**, 8–19.
74. World Health Organization (1985) *Having a Baby in Europe: Public Health in Europe, 26*, WHO Regional Office, Copenhagen.
75. Conference Report (1987) Having a Baby in the United Kingdom. *Lancet*, **i**, 989–90.

3

The practices of attendants before birth

THE BEGINNING OF ANTENATAL CARE

In the centuries before 1900, pregnancy was not a condition for which professional advice or attention was usually sought, either from doctors or from midwives. The most fertile sources of information, for better or worse, were other women who had been pregnant. The prevalence of large families and close-knit social communities ensured ready access to many with such experience.

Up till then, medical interest had concentrated on the problems of delivery, particularly abnormal delivery. Doctors knew little about the physiology of pregnancy. They did, however, share with the lay public the belief that what happened to a woman during pregnancy was important for the welfare of the fetus. At best, the general principles they advanced were those which should bring good health to everyone: adequate diet, hygienic habits, adequate exercise of a not too exhausting kind, rest in moderation and freedom from stress. Detailed advice which was not always so unexceptionable, including rules for regular purging, came to be written down in books addressed directly to women or to midwives or doctors [1].

Whether the written precepts penetrated far down the social scale in a largely illiterate society is questionable and even if they were understood widespread poverty would have made them impossible to follow. The urban poor, whose numbers had greatly increased during the 18th and 19th centuries, could not afford a diet adequate in either quantity or variety, although the rural poor fared better. Few working class women could have adequate rest or avoid heavy physical toil whether they were employed outside the home or within it, looking after their growing and too often ailing families. Primitive domestic plumbing in overcrowded dwellings made adequate standards of hygiene, even if attempted, difficult to achieve. Stress for women living in such conditions must have been constant. If they were aware of the popular theory that the mother's emotional state and mental attitude directly affected her fetus, and that adverse feelings of anger, depression or anxiety could cause it to be malformed, they were ill-placed to fill their minds with calm and uplifting thoughts to avoid the threatened disaster.

Doctors' antenatal attentions were restricted to women who could afford to pay for them and who sought relief from the transient ailments of pregnancy. For nearly all such ailments – nausea, vomiting, headaches, vertigo, insomnia, muscle cramps, varicose veins, swelling of the legs and even haemorrhage – their standard remedy before the mid-19th century was blood-letting [2]. These conditions were thought to be generated by the cessation of the menstrual blood loss, an aberration of nature whose consequences were thus to be counteracted. For a long time mothers apparently believed, or were talked into believing, that blood-letting was beneficial, an example of the immense powers of self-deception of which doctors and patients are capable. But ultimately the patients rebelled and their protests were gradually acknowledged as advances in the understanding of human physiology undermined medical confidence in blood-letting as a nostrum for human ailments. Doctors could also prescribe antidotes to pregnancy disorders from a wide variety of herbal remedies, but these would be as readily available from lay sources which would serve most women who wanted them.

EARLY INTEREST IN THE PHYSIOLOGY AND PATHOLOGY OF PREGNANCY

Before 1900, little thought was given to the possibility that complications encountered in labour might be averted or their severity mitigated by appropriate treatment during pregnancy. Exceptionally in the later years of the 19th century the French obstetrician, Adolphe Pinard, did give thought to the value of listening to the fetal heart and invented the fetal stethoscope which bears his name. He also devised a method for forestalling the greater risk associated with breech presentation. By abdominal palpation of the woman in the eighth or ninth month of pregnancy, the presenting part of the fetus could be identified and by his technique of external version a breech could be converted to the normal vertex presentation. External version came to be widely practised, although it does not always achieve a stable lie and can cause premature detachment of the placenta with life-threatening consequences. Another of Pinard's useful contributions was the development of a method still used to estimate 'disproportion', a fetal head too large for the maternal pelvis [3, pp. 26–7].

Pinard obviously had the opportunity to study pregnant women. Such opportunity was lacking in Britain when the Scottish obstetrician, J.W. Ballantyne, made his plea for a Pro-Maternity Hospital in 1901 [4]. Such a hospital would be 'for the reception of women who are pregnant but who are not yet in labour'. It would be of immediate benefit to the women who used it, but more importantly, it would be of lasting benefit to obstetric knowledge through the opportunity it would present for direct study of the pregnant state, its physiology and pathology and of the effects of treatment. He wanted it to do for medical understanding of the developmental stage what the lying-in hospitals had done for medical understanding of the delivery stage of childbearing.

Hitherto, doctors had been more concerned to save the life of the mother, but Ballantyne now wanted them to be as much concerned with the survival and health of the infant. To this end he recommended that

the maternal urine and blood should be subjected to chemical and microscopic examination as it is beginning to be realised that the condition of the foetus *in utero* is to some extent reflected in the composition and character of the maternal excretions [5, p. 148].

Ballantyne had great faith that scientific enquiry could be as profitably applied to obstetrics as to physics and chemistry and in his inaugural address to the Edinburgh Obstetrical Society in 1906 [6], he predicted with remarkable accuracy a time when it would be possible to watch the fetus within the uterus, to induce labour pharmacologically, to monitor the fetal heart, to keep the premature infant alive and to replace destructive operations with life-saving ones – predictions that were to be fulfilled in the course of the next eighty years. One prediction that had not been fulfilled within that time, however, was that antenatal care would correctly foresee and forestall all the serious complications of labour.

His plea for hospital facilities met with a prompt response. The first pre-maternity or antenatal bed to be endowed in the Edinburgh Royal Maternity Hospital in 1901 was soon followed by more [5]. The example was quickly copied by other teaching hospitals.

The occupants of the antenatal beds would already have developed complications or be in late pregnancy and tired. Ballantyne saw the advantage of consultation in early pregnancy, in time for the doctor to give advice about diet, dress, behaviour and bodily functions. He believed 'that it was better to check the beginnings of evil in pregnancy than to await until an abnormal gestation had developed into a labour dangerous for mother and baby alike' [5, p. 148].

Surprisingly, he did not make a corresponding plea for outpatient facilities, where doctors could systematically study the different stages of pregnancy and learn to detect the first signs of impending abnormality and where maternal urine and blood could be subjected routinely to the examinations he advocated.

An experiment involving regular visits to pregnant women in their homes by nurses attached to the Boston Lying-in Hospital, Massachusetts, had such encouraging results that an outpatient clinic was started there in 1911. Similar clinics had been set up in teaching hospitals in Australia in 1910 and 1912 before the first antenatal clinic in Edinburgh was opened in 1915. A few experimental clinics in London and a few outpatient dispensaries quickly followed [5].

The Edinburgh clinic was set up at the instigation, not of Ballantyne, but of Haig Ferguson, a physician who, in 1899, had co-founded a refuge for young unmarried women in their last weeks of pregnancy. He was so impressed with the finding that rest, good food, healthy surroundings and medical supervision resulted in lower pre-term delivery rates, higher birthweights and lower neonatal mortality that he advocated the provision of medical supervision at least for expectant married women as well [3, p. 51]. In due course, every obstetric hospital was to have its outpatient clinic, a facility influencing the pregnancies of far more women than did the inpatient antenatal beds.

However, for the next thirty-five years the main providers of antenatal care in Britain were the local authorities.

THE EARLY INVOLVEMENT OF LOCAL AUTHORITIES

When the public's conscience was first stirred about the persistently high infant mortality rate, the first remedies proposed were education of mothers in the care of their infants and better food for them both. By 1900, ladies from the more advantaged classes were visiting the least advantaged families to educate mothers in the virtues of hygiene and good feeding practices. These voluntary visitors were soon to be supplemented and later supplanted by professional health visitors paid for by local authorities. Following examples set in Paris and New York, some local authorities provided uncontaminated milk for poor mothers and babies. They also organized schools for mothers which offered, not only classes in domestic hygiene and infant management, but also cheap dinners for expectant and nursing mothers [3, pp. 39–45].

By 1914, more than educational and welfare interventions were thought necessary. A Local Government Board circular of that year proposed 'that medical advice, and where necessary, treatment should be continuously and systematically available for expectant mothers' [3,

p. 45]. The condition of pregnancy was not to 'be regarded as pathological, but attention should rather be devoted to the prevention and . . .
treatment of . . . minor departures from the normal' [3, p. 56]. The
antenatal care was to be provided in outpatient clinics, intended for
women who could not afford private care. They were to be staffed by
midwives and medical officers who would give advice but refer
patients to hospital or a general practitioner if treatment was required.
The proposals were consolidated in the *Maternity and Child Welfare Act*
of 1918 and 'the number of clinics increased from 120 in 1918 to 891 in
1929 and 1931 in 1944. In addition, many rural and some urban
authorities arranged for antenatal supervision to be given by a panel
of general practitioners or by home visits from municipal midwives' [7,
p. 22].

While the objectives of the antenatal movement were to remove
anxiety and discomfort, treat early complications, increase the proportion of normal labours and lower the stillbirth and maternal death rates,
there was no clear conception of the clinical practices which would
enable this to be achieved. Breaking new ground in little-known territory, the first steps in care were bound to be tentative. Actually to
detect the signs that there were 'the beginnings of evil' and then so to
treat the incipient complication that 'a labour dangerous for infant and
mother alike' would be averted was a demanding requirement which
medical science could hardly begin to meet. Doctors and midwives had
to learn their trade as they went along and their experience was only
gradually incorporated in their training programmes.

ANTENATAL SURVEILLANCE

A model maternity and child welfare record card was prepared by the
Local Government Board in 1915. Information was to be obtained by
the midwife about the mother's obstetric history (which has a tendency
to repeat itself), her medical history, her present state of health, the
adequacy of her diet and her weight [3]. From 1916, the midwives'
training syllabus included the study of pregnancy, its hygiene, its
diseases and complications, including abortion. They were to detect the
signs and symptoms of venereal disease; they could diagnose maternal
syphilis by the Wasserman test and, with foreknowledge, they could
prevent congenital syphilis in the infant by prompt treatment with an
arsenical drug.

By 1923, the midwives' practical training included external pelvic
measurement and the analysis of urine but not blood pressure measurement, although it had been known since the 19th century that raised
blood pressure, especially in conjunction with protein in the urine, is

associated with the condition then called toxaemia (later pre-eclampsia, and later still pregnancy-induced hypertension), which can lead to eclampsia, a very serious condition characterized by convulsions. When identified, this danger appeared to be reduced if the women at risk were treated by a combination of rest, diet (although opinions varied as to the correct diet) and sedation, treatments which later research showed to be of doubtful or no benefit [8]. The midwives' rule book of 1928 specified the abnormal conditions which had to be referred to a doctor [1, pp. 216–17].

In 1929 the Ministry of Health, drawing on the accumulated but un-evaluated experience, prepared a memorandum, 'Antenatal clinics: their conduct and scope', which set a basic pattern for all clinics and which is still followed in the 1990s, albeit with modifications and additions in the light of expanding medical knowledge and theories. Examinations were advised at sixteen, twenty, twenty-four and thirty weeks of preg-nancy, then fortnightly to thirty-six weeks, then weekly until delivery. The mother's health was to be checked, her urine tested and now her blood pressure measured, for a specific objective was to be the diag-nosis of toxaemia, as well as venereal and other infectious diseases. Uterine height and girth were to be measured, the fetal heart was to be checked by auscultation and the fetal lie by palpation. There is, however, a good deal of evidence that these laudable precepts were often not carried out in practice, especially in the earlier years [3, pp. 79, 80, 93, 94].

THE USE OF PRENATAL RADIOGRAPHY

The application of radiography, which did not develop rapidly until the 1920s, offered new possibilities in antenatal diagnosis, determining the position and presentation of the fetus, detecting skeletal malforma-tions, including anencephaly and spina bifida, locating the placental site and establishing multiple pregnancy. The new possibilities in diag-nosis were unfortunately not matched by new possibilities in treating the pathological conditions discovered. However, when a breech pre-sentation was diagnosed the technique of external version (pages 87, 150, 171) was increasingly used to forestall the problems at delivery associated with high fetal mortality. Version was particularly recom-mended when a potentially inadequate pelvis for the fetal head was also diagnosed [9]. Radiography, however, led to this disproportion being overdiagnosed. It drew attention away from the fact that the forces of labour can stretch the pelvic opening and mould the fetal head, so that in the event it can find a safe passage through a quite severely deformed structure [10].

As solutions were found to the technical difficulties, prenatal radiography came to be used with great abandon by doctors whose patients could afford it, in complete confidence that the infant would suffer no harm as a result. In 1937 the Director of the Radiological Department at University College Hospital, London, wrote 'It has been frequently asked whether there is any danger to the life of the child by the passage of X-rays through it; it can be said at once that there is none if the examination is carried out by a competent radiologist or radiographer' [11, p. 497]. And as late as 1954 the verdict was the same: 'Today the fear that exposure to diagnostic X-rays might injure the foetus has not been borne out by experience' [10]. This sublime confidence was not shaken until after 1956, when the results of a study showing an association between antenatal X-rays and childhood cancer were published [12]. The infants of poorer mothers, who were less likely to be cared for by doctors, were less likely to be exposed to this unrealized threat to their ultimate, if not their immediate, health.

NEW TREATMENTS

From the mid-1930s, antenatal care was benefiting also from advances in biochemistry and pharmacology. The antibiotic drugs, first Prontosil and the sulphonamides, which became available from 1936, and then penicillin, which became available for civilian use after the war ended in 1945, led to the successful treatment of venereal and other infections of varying degrees of severity, including urinary tract infections of which the incidence was relatively high [13]. It had become possible to confirm pregnancy by testing for the presence of oestrogens in maternal urine in advance of the usually recognized signs and symptoms. Recognition of rhesus blood groups in 1940 made possible treatment and then prevention of maternal iso-immunization and the dangerous haemolytic disease of the newborn. New knowledge led to the appreciation of the importance of haemoglobin in the blood of pregnant women and the treatment of anaemia, which was known to be a chronic condition, highly prevalent in women of reproductive age. As a result of the improved diet of the war years, the haemoglobin levels of women, when tested at antenatal clinics, showed a marked improvement [13], but routine blood testing was not introduced until the late 1940s.

In 1941, the discovery was made by an Australian obstetrician of the association between rubella (German measles) in pregnancy and the death or severe neurological damage of the infant, but it was not until after 1950 that preventive intervention became available [14].

WOMEN'S EARLY REACTIONS TO ANTENATAL CARE

The manifold growth in the number of antenatal clinics was matched by a manifold growth in the number of attenders. Official records were not routinely kept, but according to different unofficial estimates the proportion of women receiving antenatal care of some kind from local authority or hospital clinic or from private doctors or midwives increased from a fraction 'incalculably small' in 1915 to 80% in 1935 [15] and to 99% in 1946 [7, p. 23].

It might have been supposed that the enormous increase in the number of women attending clinics was because they found it an enjoyable and profitable experience or at least that the ultimate benefits were so rewarding as to compensate for any discomforts suffered in the process and for the financial costs incurred by individuals and the State. One inducement to attend, particularly valued in the war years, was to collect the free or subsidized dietary supplements distributed from these centres. Apart from this, evidence to support any of the supposed reasons for attendance is extremely hard to find. Credit for the result must be due to the persuasiveness of leaders of opinion in propagating faith in a theoretical ideal.

The underlying theory that serious troubles can be prevented if they can be tackled in their earliest stages is undoubtedly attractive. It is especially appealing to women of the upper and middle classes, who characteristically plan for the future. They value education, supply recruits to the professions and trust the advice of their professional peers without questioning too rigorously whether it is sound. They are the leaders of fashion and from their ranks came the politicians and medical advisors who proposed the action aimed at reducing the national infant mortality rate, action which involved a more radical change of behaviour from the working classes than from their own.

At first the attitude of working class women to antenatal clinics was one of suspicion and scepticism and their attendance was reluctant. In the early years of the century, women were becoming increasingly conscious and resentful of the disabilities, political, social, economic and medical, which society imposed on their sex. They were only too aware of the dangers of childbirth and the burden of bringing up their children. They were at last forming militant organizations to struggle for their emancipation. Working class women became actively involved in some of these organizations, for example the Women's Co-operative Guild. They were persuaded and in turn spread the gospel that it really was in their own interest to take advantage of the antenatal care provided [3, p. 65].

The providers of medically directed antenatal care were in no doubt that it was advantageous. In 1924, Dr Janet Campbell, the Senior Medical Officer concerned with maternity and child welfare in the recently created Ministry of Health, wrote

> It is the key to success in any scheme of prevention and it must be insisted upon in and out of season until it is no longer ignored or looked upon as a luxury for the well-to-do woman. . . . Until antenatal supervision is accepted by patients and their advisers as the invariable duty of the professional attendant . . . we shall never make substantial progress towards the reduction of maternal death and injury. [16, p. 74]

Recommended medicine, like cod-liver oil, is often unpalatable. Many women who attended the early clinics did not find them welcoming, reassuring places and many official reports deplored their manifest reluctance to attend [3, p. 73].

Nor did the clinics become more attractive as attendances increased. They consistently failed to live up to the standard proposed by the Local Government Board in 1915 that 'Crowding, and protracted waiting of mothers and their children, should be avoided, and the interview of the doctor with each mother and child should not be hurried' [17]. Crowding, waiting and hurried consultations were to remain perpetual sources of complaint in British clinics (pages 103–4) and the problems were not unique to Britain. In the USA, many poor women were deterred from using clinics 'because they must spend hours waiting for a 30-second examination' [18, p. 244].

ALLAYING FEARS OR CREATING ANXIETIES?

A primary objective of routine antenatal care is to reassure the expectant mother and relieve her anxiety. Health checks to some people, who do not feel unwell, may indeed be reassuring to their confidence that they are capable of looking after themselves. But to others they are disturbing reminders of their vulnerability, which tend to induce expectations of illness and threaten their self-confidence. As the Chief Medical Officer of the Ministry of Health commented in his *Annual Report* of 1933 [19, pp. 75–6],

> It is frequently found that the officers in attendance at a clinic concentrate unduly on the search for major obstetric abnormalities and tend to lay too little stress on physical discomforts, minor departures from health, undernourishment of the mother and the general hygiene of pregnancy. This attitude may unfortunately be reflected in that of the mothers who may be so impressed with the

possible perils of pregnancy and childbirth that they develop a constant sense of anxiety as to what the future may bring.

Overinvolvement of the doctor was said to bring the 'danger that, if there is a doctor's consultation at each visit, the abnormal side of pregnancy will be emphasised' [7, p. 45].

Likewise, the confidence of people who do feel unwell is not boosted by health checks which lead to advice or treatment which they find inappropriate or ineffective, such as telling overburdened working class mothers to rest or eat food they cannot afford. Nevertheless, the knowledge that their health was being monitored, that someone else was interested in their wellbeing, probably encouraged many women to take as good care of themselves as their circumstances would permit.

Antenatal care in a setting where a trusting and continuing relationship can be built up between client and adviser, midwife or doctor, a relationship which will carry through to labour and delivery, is most likely to provide effective reassurance. This could happen where general practitioners or specialist obstetricians looked after throughout their pregnancy the private patients they were booked to deliver. It could also happen where a midwife was able in a public antenatal clinic to look after women she was booked to deliver at home. But otherwise the work of medical officers and midwives in the municipal clinics was limited to antenatal care. A woman who was booked to deliver in hospital – and she would be predicted for some reason to be at highest risk – had to make the emotional adjustments to unfamiliar attendants in an unfamiliar setting at the time when she was having to make emotional and physical adjustments to the unfamiliar changes that were taking place in her body.

The transition could be just as upsetting for a woman who had her antenatal care as an outpatient of the hospital where she was to be delivered, for antenatal clinics and labour wards were usually separately organized and unlikely to have overlapping staff, an unhappy divorce that has become permanent (page 72). The organization of the maternity service has never taken into account the possibility that the fragmentation of care into discrete periods, each with its own specialist personnel, could be a factor running counter to its objective of reducing the physical dangers of birth. The emotional dangers were beyond its remit, though they were recognized by some doctors. One general practitioner [20] wrote in 1934

To separate the antenatal supervision of a patient from the conduct of the confinement is simply ridiculous. Yet this is being done regularly all over the country and is one of the most serious disadvantages of the present method of running antenatal schemes.

That emotional dangers were in fact being increased by medical management, which succeeded in fostering apprehension in the parturient woman and weakened her self-confidence, was realized also by the obstetrician Grantly Dick-Read, whose books *Natural Childbirth* [21] and *Childbirth Without Fear* [22] first appeared in 1933 and 1942 respectively. He had witnessed birth without pain, first in Flanders (page 40) and later in the home of a poor woman who refused his offer of chloroform and went on to deliver her baby without fuss or noise. Neither woman apparently expected pain, so did not fear it. Having no fear, her body like her mind was relaxed and allowed the automatic processes to be completed with the ease with which other animals reproduce. The body's response to the stimulus of fear is tension, affecting in particular the circular muscles of the cervix and causing them to resist dilatation. This causes pain and reinforces the vicious circle of fear–tension–pain.

Since her social culture had conditioned her to fear pain, the mother needed to be re-educated. Dick-Read's theory was that her fear would be alleviated if she were instructed about the physical and emotional changes associated with pregnancy and labour, about the importance of relaxation and the technique to achieve it. She should be taught how to overcome tension by deep slow breathing in the first stage of labour, followed by controlled effort during contractions and relaxation between contractions in the second stage. The deep breathing would also ensure a good supply of oxygen to the fetus. With their fears dispelled by knowledge and the technique of relaxation mastered, most women should not need anaesthesia or, indeed, any obstetric intervention. In his experience, nine out of ten women so prepared had been able to deliver without anaesthesia. He laid great stress on the personal interest of the physician in the training and on his presence during labour, which in his practice took place mostly in the relaxed environment of the home. These factors were probably critical to his success.

Not surprisingly, Dick-Read's methods were not welcomed by proponents of orthodox obstetrics either in Britain or the USA. They were time-consuming and threatened to make conventional obstetric skills redundant. The few interested obstetricians who tried to follow the method in the unrelaxed environment of American hospitals found that 'prepared' women did indeed need less anaesthesia than those not so 'prepared', but not so much less as Dick-Read predicted. The success they did achieve seemed to last only as long as the 'prepared' women were given special consideration as subjects of an experiment. When the experiments were over, the 'prepared' women were exposed to the same interventions and seemed to need as much anaesthesia as the 'unprepared' [18, p. 192], which suggests that more benefit comes from special consideration than from training in relaxation.

OBSTETRIC PHYSIOTHERAPY

Dick-Read was less impressed by the value of physical training as a preparation for childbirth than were physiotherapists, who formed the Obstetric Association of Chartered Physiotherapists in the late 1940s [23]. They believed 'that the harmonious interaction of mind and body is essential in childbirth and that training of the muscle system goes hand in hand with training of the nervous system in order to preserve this harmony' [24, p. 45].

They devised a series of exercises to strengthen muscles used in bearing down; to increase flexibility of the joints of the pelvis and improve the tone of the muscles of the pelvic floor so that the baby could pass through without damage; and to accustom the mother to postures, alien to Western behaviour but helpful to the descent of the baby.

Orthodox obstetricians greeted Dick-Read's innovations with scepticism and the programme of the physiotherapists with hardly greater enthusiasm. Nor did the new ideas quickly gain popularity with British mothers and they had little impact on antenatal care before 1950. They did, however, gain considerable popularity with American mothers who organized lay classes for preparation for childbirth, an example that was eventually to be followed in Britain (page 107).

WAS ANTENATAL CARE ACHIEVING THE PROMISED RESULTS?

To the small extent that orthodox medical treatment could alleviate the transient disorders of pregnancy, attendance at antenatal clinics should have made pregnancy more comfortable. But the objective of antenatal care was more ambitious. Ballantyne's vision had inspired the belief that all the dangerous complications of labour were preceded by signs of abnormality in pregnancy which medical science could learn to detect at an early stage and for which it could develop treatments to prevent further deterioration. If this were so, the effect of antenatal care would be directly reflected in mortality rates and changes in the trends of these would mark the progress of medical antenatal diagnosis and therapeutics. By this criterion, very limited progress had been made towards such an ideal by the mid-century (Chapters 7 and 8).

But the criterion is unrealistic. Many of the dangerous complications of labour, for example puerperal sepsis and postpartum haemorrhage, have their immediate cause in intranatal or postnatal events and are only distantly dependent on antenatal conditions. Changes in maternal mortality from such causes would mask changes reflecting the effects of improved antenatal care. The reduction after 1936 in death rates from these causes coincided strikingly with the advent of new intrapartum and postpartum treatments, curative drugs and blood transfusions (Chapter 7), but antenatal care may have played a part in so far as it contributed to improving the mothers' general health, making them less anaemic and more resistant to infections of all kinds. Such a beneficial effect may have been offset before 1936 by an increased incidence of sepsis and haemorrhage, resulting from increased intranatal interventions (Chapter 4).

In theory, antenatal care should have reduced maternal and infant mortality from toxaemia of pregnancy and consequent eclampsia through detecting the precursor signs and instituting preventing treatment, but obstetricians had to admit there was no evidence that it had done so by 1934. 'Yet considering that eclampsia is almost entirely a preventable disease, the incidence and death rate are still far too high' [15]. Indeed, obstetricians must have found it hard to explain why mortality was actually lowest among women of the lowest social class who had least antenatal care (Table 7.1). They do not seem to have tried to do so.

Death rates were high in other countries too. In New Zealand the incidence of eclampsia, a notifiable disease there, was reduced to one-half and the case-fatality rate to less than one-quarter between 1933 and 1950 and this improvement was attributed to antenatal care [5], although there were coincidental improvements in other possibly causative factors, including the standard of living. In a maternity hospital in Sydney, Australia, an intensive preventive campaign in 1948 coincided with a nearly forty-fold reduction in incidence [5]. Figures of incidence in Britain are not available. No intensified prevention campaign was reported, but mortality from toxaemia, which for years had changed little, began to fall after 1937 to reach one-third of its level then by 1950 (Chapter 7). 'How much of this improvement is due to better antenatal care and how much to better management of eclampsia can only be conjectured' [5, p. 155]. The reduced mortality may have been in part due to improvement in maternal health, independent of medical care as later experience suggests.

The detection of abnormalities is advantageous only if it is accurate and can be followed by treatment which reduces the danger. Accurate detection can be extremely difficult. Zealous antenatal investigations are always liable to overdiagnose, to misinterpret conditions which are in fact transient and self-correcting as signals of impending disasters which can be averted only by obstetric interventions of some kind. Interventions, however, bring risks of their own (Chapter 4). Overdiagnosis, identifying risks which do not exist, followed by intervention must increase, not reduce, the dangers in these cases. In half the cases in one study where labour was induced for disproportion, the condition was found to be wrongly diagnosed [25]. If such overdiagnosis happens often enough, there will be a net disbenefit from antenatal investigations.

Women of the highest (and healthiest) social classes were the most likely to be attended by doctors, to have most antenatal care and more interventions, including more anaesthesia and analgesia; '. . . regular consultation with a doctor, rather than a midwife, tends to turn every pregnancy from a physiological process into a pathological one' [7, p. 45]. Yet an official analysis of mortality over the years 1930–2 confirmed the results of past centuries in finding that these women, despite their better health and physical development, had a higher maternal death rate, in total and for most specific causes besides toxaemia, than women in the lowest social class, those least likely to be attended by doctors antenatally or intranatally (Table 7.1 and page 282).

The opposite danger to overdiagnosis is underdiagnosis. One reason for underdiagnosis arose because, contrary to the initial standards proposed in 1915 by the Local Government Board, clinic staff had too little time to examine the large number of women attending at each session and listen to their problems. A Professor of Obstetrics admitted in 1934 that 'examinations are too infrequent, perfunctory and unskilled to accomplish anything useful' [15]. The same criticism was repeated twelve years later in 1946 when it was found that because hospital doctors tended to see every patient at each clinic session, they could spend less than three minutes with each, resulting in hurried, superficial consultations, unlikely to reveal any but the most obvious signs of abnormality [7].

Another reason for underdiagnosis was that most of the women did not have signs or symptoms of abnormality, so that attendants could become complacent and miss the unexpected indication: '. . . the constant watchfulness of those in attendance tends to slacken as in so many cases nothing abnormal occurs' [26].

Net disbenefit will result even when the danger signals are correctly identified unless the risks of the intervention are known, not just assumed, to be less than the risks of the anticipated complication. Risks from the induction of premature labour and caesarean section were said to be as great as the risks from the obstructed labour which the interventions were to prevent [15].

Reasons such as these, together with the probability that those most likely to have problems did not seek medical care, would help to explain why, twenty years after antenatal clinics started, death rates for mothers, fetuses and neonates were as high as ever. This experience was exactly paralleled in the USA and Australia, despite their early introduction of antenatal care. Two American studies in 1933 and 1934 found the same reasons why antenatal care failed: on the one hand because it underestimated or overlooked complications and on the other because it led to excessive intervention, for nearly half the women died after an unnecessary operation [18, p. 161].

When the downward trend in mortality did start, in Britain quickly for mothers after 1936, slowly for fetuses after 1935 and for neonates after 1940 with similar trends in other countries, there is no evidence that these changes coincided with changes in the quantity or quality of the medical element of antenatal care to which improvements in outcome could be attributed. That means that the eventual decline in mortality was not caused by benefits from obstetric antenatal care. The effect of changes in obstetric intranatal care on maternal and perinatal mortality will be discussed in Chapters 7 and 8.

SOCIAL FACTORS

The essential link between nutritious diet and good health at all stages of life has been recognized throughout the ages in all countries. Death rates are always higher in the poorer countries and the poorer districts within countries where the people cannot afford an adequate diet. The obvious first step to improve the standard of health and reduce death rates would be to improve the standard of nutrition among the populations, or sections of the populations, where it is deficient. The practical politics of doing so, however, often seem to be strangely difficult. It seems easier to devote resources to providing high-cost medical treatment when illness has occurred than to providing social conditions which would prevent the illness from occurring.

The first efforts to reduce infant mortality around 1900 in Britain and other countries had been to improve the nutrition of expectant and nursing mothers. But faith that this kind of social intervention would be enough was weak and was soon overtaken by the conviction that surer salvation would lie in taking steps to improve the quantity and quality of medical care in pregnancy and labour.

As in many other countries, the British economy recovered only slowly after the First World War and suffered a devastating set-back with the depression of the 1930s. The poverty caused by the high level of unemployment was slightly mitigated by income supplements from the compulsory insurance schemes introduced in 1911. But even for those in employment wages were low, so that in 1936 about half the population was estimated to be too poor to buy an adequate diet and up to one-third to suffer from serious dietary deficiencies [3, p. 91]. Yet even these proportions were probably lower than they had been in the early 20th and 19th centuries.

Unemployment was particularly high and wages were particularly low in inter-war Wales. Accompanying the ensuing poverty was a high rate of maternal mortality. In 1934, a campaign was funded by the National Birthday Trust, a charity which has supported the work of the Royal College of Obstetricians and Gynaecologists, to increase the amount and coverage of specialist antenatal care in the Rhondda area. Despite this extension of medical care, maternal mortality increased. Then in 1935 and the first half of 1936, the experiment changed to providing free food – beef extract, dried milk, Ovaltine and Marmite, a yeast preparation found to be useful in the treatment of pernicious anaemia of pregnancy. The maternal mortality rate fell by more than half [27]. This decline may have been assisted by the easing of the economic depression and in 1936 by the first use of the sulpha drugs in intranatal care (page 284), but the experiment indicated that maternal mortality was prevented far more by better antenatal nutrition than by more antenatal medical care.

This finding on a local scale was to be fortified on a national scale by British experience during the Second World War (Chapters 7 and 8). The importance of nutrition to the welfare of mothers and infants of the next generation was early recognized by those in charge of policy when food had to be rationed. From mid-1940, expectant and nursing mothers were enabled to buy a pint of fresh milk a day at less than half price or receive it free subject to a means test. Dried milk for infants was similarly subsidized, as were supplements of vitamins A and D, in the form of cod-liver oil or tablets, and vitamin C in the form of concentrated fruit juice or rose-hip syrup. In addition, extra amounts of rationed foods, such as eggs, could be bought and these mothers and young children had priority when occasional shipments of 'luxuries' like fresh oranges arrived. The dried milk and vitamin supplements were distributed through maternity and child welfare centres, which encouraged expectant mothers to attend antenatal clinics regularly.

The advice of expert dieticians was used in managing the restricted food supplies of war-time, so as to give everyone adequate nourishment. Flour for bread became progressively less refined; the weekly rations of sugar, fats and meat were small, potatoes and carrots were plentiful and the consumption of home-grown vegetables increased. Partly because scarce basic foods were rationed and their prices controlled, and partly because the level of employment and family incomes rose, a far greater proportion of the population than ever before came to enjoy a healthy diet and a good standard of nourishment. This was reflected in lower death rates for every subgroup in the population, including at last childbearing mothers and their babies.

The reduction in mortality took place at a time when the medical service available for the civilian population was considerably reduced, following the withdrawal of many doctors for military service. Fewer of them, including fewer of the younger graduates whose training in obstetrics had been improved, were left for maternity work including antenatal care. Moreover, personal anxieties, air raids, evacuation and the social privations of war-time must have introduced disturbing complications for many pregnancies and deliveries. Yet these factors did not halt the fast decline in maternal mortality nor prevent an unprecedented decline in the stubbornly high rate of stillbirths and neonatal deaths, welcome developments which will be described in detail in Chapters 7 and 8.

THE EXPANSION OF ANTENATAL CARE AFTER 1948

Changes and lack of changes in the organization of clinics

In 1946, local authority clinics provided some antenatal care for over half of the 99% of the childbearing women who were then receiving it [7]. But this predominance was soon to be eroded once the National Health Service was instituted in 1948, for now all mothers could, without charge, book a general practitioner as well as a midwife for complete maternity care. With additional reimbursement for their maternity work and without the contractual obligation to attend the actual delivery, many doctors willingly collaborated with midwives to provide antenatal supervision, usually leaving the conduct of the delivery to the midwife.

At the same time, more serious competition came from the obstetric hospitals as the desirability, not only of giving birth there, but also of having antenatal care in the attached clinics, was being persuasively advertised from all sides. By 1958, 49% of women were choosing to have all or part of their antenatal care in hospital clinics, while 30% chose general practitioner clinics, which left only 19% to depend mainly on local authority clinics [28, p. 66]. These trends continued, so that by 1970 64% of expectant mothers had all or part of their antenatal care in hospital clinics, 73% used GP clinics and only 3% municipal clinics [29, p. 10].

Obviously, many women attended more than one kind of clinic. Each offers its own attraction. The hospital clinics are staffed by the experts in pathology and have the technological equipment necessary for the widening range of diagnostic tests and procedures. Thus the physical elements of monitoring are well provided for. The provision for the social and emotional needs of the pregnant woman is less satisfactory.

The preference of medical planners has been increasingly to concentrate deliveries into larger units where expensive technological equipment can be more economically provided. Large units have extensive catchment areas, so that for many mothers travel is expensive in time, money and stress. Many of them have found the accommodation unattractive, uncomfortable and inconvenient, with inadequate facilities to distract them or the young children they have to bring with them during their frequent long waiting periods, or for privacy during their medical consultations and examinations. The large throughput deprives the women of their sense of individual importance and discourages them from taking up the precious time of the obstetrician in listening to their worries and answering their questions. The larger the clinic, the more staff members and staff changes there are, so that the women, seeing many doctors and midwives, are not able to build up a personal relationship with anyone, which does not create a sympathetic atmosphere in which it is easy to discuss their personal problems and anxieties. For many women, a clinic visit is more an upsetting than a reassuring experience, even when no physical abnormality is diagnosed. Not surprisingly, some of them fail to keep all their appointments and earn the condemnatory description 'defaulter'. But most have been persuaded to believe that, however unpleasant the experience, it is in the interest of the child that they should attend as often as instructed and this they do.

The social and emotional shortcomings of antenatal clinics, recognized as early as 1915 (pages 93–4), seem to have defied reform. In 1961 an official committee [30] reported

The commonest cause of dissatisfaction during the antenatal period seems to be the long waiting times, often hours spent in poor overcrowded premises, followed by a rapid examination with no real privacy. Another frequent complaint is either the lack of explanation of abnormalities which have arisen . . . or a partial explanation which gives rise to worry.

Nineteen years later, the House of Commons Social Services Committee [31] still found strong criticisms about '. . . long waiting times, difficult access to clinics, lack of continuity of care, lack of opportunity to discuss things that women themselves are worried about . . .'. The complaints were acknowledged by the Royal College of Obstetricians and Gynaecologists [32] and reforms were recommended. Nevertheless, a consumer watchdog body was able to entitle its 1987 review of the unsatisfactory conditions as Antenatal Care: Still Waiting for Action [33], and the same complaints were made to the House of Commons Health Committee in 1991–2 [34, paras 37–40].

Some measures have been taken to improve the attractiveness of the physical environment, to provide more amenities for small children, to organize appointment systems and to supply educational films or reading material (which emphasize the virtues of obstetric management and technological interventions and so make profitable use of the inevitable waiting time to spread propaganda). But the more serious problems are inherent in the size of clinics, the large number of clients and the large and changing number of staff. Their solution seems to lie in strategies to break down the large clinics into smaller and more continuing units, so that positive, personal relationships become possible. Such a strategy, the 'Know Your Midwife' project, was devised by Caroline Flint, a research midwife at St George's Hospital, London, in the 1980s and shown to be both feasible within the hospital system and beneficial [35].

Shared care

Although obstetricians mistrusted general practitioners to ensure as thorough antenatal care as they provided in hospital clinics, the practical realities of crowded clinics led to some disenchantment. As they moved towards their goal of hospitalizing all deliveries, the specialists found themselves

> . . . unable to provide enough staff or hours for the sheer volume of antenatal and postnatal work required. Much of what they did provide was seen to be inappropriate, or inadequate, or even inhumane by many women. Not only did the sheer volume of care overwhelm them, but specialists became increasingly weary of huge clinics of perfectly normal women, performing for the most part a perfectly normal physiological function. They found that their highly specialised, pathology-oriented training rendered much of what they were doing extremely boring. [36, p. xiii]

So for their own interests, as much as for those of their patients or their generalist colleagues, obstetricians were disposed to accept the obvious strategy for overcoming the disadvantages inherent in large clinics, by sharing antenatal care with general practitioners in their practice clinics and so reducing the number of attendances at the hospital clinic. Within the hospital clinic, they were prepared to lighten their work load by passing more responsibility to midwives. The antenatal supervision they were prepared to delegate was of women judged to be at suitably low risk as assessed from information elicited at their first attendance (page 110), selection criteria too non-specific accurately to predict the future occurrence of complications [37] or their non-occurrence. Obstetricians did, however, retain their status as the senior partners of any collaboration; as one Professor testified to the House of Commons Health Committee in 1991, 'Within the hospital antenatal clinic, I see no difficulty in routine, low risk antenatal care being supervised by midwives provided that the line of responsibility is to the Consultant in charge of that clinic' [38, p. 314]. They had to be consulted about any deviation from the expected normality and usually took over the further control of the case, whatever the diagnosis. Programmes had to be agreed of the detailed content of care to be given by each of the providing partners and a record document was devised which the mother would take to each clinic for their mutual information.

Family doctors, whose role is to give medical care to the whole family throughout their lives and who see pregnancy as a uniquely significant episode in that cycle, value the opportunity that antenatal care, even shared care, affords them of getting to know and understand the developing unit. Surveys have found the general practitioner clinics to be more popular with women, more accessible, less time-consuming, more comfortable and intimate, with better opportunities for developing continuing relationships and discussing problems [39, 40]. Especially appreciated are those clinics which have attached community midwives who can take their care further by visiting the women in their homes. This personal attention may help to overcome the distrust of the medical establishment felt by some women, particularly the least privileged ones whose needs are greatest but who are most reluctant to co-operate with medical management.

Community-based clinics

Yet another strategy for avoiding the disadvantages of the crowded central hospital clinic is to 'decentralize' the obstetrician. In some districts, large enough to ensure a substantial flow of births, probably over a hundred a year, community-based clinics have been set up in health centres, large group practices, welfare clinics or other suitable premises. They are staffed by community midwives and local general practitioners who wish to participate. A consultant obstetrician from the central hospital attends at frequent intervals, primarily to advise on problem cases, for which he may be consulted between visits by telephone. The system generates good relationships and mutual understanding between the consultant and clinic staff, making communication easy and profitable. Women find the same advantages as they do from the general practitioner clinics, with the additional bonus of rarely being referred to the hospital clinic in the event of complications. Excellent results have been reported with lower than expected proportions of preterm deliveries, low-weight babies and caesarean sections [38, p. 305, 41–43].

Another variant of the community-based clinic, inspired by Flint's 'Know Your Midwife' scheme, was introduced in 1989 by the Riverside District Health Authority (London). Based on local authority clinics near the mothers' homes, four teams each of six midwives would care for women during pregnancy and one of the midwives, by now a familiar friend, would attend each mother in labour, taking her into hospital for delivery and home again soon after. Midwives and general practitioners provided the sole care for the 30–40% of women in the district deemed to be at low risk. Rates of spontaneous delivery were relatively high, rates of perinatal mortality relatively low.

The scheme was very popular with mothers and midwives but not so with other birth attendants. There was disagreement on the definition of low risk, midwives considering that as many as 70% of women are suitable for midwife-only care throughout, but obstetricians being unwilling to cede so much of their market and power. Some general practitioners have been antagonistic to midwife teams. Midwives in turn have co-operated reluctantly in the training of medical personnel, preferring to turn directly to consultants or senior registrars when complications arise and so denying junior medical staff important learning experience [44, p. 738].

Midwives clinics?

In general practitioner and community-based clinics, midwives may perform a role more commensurate with their professional capabilities than the one usually assigned to them in hospital clinics where they do not act as specialists in their own right but rather as handmaidens to the obstetricians and their contribution is limited to carrying out routine tests of physical conditions. But they would like to go further and detach themselves more distinctly from medical influence and medical management. Approaching maternity care from their different philosophical point of view, they believe that they have much more positive contributions to make to the welfare of pregnant women. To facilitate offering this differently oriented service, they have proposed setting up, under midwives' own control, small, conveniently sited, low technology, low cost clinics where the great majority of women who do not in fact develop physical complications could have their emotional and social needs satisfactorily met, their questions answered and their confidence in their normality reinforced [45] (page 76). Since the 1920s midwives' training has developed to equip them to detect signs of abnormality without reliance on high-technology screening and any such affected cases they would directly refer for obstetrician's advice. Though a few of such clinics have been set up, the proposals, like the 'Know Your Midwife' scheme for hospital clinics, have not yet been considered as positively as they deserve by most Health Authorities and, as in the Riverside Scheme, have to face opposition from other professionals whose interests are challenged.

ANTENATAL CLASSES

In addition to the medically oriented clinics, classes to prepare women, physically and mentally, for childbirth and childrearing are organized by local authorities, hospitals, health centres and private consumer bodies, such as the National Childbirth Trust in Britain [46] and several organizations in the United States [47]. The classes attract principally first-time mothers and others anxious not to repeat an earlier unpleasant experience. How wide participation is overall is not known, but probably covers fewer than half the pregnant women at any time. In England attendances at the public community health classes, relative to the number of births, increased from 18% in 1970 to 34% in 1985 and was still around that proportion in 1987–8 [48]. Enquiries have established that it is the women of lower social class and with shorter formal education who are less likely to attend. For some the reasons given are the inconvenient location or timing of the classes and the higher priority of their other commitments. Others felt that they had already learned all they needed to know from their own previous experience or from reading and talking to other women [44, p. 685, 49]. They might have had even more productive opportunities for mutual education and moral support as members of an antenatal class where they could get to know other women, probably living nearby, with the same immediate and prospective interests.

After a time lapse of some years, following the ideas put forward in the 1930s and 1940s by Dick-Read (page 96) and the psychoprophylactic method developed and popularized by Lamaze in France and America in the 1950s [50], instruction is now given about the physiological changes to be expected in the course of labour and in the breathing and relaxation techniques intended to help the process. Fathers also may now attend the classes and learn what their partners are supposed to do, so that they can coach and support them in labour, physically as well as emotionally.

The opportunity is taken, particularly in hospital classes, to familiarize the women with the intranatal interventions which they are likely to encounter and to allay apprehension of the hospital setting, with its connotations of illness and emergency, the impersonality of its technological equipment and its sterile bustle. The women have to be persuaded that these off-putting features are necessary and a small price well worth paying for the promised advantage of greater safety in an event fraught with danger. Thus the hospital antenatal class presents an unrivalled opportunity for putting across obstetric propaganda from authoritative sources to the target population, the women most immediately concerned, most likely to be influenced and most unlikely to ask for the evidence which would justify the propaganda. What women are taught in community-based classes depends on the philosophy of the teacher: some may teach techniques for coping, not so much with labour itself, as with the obstetric management of labour, and how to incorporate their personal wishes, if these do not conform to standard practice, in their own 'birth plans', which may or may not be respected by hospital staffs.

Whether on balance women are mentally reassured or physically helped by what they are taught about the birth process in antenatal classes, conducted either by consumers or providers of maternity care, has proved difficult to establish. In comparisons between 'prepared' and 'not prepared' groups, it is not easy to standardize satisfactorily for other variables, including motivation, which might bias outcome. However, more of the trials carried out seem to show that 'prepared' women need, or actually take, less pharmacological pain relief [51], so that infants are less harmed. No single element of the preparation course has been identified as being unequivocally beneficial.

It is indeed possible that structured antenatal preparation for structured behaviour in labour does not make it easier for a woman to yield to the primitive instincts deep inside her and let them dictate her physiological responses to the processes of parturition. For this, according to the insight of Michel Odent [52], is the surest way for her to attain complete relaxation and give birth with the normal efficiency of other animals.

MODERN ANTENATAL PROCEDURES

In the course of the decades since antenatal care was introduced, the health states of pregnant women in the more prosperous countries changed markedly for the better. Undernutrition and malnutrition became much less widespread, so that resistance to infections improved and developmental damage lessened, which changed the nature of the health problems to be tackled by the antenatal care service. But that there were problems still to be solved and that, whatever their cause, their solution lay within the burgeoning capacity of the medical profession was not doubted. The crusade was pursued with undiminished zeal.

The outstanding success of antibiotics encouraged the introduction of other drugs to treat the ailments of pregnancy. But after the disastrous malformations which followed the use of thalidomide in the 1950s were realized, the possible teratogenicity of other drugs became suspect and caution in prescribing came to be exercised. The spirit of innovation was not, however, inhibited.

When antenatal care started early in the century, the primary concern was to safeguard the life and health of the mother. By the 1950s, great progress had been made towards reaching this objective, though very little of it as a result of medical antenatal care (Chapter 7). Primary concern then turned to safeguarding the life and health of the infant. The antenatal regimen was progressively extended with the introduction of screening and diagnostic techniques of great sophistication, the most frequently used of which have so far been ultrasound scanning, amniocentesis and electronic monitoring of the fetal heart. These technological advances have enabled obstetricians to learn a great deal about normal fetal growth and hold out the promise of detecting otherwise unrealized deviations from normality. Visualizing the fetus by means of ultrasound, probing its uterine environment by analysing the amniotic fluid, and investigating its physiological welfare by means of monitoring its heart and other biophysical and biochemical tests seemed to offer the key to Ballantyne's vision that antenatal care would one day foresee and forestall all the serious complications of labour (page 88).

How far has the vision since been realized? Indeed, in the light of evaluated experience is the vision capable of being realized? Can all the complications be foreseen and if foreseen, can they be forestalled?

Unfortunately, ingenuity in inventing diagnostic techniques has far outstripped ingenuity in developing curative therapies; the new powers to diagnose have not yet been matched by new powers to cure [53]. By the 1980s it still had to be accepted 'that, whatever the method(s) of screening, the prediction and detection of problems by current antenatal procedures remain unacceptably inaccurate' [54]. The perpetual problems of underdiagnosis and overdiagnosis remain unsolved. Even more sophisticated procedures have been developed for using Doppler ultrasound to measure blood velocity in the maternal–placental–fetal circulation, decreased velocity being associated with fetal morbidity [55]. But whatever problems can thereby be detected and predicted with greater accuracy, the positive value of most of the therapies provided to cope with the problems remains very uncertain.

In 1980 an obstetrician summed up his profession's attainments in the field of antenatal care:

> . . . we use a variety of drugs (the efficacy of none of these is well established). We assess maternal and fetal welfare by a variety of tests all of which are still *sub judice*. With the significant exception of Rh disease [administering anti-D immunoglobulin to women with rhesus negative blood which significantly reduces the incidence of iso-immunisation during pregnancy], we have no specific form of therapy for prenatal disease. In general obstetric practice rests on two modalities of treatment – hospitalisation for bed rest and observation and timed delivery. [56]

This comment is still valid. There is strong reason now to doubt that even the two modalities are of benefit, while since 1980 some drugs and procedures have been evaluated and found actually to do more harm than good [57].

WHY ATTEND FOR CARE EARLY?

The new diagnostic facilities needed their own special clinics and inpatient accommodation, as well as laboratories to analyse material collected and interpret results, and they imposed changes in the pattern of traditional outpatient clinics.

The programme set out in 1929 (page 91) had proposed ten visits between the 16th and 39th week of pregnancy. In due course an inverse relationship was observed between the number of antenatal attendances and perinatal mortality and this was used to exhort women to start their antenatal care as early as possible, although investigation showed that this correlation was not causal but spurious (page 268), being explained by an intermediate factor: it was the healthy married women of higher social class, those most likely to bear healthy full-term infants irrespective of antenatal care, who attended most − the number of attendances before 16 weeks, and so in total, increased greatly. Since in any case several morbid conditions originate before the 16th week, early measurements can be made which serve as critical baselines for the detection and management of existing or future complications. An early measurement of blood pressure before it is affected by the pregnancy makes it possible to judge the significance of future changes and hence, in the light of another baseline measurement − duration of gestation − best made early using ultrasound, to prescribe treatment considered appropriate (page 113).

On the other hand, earlier diagnosis may increase the risk of over-diagnosis and encourage unnecessary interventions. Analysis in 1991 of data from the 1970 British Births Survey found no association between delayed or irregular antenatal attendance and adverse outcomes, indeed in some respects the reverse [58]. Patterns of attendance for antenatal care vary considerably from country to country, without correlation with the relevant national maternal or perinatal outcomes.

From information gathered at the woman's first visit, including her age, how many children she has had and her obstetric and medical history, an assessment is made of her risk status. Specialist care is planned for those deemed to be at higher risk. The risk criteria are based on unbiased epidemiological findings that certain characteristics and experiences are associated with higher maternal and perinatal mortality rates than are others. Over the years, despite improvements in the average level of health, high-risk status has become more liberally defined to include more women. The decision about the kind of care needed is based on the biased assumption, which has never been supported by evidence (Chapters 7 and 8), that obstetric management, using the technological aids, is especially advantageous in cases of high predicted risk. While the epidemiological findings indicate that the chance of death is greater in the presence of certain characteristics, the vast majority of babies will be delivered safely even when the predicted risk is high, while a few babies will die even when the predicted risk is low, whatever kind of maternity care they receive. In fact, half the perinatal deaths occur among the women at low predicted risk [59]. There is as yet no known system for reliably predicting the minority of pregnancies which finish up with problems. Labelling women 'high risk' early in pregnancy, because of past conditions they cannot change, can hardly boost their self-confidence; the process of self-fulfilling prophecy is insidiously initiated.

WHY ATTEND FOR CARE FREQUENTLY?

The extra burden of early attendances has not been offset by any reduction in the conventional programme of later attendances, despite research findings of the low productivity of these in detecting latent dangers. Doubt was cast on the value of the established programme of attendances by the findings of the retrospective examination of a large sample of cases in Aberdeen in 1975 [60]. There was both considerable underdiagnosis – failure to detect pathology which did exist and failure to forecast complications which did arise – and considerable over-diagnosis – detection of pathology which did not exist. These were the same faults which characterized antenatal care in earlier decades, despite more accumulated knowledge, more technological aids and improved medical training, and which have continued to characterize antenatal care ever since.

The obstetrician researchers concluded that many routine visits were unproductive and the number of these could be safely reduced to almost half for the majority of women who are normal, leaving clinic staff time to deal at greater depth with the minority who do have problems. However sound and sensible this proposal is, it has not yet been widely adopted, although a revised scheme was introduced in Aberdeen in 1980. Ironically, women who might have been expected to embrace enthusiastically this release from an experience few enjoyed have been found to cling to their indoctrinated conviction that antenatal care must be beneficial and to feel deprived if their ration of it is cut down [40, p. 88].

Later research by the same obstetricians confirmed their conclusion that inflexible adherence to outdated routines means that women with uncomplicated pregnancies are seen more frequently than is necessary or beneficial. They recommend that women should attend only when they themselves feel they would benefit from advice [44, p. 779, 59]. But this recommendation is opposed by many obstetricians in whose eyes the valuable role of antenatal care is precisely to detect the early signs of morbid conditions of which the woman is not herself yet aware.

DIAGNOSING HYPERTENSION

One such condition, not usually accompanied by early symptoms, is maternal hypertension, which may dispose to pre-eclampsia and eclampsia. These conditions bring dangers, both to the mother and her child, which obstetricians have always been anxious to avert by detecting signs of rising blood pressure and the presence of protein in the urine of the pregnant woman (pages 90–1). Pre-eclampsia is much more likely to affect first than later pregnancies and it is now known that a serious outcome is much more likely to follow when blood pressure rises in mid-pregnancy, when other problems and so recommended clinic visits are few, than in late pregnancy when recommended visits for other reasons are frequent. Only if the value of reducing the risk of a serious outcome for a small minority of pregnancies is judged to outweigh the low productivity in detecting this and other latent dangers in mid-pregnancy, should there be more, not fewer, antenatal consultations than the number conventionally prescribed [61]. Possible congestion in clinics would, however, be eased if measurements of blood pressure and proteinuria were carried out in the mother's home, as has successfully been done in some places, with no less reliability [62]. Indeed, blood pressures tend to be lower when measured in the more relaxed atmosphere of the home, rather than in the less relaxed atmosphere of the antenatal clinic, a finding which has caused prudent obstetricians to revise downward their whole conception of the incidence and prevalence of hypertension in pregnancy.

Blood pressure is affected by many factors besides emotional state, including age, parity, race, level of activity, posture, and even time of day. This subjective variability is in turn compounded by variability in techniques practised by the persons doing the measuring, who may have a bias towards detecting the abnormal [63]. Because of inconsistency and bias, raised blood pressure noted in the antenatal clinic constitutes an unreliable basis for prescribing treatment. Moreover, as often as not the condition is found to settle by itself and create no later problem [40, p. 30].

Treating hypertension

This is fortunate because a century of assiduous study has not led to the understanding by orthodox obstetricians of the real nature and effective causes of pre-eclampsia and eclampsia [61]. Such an understanding might have led to the development of effective treatments, instead of ineffective efforts to treat symptoms. Severe hypertension impairs the maternal–placental–fetal blood circulation and so the source of nourishment and oxygen for the fetus (page xiii). Various drugs, diuretic, antihypertensive and antithrombotic, and various regimens, bed rest and biochemical and biophysical tests, have been favoured at different times without proven benefit. Certain drugs, like methyldopa, reduce hypertension and the ultimate maternal risks of cerebral haemorrhage, prenatal hospital admission and emergency delivery, but not the risk of retarded fetal growth or perinatal death [64, 65].

Inappropriate treatment almost certainly does more harm than good and by the 1980s the verdict was that 'no medical or other manoeuvre has been shown to prevent or significantly alter the course or decline of the disease [pre-eclampsia].' [8, p. 193] By 1992 there was still wide disagreement among British consultant obstetricians and general practitioners about what treatment was the most appropriate [66, 67]. It is therefore still as unjustified as it was in the 1930s (pages 98–9) to claim a causal benefit in this respect from medical antenatal care.

Adequate maternal–placental–fetal blood flow may be maintained if the ability of the blood to clot is lessened and early studies were raising hopes that aspirin in low doses could achieve this [68, 69]. These hopes were supported by a randomized controlled study of women identified in early pregnancy as being at high risk of pregnancy-induced hypertension. This found that the group taking regularly a low dose of aspirin were significantly less likely to develop proteinuria and to deliver low-weight babies, without suffering harmful side-effects, than the control group taking placebo (inactive) medication [70]. These findings were repeated in a similar, but wider, multicentre randomized controlled trial of high-risk mothers in France, using a larger dose of aspirin [71]. Even wider international trials (CLASP), covering 9364 pregnant women, were conducted in the early 1990s to evaluate this simple, non-invasive, low-cost treatment. Disappointingly the results, reported in 1994, did not show significantly better outcomes and so support the hypothesis that a beneficial therapy had at last been found [76].

But as far as the mother's risk of pre-eclampsia is concerned, the hoped for cure looks like arriving too late to have a spectacular effect on the experience of pregnant women in general. Unlike in the 1930s, there is now good evidence from Britain and other prosperous countries, like New Zealand and Sweden, that, since the 1950s for reasons unknown, the incidence of eclampsia has fallen to only about 1 in 2000 deliveries, and case-fatality rates have likewise diminished to a very low level [72]. The history of pre-eclampsia is similar: despite probable overdiagnosis, there has been reduced incidence [40, p. 30] (page 98 and Chapter 7), and reduced associated mortality. The downward trends in specific mortality are in line with the contemporaneous downward trends in overall maternal and perinatal mortality and probably have the same causes – improved maternal nutrition and health status.

Forestalling pre-eclampsia

Support for the conjecture that pre-eclampsia is related to nutrition comes from the work of an American obstetrician, Tom Brewer, who observed its much higher incidence among his poorly fed public patients than among his better fed private patients. He started prescribing a liberal, high protein diet for his public patients in a deprived district of New Orleans and claimed that this, with nutrition counselling, completely eradicated eclampsia and virtually eradicated pre-eclampsia from his practice. This result has not been confirmed in scientifically designed trials [73], but it has been confirmed by many women in many places who, despairing of the ineffectiveness of the advice and treatment provided at their orthodox antenatal clinics, like restriction of salt intake or prevention of maternal weight gain, have chosen instead to follow the Brewer diet (page 238). The scientific explanation of the biological link between the mother's diet and the efficient nourishment of her fetus seems persuasive to the layman (pages 121–2).

Another link between diet on the one hand and pre-eclampsia and low-birthweight babies on the other has been inferred by comparing the relatively low rates of these conditions in the Faroe Islands and Greenland with the higher rates in the related country, Denmark. An important difference between these countries is that the diet in the Faroes and Greenland is much richer in fish oils, which seem to improve the blood flow between mother and fetus, and it is to the effect of this abundance that the better health outcomes are attributed [74, 75].

The possibility of a causal relationship between poor diet and the manifestations of severe hypertension is strengthened also by the stubbornly high prevalence of these conditions among poorly fed mothers in the underdeveloped countries compared with the diminishing prevalence in developed, better fed, countries (page 305, Chapter 7).

The scope of obstetric antenatal care in forestalling pre-eclampsia is further limited in that 'in as many as 30% of cases, pre-eclampsia presented for the first time in labour or the puerperium: in other words either the condition did not manifest itself until then, or it was not ascertained by the traditional frequency of antenatal care (weekly visits in late pregnancy)' [40, p. 30]. Later retrospective inspection of case histories found that less than 10% of unpredicted complications in labour could have been predicted by better antenatal care, even if carried out by a consultant obstetrician [59]. Some complications are actually generated by certain of the intranatal or even late antenatal practices prescribed by obstetricians (Chapter 4). Clearly, experience to date gives only very qualified support to Ballantyne's visionary hypothesis that 'dangerous labours' are preceded by 'abnormal gestations' (page 90).

FORESEEING AND FORESTALLING BIRTHS OF LOW WEIGHT

Apart from the few healthy ones who are small through genetic inheritance, babies of low birthweight or short gestation are at higher risk of perinatal and infant death and illness. Therefore, a primary objective of antenatal care should be to prevent the occurrence of such disadvantaged births. So far this objective has eluded attainment.

In the British 1958 perinatal survey [28], 6.7% of births weighing under 2500 grams caused 53.3% of all deaths, while 9.4% of births under 38 weeks' gestation caused 46.2% of deaths and 3.4% of births of both low weight and short gestation caused 37.9% of deaths. By 1990 6.8% of births were at this low weight and caused 59.3% of deaths [77] (length of gestation is not recorded in routine official statistics). Manifestly, thirty years of medically directed antenatal care, followed by obstetric intranatal and neonatal care, had failed to reduce either the incidence of low-weight births (and presumably preterm deliveries), or the proportion of perinatal deaths they cause.

The birthweight of babies may be low, 2500 grams ($5\frac{1}{2}$ lbs) or less, because they are born preterm before their uterine development is complete, or because their uterine growth has been retarded, or for both reasons. Whatever the reason, many of the associated risk factors are the same and include multiple births, short interpregnancy intervals, small, thin mothers from poorer backgrounds or of Asian race. But most mothers with these characteristics bear children of normal weight.

Preterm births

Some babies are born preterm spontaneously. The basic reasons for this happening can be both physiological, often the consequences of the mother's inadequate nutrition during pregnancy, and psychological, the consequences of the social stress she has suffered during pregnancy.

Such deprivations and stresses are suffered more frequently by women in the lowest social classes [78, 79] and the experience may well have preceded the present pregnancy and indeed the present generation (pages 33–4, 361).

The successful reproductive system has evolved to ensure that the fetus is nurtured until it has developed sufficiently to embark on independent existence. The fetus derives its nourishment via the maternal–placental–fetal blood supply. As the pregnancy progresses, the mother's blood must increase appropriately in volume and this is achieved so long as her diet supplies her liver with an adequate input of protein. If the blood volume stops increasing or drops, the body reacts via the kidneys to limit the loss by constricting the blood vessels, which causes a rise in blood pressure. Ultimately, and apparently perversely, the kidney starts excreting protein in the urine, the symptom of pre-eclampsia. The outlook for the fetus is most prejudiced when the rise in blood pressure takes place in mid-pregnancy, so leaving a longer time for undernourishment.

An adequate blood volume is necessary to maintain a healthy placenta, one of whose functions is to produce the muscle relaxant which keeps the uterus quiescent during pregnancy instead of forcing out the foreign body, the fetus. Premature inadequacy of blood volume may be the trigger which stops this harbouring function and precipitates labour. Inadequate blood volume may cause the pool of maternal blood to clot behind the placenta, causing it to detach with maternal bleeding. Certainly, mothers who suffer bleeding in pregnancy are known to be at greater risk of preterm labour. Another known predictor is a previous low-weight birth, which, of course, may have resulted from the same causative factors [79].

Interventions to delay preterm birth

In many preterm births the babies do not give reliable physical signals well in advance of their impending arrival, so medical efforts to postpone birth have to depend on the emergency administration of drugs. Synthetic derivatives of the naturally occurring hormones, oestrogen and progesterone, have been used on the hypothesis that deficiency or imbalance of these causes premature labour. Also used are betamimetic drugs to relax uterine muscles and discourage contractions and drugs to inhibit the synthesis of prostaglandin, a natural hormone of crucial importance in the initiation and maintenance of labour. These have had some success in postponing delivery, but they may harm the infant and by themselves have not been shown to improve its chance of survival, though the time gained may allow other life-saving measures to be attempted. Other drugs have been used, but none has delayed delivery to a useful extent and none has been shown to benefit the infant [80].

Premature delivery is sometimes blamed on an 'incompetent' cervix, one unable to act as an effective sphincter through weakness or damage. To compensate, obstetricians can insert a reinforcing suture, cervical cerclage, which can be removed near term or when labour starts spontaneously. The operation is widely used, notably in France, and those who do so must believe it to be effective. Its success seems to depend on the reasons for which it was done. A multicentre randomized controlled trial showed that delivery was usefully delayed to the benefit of the infant in one in twenty cases of previous mid-term abortion or preterm delivery. Otherwise the many associated complications weighed heavily against any benefits [81].

Rest in bed, one of the modalities relied on by obstetricians (page 109), is traditionally believed to enable the body to conserve its strength, the better to withstand the extra demands of any attack on its good health, so it seems a reasonable and safe precaution to take against any deviation from the course of normal pregnancy, such as threatened preterm delivery in both singleton and multiple pregnancies or developing hypertension. It is hoped that blood flow will be concentrated through the placenta to the fetus (or fetuses) and not dissipated to meet the needs of active maternal leg and back muscles. Obstetricians, probably with good reason, do not trust women who may feel quite well and have other responsibilities, to carry out the restrictive prescription of bed rest unsupervised, so the policy of antenatal hospitalization has been favoured. Many women do not find a stay in hospital restful and there is no evidence that bed rest, which brings its own risks, has ever succeeded in maintaining threatened pregnancies or stimulating faltering fetal growth [82–84]. Nevertheless, many women have had an enforced antenatal stay in hospital for this reason. They may also be hospitalized for observation when they have hypertension and so that other diagnostic tests can be conveniently carried out. The limited data available indicate that, despite the absence of evaluated evidence that it effectively improves the welfare of mothers or babies, obstetricians resorted to antenatal inpatient care with increasing frequency.

Published records for all NHS hospitals [85, 86] estimate the 'undelivered discharges' (meaning antenatal admissions), but not how many women are affected since one woman may be admitted for more than one inpatient spell. Moreover, data for later years may not be strictly comparable with data for earlier years, but these limitations do not disguise the relative increase in the use of antenatal inpatient care. In 1973, 13% of all maternity discharges were undelivered, in 1985 24%. For every 'discharge undelivered' there were 6.7 deliveries in 1973, but only 3.0 in 1985. Between 1973 and 1985, the number of hospital deliveries decreased by 3%, but the number of 'discharges undelivered' increased by 119%. Beds were kept occupied. The percentage of women delivered who were admitted prior to labour fell from 46 in 1973 to 31 in 1985. This may reflect a change in obstetricians' policy or, more likely, the development of women's strategy to escape having labour induced. The rate of antenatal admissions varied considerably between the Health Regions of England – between 9% and 16% in 1973. The rate increased everywhere, but the variance was only slightly less in 1985 – from 20% to 28% – illustrating differences either in the incidence of diagnosed pathology or in prescribed treatment.

Unfortunately, comparable records have not been collected and published since 1985 [87, p. 574]. Thus it is not possible to see whether more recent trends reflect the later research findings that antenatal inpatient care in hospital definitely does not improve fetal outcomes nor prevent the development of proteinuria in hypertensive women. The need for inpatient stays and medical interventions has been shown to be greatly reduced by supervision at home or in a hospital day unit, at much lower cost to the service and greater satisfaction to the mothers [88].

The risk of premature delivery is greater in the presence of vaginal infections, including sexually transmitted diseases, which may or may not give rise to symptoms in the mother but which routine screening should uncover [89–92]. Treatment with antibiotic drugs should in most cases be effective in clearing the infection, but that it continues to be found, and much more often in preterm than in term births, suggests that this is an area in which antenatal screening could profitably be more thorough.

If obstetric interventions to delay preterm delivery have so far had little success, new interventions hold out much more hope of reducing its dangers for the baby. Over half the babies born preterm, especially those at less than 34 weeks' gestation, suffer respiratory distress, for many of them a very serious or fatal illness. Recent controlled trials have shown that administration of corticosteroids to the mother in the period before birth reduces the incidence of this condition for the infant by 40–60%. The optimum predelivery period is between twenty-four hours and seven days, but some benefit follows administration outside these limits even for the least mature.

For probably interrelated reasons, corticosteroids also reduce the risk of other life-threatening morbidity – haemorrhage affecting the neonate's brain and necrotizing enterocolitis affecting its digestive tract. This reduced morbidity leads to reduced mortality and shorter periods of intensive care for the survivors: the average cost per survivor is reduced, but the greater numbers of survivors mean that total costs and pressure on accommodation in intensive care units is increased (page 233). Since this therapy does not seem to bring adverse consequences, either short or long term for mother or child, it must be welcomed as one of the few real advances in medical antenatal care [93, 94].

Psychological reasons for preterm birth

The other basic, and no less important, underlying reason for spontaneous preterm delivery is the psychological consequence of stress. There are many depictions in lay literature of dramatic events in late pregnancy culminating in premature birth, but stress from unfavourable life events throughout pregnancy may have just as, if not more, damaging an effect. Medical antenatal interventions are clearly an inappropriate remedy for social problems. Prevention is more likely to be achieved by successful efforts to relieve the stress and much can often be achieved simply by the giving of kind friendly support by professional workers to women who cannot find such comfort from their family or personal associations.

It has been constantly observed in several countries that the proportion of preterm, low-weight births is smaller where antenatal care is provided entirely by sympathetic midwives [35, 95–98]. Harassment by providers of orthodox antenatal care to conform to their standards of what is desirable and the constant exaggeration of the potential risks of childbirth, which so often characterizes professional advice, cannot possibly contribute to reassuring women of their competence to complete a normal physiological function and can only aggravate the stress of those already suffering it.

A few local schemes have been set up by Health Centres in Britain in districts of social deprivation where preterm labour is more likely to happen, in order to ensure continuous social as well as medical support to the women who most need it. These seem to have achieved some positive effects and in at least two cases were able to report rewarding reductions in the incidence of preterm labour and low-weight births [41, 95, 96].

A systematic review of thirty-eight studies of social or dietary support undertaken in several countries had led to the conclusion

> that there is considerable evidence to suggest that intervention programmes aimed at improving the social side of antenatal care are capable of affecting birthweight. . . . It is suggested that traditional professional approaches to pregnancy which divide the medical from the social perspective have acted to prevent recognition of this evidence and its relevance to medical policy. [98]

However, several randomized controlled trials, carried out in different countries including Western Australia, the USA, France and England failed to find that their particular support measures, always additional to normal conventional antenatal care, significantly reduced the proportion of low-weight births in the subgroups of their selected populations which were randomized to intervention [99–104]. The numbers of subjects in the trials were fairly small and the kind of social support which it was possible to give was very limited, but nevertheless resulted in some benefits which were appreciated by the supported mothers and no disbenefits [99]. More convincing improvements might have been demonstrated if normal antenatal care had been compared with a package of more generous social interventions, combined with fewer medical interventions, that is, if the existing balance between medical and social care had been reversed.

The growth-retarded fetus

For some babies born preterm their birthweight, though low, is appropriate for their gestation. For other babies their birthweight is low because some interruption in the quantity and quality of nourishment brought to them from the placenta has impaired their growth during gestation. For yet others birthweight is low because of both factors, shortened gestation and retarded growth. Many congenitally malformed babies, still and live born, are also growth retarded. The impairment may have started early, in which case the growth of all organs may be equally depressed (symmetrical retardation), or late, in which case growth of the head and brain tends to be maintained at the expense of the rest of the body (asymmetrical retardation). Several of the causes of retarded growth are the same as those already described as causing preterm birth, including maternal stress and inadequate diet, and the same mothers are most likely to be affected [105].

Smoking – a response to stress

A popular way of coping with stress is smoking. Smoking does the same damage to the maternal–placental–fetal vascular system as it does to all vascular systems. The blood flow is impaired and the fetus is deprived of food and oxygen. Birthweight is lowered and there is evidence that the damage may persist after birth [106, p. 162]. Mothers who smoke less or not at all have heavier, healthier babies. The only contribution that the providers of orthodox antenatal care can make towards achieving this desirable outcome is to persuade mothers to cut out or cut down their smoking, make them aware of helpful techniques for overcoming an addiction and give them constant encouragement and support while they make the effort to do so. Such care is more likely to be given by midwives in an informal setting than in the usual antenatal clinic.

Since harm comes also from passive smoking, strategies to persuade women to smoke less would benefit if they were accompanied by strategies to persuade their partners, or those with whom they share their home, to do so too. Since the chance of low birthweight is greatly increased when mothers who smoke also drink much alcohol or use opiates, help in overcoming these habits would likewise be beneficial.

Maternal diet

Common sense favours the view that the diet which keeps non-pregnant people healthy should keep the pregnant woman healthy and prepare her child for its postnatal environment. Some women, however, are not able to enjoy this healthy diet because of their economic or social circumstances. Even so, the growing fetus is biologically pro-grammed to absorb the nourishment it requires, if necessary at the expense of its mother's reserves, so that only when the mother is suffer-ing from a serious lack of food and depleted reserves do additions to the diet achieve useful increases in birthweight.

Evaluating diets is notoriously difficult. It is virtually impossible to isolate the effects of the chemical interactions of the different foods people eat in different quantities; it is difficult, too, to distinguish the effects of diet and other aspects of their lives. Consequently, scientific trials to test any hypothesis are very difficult to organize. Nevertheless, Brewer's observations in America in the 1960s were that the diet of poor mothers, before intervention, was critically deficient. This was also the finding of a 1989 study in a deprived London borough of the food intake of women at the time of their first antenatal visit and before they received any dietary advice, so probably representing their normal prepregnancy diet. The food intakes were analysed in terms of forty-four nutrients, calories, proteins, fat, carbohydrates, the main vitamins and ten minerals. When the birthweights of the babies were related to their mothers' recorded dietary intake, it was found that the mothers of babies weighing under 2500 grams had a lower intake of forty-three of the forty-four nutrients, than the mothers whose babies weighed between 2500 and 3000 grams. These mothers in turn had lower intakes than the mothers of babies weighing over 3000 grams, who in turn had intakes similar to those of women in a neighbouring well-to-do suburb. Intakes were not significantly different for the mothers of preterm and growth-retarded babies. There was a very strong correlation between a small intake of vitamin B1 and low-weight babies [107].

While most problems seem to be avoided by a varied diet in quan-tities best dictated by the mother's appetite, diets sufficient in quantity may be deficient in certain essential elements. Unfortunately, scientists have not been able precisely to define these, nor to trace most of the unsatisfactory outcomes to specific deficiencies [73, 108].

It has been assumed that certain unsatisfactory outcomes are caused by lack of iron, but the dietary supplementations thought appropriate in these cases have proved ineffective [108]. Indeed, since severe anaemia is rare among adequately fed women, extra doses of iron may do more harm than good, as may happen also with an excess of any nutrient which the body cannot easily get rid of. Fetal abnormalities have been found to be associated with an excessive intake of vitamin A, which is needed in appropriate amounts for the development of sight and other organs, and British pregnant women in the 1990s have been officially, but not in all cases wisely, advised not to eat liver, a source of many nutrients, in the off chance that the animals have been overfed with vitamin A. On the other hand, malformations of the neural tube, anencephaly and spina bifida, are associated with a lack of folic acid (one of the vitamin B group). A large multicentre randomized controlled trial of births at high risk of neural tube defects showed that the incidence of these was 72% lower in the group with folic acid supplementation, without adverse side-effects [109]. Folic acid supplements for all pregnant women might well safeguard against any chance of neural tube defects, but unrestricted prescription would be inadvisable without the maximum safe dosage having been established, which no trial so far has been designed to do.

Fetuses may suffer damage also if their mothers develop an infectious illness from certain foods they eat. In the 1980s British pregnant women have been warned against eating insufficiently cooked eggs, lest they contract salmonella (assuming an unproven causal relationship), and insufficiently reheated pre-cooked meals and certain dairy products like soft cheese, lest they contract listeriosis.

Diagnosing and treating growth retardation

There is no simple technique for measuring fetal size objectively [110] and identifying growth retardation is inevitably approximate. Routine abdominal palpation, the simplest traditional technique, and deductions from serial measurements of maternal weight gain yield estimates which correlate imperfectly with actual birthweight. Serial measurements of fundal (uterine) height might yield more useful estimates, were it not for the known inconsistency between measurements by different people and even by the same person at different times. More reliance is now placed on changes in ultrasound measurements of fetal bone length and abdominal circumference. However, a study which compared these latter two methods of screening found that each had a false-positive rate of 60%, which means that more than half of the infants diagnosed as light for gestational age proved in the event to be of normal weight for their gestation [111]. On this evidence, neither test would save many fetuses from wrong diagnosis and inappropriate treatment.

Deprivation of nutrients and oxygen leads to fetal distress. The heart rate of a healthy fetus varies in response to fetal movements or uterine contractions. Reactions considered inappropriate or outside the normal range (Table 6.4) may indicate fetal distress. Doubt about fetal welfare may be confirmed by an abnormal heart rate pattern which may be revealed by the biophysical test of cardiotocography – continuous electronic monitoring of the fetal heart (Chapter 4, pages 177–9). This test may be applied antenatally to women as outpatients or, more intensively and more expensively, as hospital inpatients. Although it has been widely used, evaluative studies have found the results to be very unreliable, on the one hand wrongly detecting distress and predicting a poor outcome, and on the other hand failing to detect distress and predict the poor outcome that actually followed [54, 112]. Overdiagnosis of distress leads to the dangers of unnecessary operative interventions.

A well-designed, randomized trial found antenatal monitoring of no benefit in terms of mortality, morbidity or neonatal condition and irrelevant to almost all of the perinatal deaths in the study, which in the event were not due to chronic placental failure as had been supposed. Ironically, despite the strongly dissuasive results, this trial was followed in the same hospital by a sixteen-fold increase in antenatal monitoring! [113]. And despite similar evidence from every quarter, 'despite the fact that no prospective study has shown it to be of any value' [112], hospitals which have invested in the technical equipment continue to ensure that it is much used for the antenatal monitoring of fetuses.

Obstetricians have devoted much effort to devising a more reliable technique for identifying growth-retarded fetuses and placed great hopes on using pulsed Doppler ultrasound to measure blood velocity wave forms in the fetal umbilical artery, since decreased velocity is associated with fetal hypoxia and other morbidity. So far, this technique has offered no major advance over other ultrasound or other biophysical tests in predicting fetuses which are growth retarded or small for gestational age [114].

Even if growth retardation could be accurately diagnosed, the accruing benefits from this knowledge would not be great. No technique is as yet available for reversing the impediment to uterine growth. The only possible intervention is to advocate delivery and substitute an intensive care cot for the mother's womb.

Iatrogenic preterm birth

Some babies are born preterm, not spontaneously but by intranatal intervention when obstetricians judge that curtailing their uterine life is in their or their mother's best interest. Advancing delivery is relied on as the ultimate escape from threatened pre-eclampsia to forestall the mortal danger to both mother and infant, though ending the pregnancy to save the mother's life may be at the risk of delivering an immature, or even a very immature, infant. When obstetricians plan to curtail the pregnancy in the interest of the child, as when they suspect that its uterine environment cannot sustain the minimum desirable rate of growth, their decision rests partly on their estimate of its maturity, assumed from the gestational age derived from the visual evidence of early ultrasound (page 127), and in particular on the maturity of its lungs. In the latter case, there is a fairly, but not wholly, reliable predictive test for lung maturity which involves measuring whether the ratio between two substances in the amniotic fluid, lecithin and sphyngomyelin, has reached about 2 : 1 [54]. The advent of the last minute corticosteroid therapy to promote lung maturity has now reduced the dangers of mistaken judgement.

Probably now that its safety and cost-effectiveness have been tested, this therapy will be more widely used, and where necessary complemented with a second new, though expensive, therapy to reduce respiratory distress, the postnatal administration of surfactant to the baby (Chapter 5, page 233). Together, these should reduce the number of babies who, despite the application of other scientific technology, have been born in a less mature state than expected [115] and who have depended for survival on the even more advanced technology for resuscitation and maintenance care of neonatal paediatrics, which in turn is followed by a higher than average rate of childhood morbidity [87, pp. 383–4, 116] (page 363).

However plausible it may seem to obstetricians that the strategy is beneficial, by the 1990s no study had confirmed that on balance the rate of healthy survival, either perinatally or later, is increased by cutting short the uterine development of suspectedly unhealthy fetuses. Thus no study has produced evidence which justifies the other modality – timed delivery – on which obstetric management has relied (page 109). Perhaps the new therapies will shift the balance in favour of intervention, unless the need for iatrogenic intervention has been forestalled by other less invasive, less expensive therapies, such as low-dose aspirin, improved diet, midwives' antenatal care and social support, including influence to cut down maternal smoking.

DETECTING CONGENITAL MALFORMATIONS AND CHROMOSOMAL ANOMALIES

Obstetricians' antenatal interventions cannot prevent these causes of death and disability, but their modern technology and biochemical discoveries enable affected fetuses to be identified and termination of the pregnancy can be offered. It was discovered by 1970 that some neural tube defects, like anencephaly and spina bifida, can be identified if an abnormally high concentration of alphafetoprotein, a substance produced in the fetus, is found in the maternal blood stream. The diagnosis may be confirmed by an ultrasound scan at between sixteen and twenty-two weeks' gestation when the defects are directly detectable. Further confirmation may be obtained by the technique developed in 1969 of amniocentesis [117] – withdrawal of a sample of fluid from the amniotic sac for analysis of fetal cells. However, this withdrawal can impair development of the fetal lungs and increase the risk of neonatal respiratory difficulties. The operation also slightly increases the risk of miscarriage. The procedure is only worth the costs, in money and physical side-effects, where there is reason to suspect increased risk of the defect, as when there is a family history of congenital malformation or the mother is older. The operation is most safely done after the pregnancy has accumulated sufficient fluid, hitherto judged to be after sixteen weeks, and under ultrasound cover. Culture of the sample takes two to three weeks, so that, besides leaving an anxious interval while results are awaited, termination if desired has to take place at a fairly late stage of gestation.

In view of these drawbacks and of the increasing expertise of ultrasonographers in identifying these defects at an earlier routine scan, there is an incentive to find out the earliest date for amniocentesis with acceptable safety for the developing fetus. An alternative technique for analysing fetal cells has been developed, chorionic villus sampling (CVS). This involves taking a biopsy, under ultrasound guidance in the first few weeks of pregnancy, of the villi, which are folds of the chorion, the membrane which totally surrounds the embryo from the time of implantation. Earlier knowledge would obviously be an advantage, if it were not outweighed by other disadvantages.

To assess the balance of advantage between CVS in the first trimester and amniocentesis in the second, a large-scale randomized controlled trial was carried out and its results were reported in 1991 [118]. It was found that CVS led to more diagnoses of abnormality, hence more terminations, to more spontaneous fetal deaths before twenty-eight weeks, to more neonatal deaths because more liveborn babies were very immature, and so to the longer hospital stays they needed. One explanation of the apparent excess of abnormality is that nature would have spontaneously aborted many of the malformed fetuses before the time of amniocentesis. Another study had found an association between CVS at eight to nine weeks and limb deformities [119]. The conclusion of the trial was that CVS was potentially less safe and more prone to error than amniocentesis. It is, nevertheless, a risk which some women would prefer to take.

Fetal cells can give advance warning also of chromosomal anomalies. In contrast to neural tube defects, Down's syndrome in the fetus is associated with an abnormally low concentration of alphafetoprotein in the mother's blood [120]. Although the risk of bearing an infant with Down's syndrome is higher for older than for younger mothers, the majority of affected babies are actually borne by younger mothers. Amniocentesis for all would have prohibitive disadvantages. Abnormal concentrations of alphafetoproteins and two other serum markers in the blood of mothers carrying affected fetuses have been observed and the so-called triple test has been proposed, to narrow down the small subgroup of pregnancies at higher risk for which the costs of amniocentesis are likely to be less than the lifetime costs, human and financial, of looking after handicapped children [121]. Though useful, this biochemical test, which is not by itself diagnostic, is still far from identifying all fetuses with Down's syndrome, and only these, and its proposal met with initial objections, because it identified many fetuses falsely and so created unnecessary anxiety. An even newer technique, still awaiting further evaluation, has been devised for speeding up the detection of Down's syndrome from fetal cells in amniotic fluid, which would reduce the anxious wait for results [122].

Yet another test which would give information earlier is being pioneered by Professor K. Nicolaides, King's College Hospital, London, as a development of his studies of ultrasound images, which has enabled him to detect markers of fetal chromosomal anomalies. One of these, seen in scans made with very sophisticated equipment at about eleven weeks' gestation, is a large black 'space' behind the neck of the fetus which appears to be present in about 90% of those with Down's syndrome. Scans at such an early stage of fetal development may, however, carry risks of their own (page 129).

Through offering termination, obstetricians do their best to reduce the mortality due to congenital mistakes. Their efforts inevitably concentrate on the fetus and the mother. The preconceptional contribution of fathers to malformation should not be overlooked. There are many known associations between damaged sperm and places of work, contacts with materials, radiation, smoking, alcohol consumption and other personal habits.

ULTRASOUND

First invented in 1960, ultrasound scanning was being recommended as a routine antenatal procedure by 1980 and quickly became so. Its first and most frequent use is to date gestation more accurately than by conventional means though a margin of error remains [123]. Accurate dating is relevant if elective delivery is desired and it has often restrained intervention to deliver babies wrongly estimated to be post-term. Its later use is in the monitoring of fetal development, using tests which have different significance at different gestational ages, and so to alert obstetricians to conditions which, they believe, their interventions can improve.

Breech and other malpresentations can be clearly identified. Increasingly, for the minority which do not convert spontaneously to vertex, these lead to elective caesarean section, in preference to antenatal external version and intranatal breech delivery, though evidence can be adduced to support both options (Chapter 4). Also identifiable are ectopic pregnancies and whether the fetus has survived an antepartum haemorrhage. They can show up the placental site, so that appropriate treatment, usually caesarean section, can be arranged for the few which remain low, as placenta praevia. Multiple pregnancies can be detected earlier and more accurately than by clinical examination, but this knowledge does not alter management or improve outcome. Fetal breathing movements can be observed, but these turn out to be poor predictors of neonatal respiratory difficulties. Most fetal skeletal abnormalities can be diagnosed and for some of them visual control opens the possibility of carrying out corrective, although risky, operations on the fetus, as well as avoiding mishaps in amniocentesis and CVS.

By relating ultrasound measurements of the biparietal diameter of the skull and abdominal circumference, estimations of fetal growth in later pregnancy can be refined. Changes can be distinguished in the pattern over time which indicate the onset of retardation and whether it is symmetrical or asymmetrical. Nevertheless, detection of growth retardation has been very unreliable with many false positives, who have to share the recommended remedy – curtailment of gestation – without hope of benefit.

Ultrasound examination has revealed that the appearance of the placenta changes with advancing gestational age. A prematurely aged placenta may predict an increased risk of a poor perinatal outcome [124]. Whether knowledge of the state of the placenta can reduce this risk, without creating offsetting others, depends on a possibly preventive treatment being available. This is improbable, for although doctors have hailed ultrasound scanning as without doubt 'the most useful development in the last decade in obstetric practice' [125, p. 71], there is no evidence that it has in fact made most viable births safer [126, 127]. The risk is unlikely to be reduced in low-risk births and it was not reduced in two randomized controlled studies where the use of frequent scans to monitor pregnancies at high predicted risk of preterm labour and low birthweight respectively found more preterm births in the first and higher perinatal mortality in the second among the sub-groups that were scanned [128, 129].

British obstetricians have always advertised ultrasound enthusiastically, to women in antenatal clinics and in both the medical and lay press, as being totally harmless. They have, however, never had indisputable evidence to support this claim, for although the Medical Research Council had by 1981 considered conducting a trial to assess the benefits and hazards of ultrasound before its use became general, their proposal was never implemented. Apparently they were persuaded that only subtle anomalies were likely to be found and these might have other causes [130]. This obviously happened before their acceptance of the powers of the randomized controlled trial to identify causal associations (page 257). The opportunity was lost to evaluate a procedure while opinions about its value were still open and a fair trial was possible. That opportunity has now passed, but obstetricians seem happy to believe that the safety of ultrasound is self-evident and impartial evidence is not necessary.

The worst fear of a potential link with childhood cancer, as happened with X-rays [12], was allayed by the follow-up studies of children scanned in the 1970s, which found no such association, at least in the short term [131, 132]. This specific reassurance was overgenerously interpreted as applying to all risks, long term as well as short. Unlike the USA's National Institutes of Health, the USA Food and Drug Administration and the World Health Organization, which recommend selective use, and indeed contrary to the Department of Health's stated policy in 1984 [130], the Royal College of Obstetricians and Gynaecologists felt justified in recommending routine scans for all at around sixteen weeks' gestation [133]. It now apparently sees no objection to as many additional scans as practitioners consider helpful, not simply for the management of an individual case, but for the general study of fetal development. As a result of this indulgence, many women have several scans, some upwards of ten.

It has never been tested whether there is an upper safe limit to the number of scans though there is now some evidence that birthweight is lower after several scans [134]. Nor is it known whether safety is related to a scan's duration, which can vary widely in length, or to the power of the instrument used, which also varies widely between models, newer models usually being much more powerful than the older ones used in the 1970s. More abnormalities are likely to be picked up on longer scans and by more powerful instruments, so safety may have to be traded for more information. The imaging electronic fetal monitors, as well as the acoustic continuous and pulsed wave Doppler monitors and hand-held sonic devices, also use ultrasound energy. No records are kept of the total exposure for an individual baby, which obviously could be considerable. The exposure is probably augmented when, instead of the transabdominal instrument, the more recent invention is used, the quicker transvaginal probe which gets nearer to the fetus, bypassing the protection of the mother's body [130].

The studies which reassured about safety were carried out in the years when most scans were single events done at around sixteen weeks, after the major fetal organs had formed. The newer investigation of CVS and most recently detection of Down's syndrome (page 126) needs ultrasound participation around nine or eleven weeks, the critical period of organ formation when the risk of external factors causing malformation is greatest. Development of the neurological system continues as gestation progresses and some experts fear that cells and nerves may be irreparably damaged, though perhaps only subtly, by later scans. So far, however, no major damage has been traced to antenatal ultrasound.

Interpreting ultrasound images obviously requires considerable skill, but there is no recognized training which all operators, who may be general radiographers or doctors or midwives, must take before they practise. They ought to have a good grasp of the technology involved and ability to adapt to the frequent innovations. With the rising demand for scans, many operators have to learn quickly on the job. Inevitably there will be variations in the quality and accuracy of the diagnoses they make and on the reliance that can be put on these as bases for further treatment.

Radiologists are less confident than obstetricians about the complete safety and usefulness claimed for ultrasound. In 1988 a working party of the British Medical Ultrasound Society counselled limited output levels and exposures as brief as possible, with regular upgrading for radiographers. In his review 'The safety of diagnostic ultrasound' in the *British Journal of Obstetrics and Gynaecology* in 1987, an eminent consultant radiologist was bold enough to write:

The casual observer might be forgiven for wondering why the medical profession is now involved in the wholesale examination of pregnant patients with machines emanating vastly different powers of an energy which is not proven to be harmless to obtain information which is not proven to be of any clinical value by operators who are not certified as competent to perform examinations. [135]

Whether or not ultrasound is harmless, it is certainly costly with its expensive equipment which needs frequent updating and should have highly trained staff to operate. Therefore there is no justification for dedicating resources, which might be advantageously used for other purposes, to making ultrasound a routine procedure from which most babies will not benefit. It should be reserved for use in those complications where it might help and for educational and research purposes. Even here the ethical issues are not clear cut: submitting normal fetuses to lengthy or repeated observation, from which they derive no direct benefit, certainly can add to the understanding of fetal development, but it is morally unjustifiable unless there is proven evidence that they can sustain no harm.

WOMEN'S ATTITUDES TO SCREENING TESTS

It is undoubted that women want healthy babies and have by now been thoroughly persuaded that antenatal care, with its investigations and interventions, is the necessary preliminary to their production. From its early days, however, it was realized that antenatal care was likely to create as much anxiety as reassurance (page 94) and anxiety makes safe reproduction more difficult. That likelihood increased as the range widened of tests to screen pregnancies for the disturbing complications which, happily, affect only a small minority of them. Nevertheless, the lurking fear lest they be in that minority is implanted in all women and is not relieved until they receive a favourable test result, and even then a shadow may remain, in case the test has not actually identified the abnormality sought, which occasionally happens.

Nor is the fear avoided by refusal to undergo the tests, which are not compulsory but which most women feel under medical or social pressure to comply with. They worry in case there should be an adverse outcome, for they know that they will then feel guilty and irresponsible for not having taken action which might have averted it. It is difficult to ignore with equanimity possibilities once they are known to exist.

Anxiety is the greater the longer women have to wait for results. The waiting period varies for different tests. The first results will give most women the reassurance they hope for, but for some they will be equivocal and indicate the need for further tests, which generate further anxiety, while for the small minority they will confirm the woman's worst fears, leaving her to make very painful decisions. Stress is less likely to be aggravated if birth attendants take the trouble to communicate the results, good or bad, as promptly and sensitively as possible to the woman. Some women are clearly informed about the purpose of specific tests or about action open to them in response to adverse results. Some women are not clearly informed about the physical dangers of the tests themselves. But it is not known whether inadequate information leads to more or less stress, while results are awaited or once they are received [136].

In the case of ultrasound examination, it is because they trust the assurance of their professional advisers that it is absolutely safe that most women consent so willingly to it. Indeed, impressed by the wonders of technology which enables them, and often their partners, to share in seeing the developing creation in their bodies and feeling their interest quicken, some of them have come to consider it an indispensable procedure for safe childbirth. And because it is a routine procedure for everyone, they are not unduly apprehensive about the findings, as they would more probably be if the test were offered only in cases of suspected abnormality. For most of them normality will be confirmed and their pregnancy will continue even more happily in this knowledge; for a very few the favourable verdict may in the end be reversed, and their inspired false confidence may possibly make their ultimate grief the greater. For a minority, an abnormality will be correctly diagnosed and if it is serious enough, termination of the pregnancy may be accepted as the least distressing course. For another minority, abnormalities will be incorrectly diagnosed, while some abnormalities, like the position of the placenta or presentation of the fetus, will be diagnosed which, though apparent at the time of the scan, will in many cases have righted themselves before delivery without intervention, but not without causing the mother anxiety in the meantime.

This imposed burden of emotional stress, which certainly increases the physical risks of childbirth, has to be set against the power of screening tests to reduce the physical risks. This power is limited, since most of them cannot be followed by remedial therapies for abnormalities identified.

SHOULD MATERNITY CARE START BEFORE CONCEPTION?

It is obvious that, in the human race as in all other living species, healthy offspring are in general produced by parents who are healthy before they embark on parenthood. Many factors interact to make people healthy or unhealthy, but the most important of these are social, environmental and behavioural and on these maternity care has little direct influence. Of the factors, poverty has been identified as the most critical, because it imposes material and psychological deprivations, inadequacies of diet and shelter, less healthy places and conditions of work, less education, less security and more stressful life-styles. Their lesser poverty probably explains why pregnant women in paid employment have fewer preterm and low-weight babies with fewer first week deaths than do full-time housewives [137]. To compensate for its frustrations, poverty encourages its victims to adopt habits like smoking which add to ill health. Children suffering the disadvantages of being born to impoverished parents have a greater than average chance of growing up to be impoverished parents themselves and to pass on the disadvantage to future generations.

The problems of poverty have defied political solution throughout history; the worst privations of absolute poverty have been eased by general improvements in the standard of living in the economically prosperous countries, but the problems of relative poverty remain. The House of Commons Health Committee began its Inquiry into the Maternity Services in 1990–1 by examining the issue of preconception care and reached the conclusion that:

> Encouraging and enabling people in low socio-economic groups to improve their standard and quality of life are one of the most difficult, but important, challenges facing government. Steps taken to alleviate social deprivation will make a significant contribution to improving the outcome of pregnancy. [138, para. 47]

The Committee did, however, recommend [138] several measures to secure, through health education from childhood onwards, that prospective parents were better informed about what they could do before conception to produce healthier babies, precepts similar to what they could do after conception but probably more effective, for example giving up smoking and avoiding sexually transmitted infections (page 120). The role of family planning in sparing the mother from the exhaustion of too closely spaced pregnancies and the risk of a low-weight baby (page 115), and the suitability of such clinics for dispensing preconception advice were recognized. Acknowledging this aspect of maternity care, the RCOG broke new ground in 1993 and established its own Faculty of Family Planning.

Some parents fear that their babies will be unhealthy because they inherit a genetic disorder. The Health Committee recommended improving the availability of genetic advice and counselling, but it stopped short of recommending the provision of specific preconception clinics, for they doubted that these are really required or desired by the majority of parents, or would indeed be used by the majority of those parents whose need is greatest.

IN WHOSE INTEREST?

In the name of promoting the safety of birth for mother and child, pregnant women have been persuaded in the course of the 20th century to comply with an ever wider range of medically organized regimens, procedures and treatments. Many of these are inconvenient and disagreeable and, when they are tested, few are found to provide the promised benefits without counteracting disbenefits, which implies that most could be abandoned without prejudicing safety. Whether satisfaction would be prejudiced would depend on whether women could be weaned from their indoctrinated, but unjustifiable, beliefs that, though they may dislike much of it, antenatal care as provided is essential to safe delivery.

Why does reform not happen? Why indeed is there pressure to apply the discredited or unproven therapies and procedures routinely to all women, irrespective of predicted risk? And why is this done at a time when childbearing women in countries where absolute poverty has become rare are healthier than they have ever been?

Healthy women, like other healthy mammals, have evolved to take pregnancy in their stride without medical mediation – the mediation that obstetricians have been at such pains to organize themselves to provide. If mediation is needed, then it should take the form mainly of social and personal support, which midwives and sympathetic general practitioners could readily provide, once they have dared to discard the medical model which they have increasingly chosen or been obliged to copy.

The obstetric profession has grown so powerful that it is not likely to acquiesce willingly in its redundancy. In self-defence its professional body continues to preach unremittingly that birth is essentially dangerous and only under obstetric management can the dangers be avoided. If normal pregnancy and delivery do not need their help, obstetricians have to convince everyone that the process cannot be relied on to stay normal [34, para. 225]. They have to search for signs of abnormality of which the mother is unaware and in an age that worships science this is most persuasively done through the magic of advanced technology, even before this technology has been evaluated.

If obstetricians want to dominate intranatal care, they do this best by first dominating antenatal care and starting as early as possible to instil apprehension and undermine women's self-confidence in their own reproductive competence. The public claims to believe that prevention is better than cure. Obstetrically directed antenatal care is popularly represented as the perfect example of preventive medicine and a sound financial investment. At no time have results justified this claim and many of the modern technological procedures cannot justify their cost.

Routine antenatal care for all was started to serve primarily the interests of mothers and babies. Its relative lack of success over eighty years means that it is continued in its present form to serve primarily the interests of organized obstetricians. In recent years, however, several eminent obstetricians have broken ranks and publicly criticized present arrangements (pages 109, 122). Their submissions to the House of Commons Health Committee for its Inquiry into the Maternity Services included the following statements: 'Present schedules of antenatal care are almost certainly not cost effective. . . . Specialist obstetricians should not undertake routine care' [44, p. 780]. 'There is little or no evidence that antenatal care and delivery in a consultant unit carries any benefit to the normal pregnant woman or her baby. . . . There is, however, accumulating evidence that such care is expensive. . . . There is little evidence that having each pregnant patient seen by a consultant once in the pregnancy improves the recognition of abnormal pregnancies or the management of low risk pregnancies' [44, pp. 677–8] . . . 'Antenatal care . . . badly needs re-examination and trimming back for most women' [44, p. 818] . . . 'In general, doctors, midwives and patients like technology and come to equate the use of technology with good care. . . . This love of technology means . . . that it is often introduced without proper evaluation. There is a temptation to do many tests, such as scans, when frequently they may be of little or no value other than to make the patient or her medical attendants feel happier' [44, p. 757].

Weighing the large amount of evidence it received from many angles, the Committee was persuaded

> that the present imposition of a rigid pattern of frequent antenatal visits is not grounded in any good scientific base, and that there is no evidence that such a pattern is medically necessary. The identified needs of women for information and support during pregnancy can be met more effectively than happens at present. There is widespread agreement that this requires a more flexible system which is based in the community, not in the hospital. The present system of shared care between hospitals and the community should, by and large, be abandoned. Hospitals are not the appropriate place to care for healthy women. [34, para. 208]

It remains to re-educate both the receivers and most of the providers of antenatal care, including the service administrators, and inform them about the facts.

REFERENCES

1. Towler, J. and Bramall, J. (1986) *Midwives in History and Society*, Croom Helm, London, Chaps 1–6.

2. Siddall, A.C. (1980) Blood-letting in American obstetric practice 1800–1945. *Bull. Hist. Med.*, **54**, 101–10.
3. Oakley, A. (1984) *The Captured Womb*, Blackwell, Oxford.
4. Ballantyne, J.W. (1901) Plea for a pro-maternity hospital. *Br. Med. J.*, 6 April, 813–14.
5. Browne, F.J. (1954) The initiation and development of antenatal care, in *Historical Review of British Obstetrics and Gynaecology, 1800–1950*, (eds J.M. Munro Kerr, R.W. Johnstone and M.H. Phillips), Livingstone, Edinburgh, Chap. XXII.
6. Ballantyne, J.W. (1906–7) The future of obstetrics (inaugural address). *Trans. Edin. Obstet. Soc.*, **32**, 3–28.
7. *Maternity in Great Britain* (1946), (survey undertaken by a Joint Committee of the Royal College of Obstetricians and Gynaecologists and the Population Investigation Committee), Oxford University Press, Oxford.
8. Redman, C. (1982) Management of pre-eclampsia, in *Effectiveness and Satisfaction in Antenatal Care*, (eds M. Enkin and I. Chalmers), William Heinemann, London, Chap. 12.
9. Johnstone, R.W. (1954) Labour, in *Historical Review of British Obstetrics and Gynaecology, 1800–1950* (eds J.M. Munro Kerr, R.W. Johnstone and M.H. Phillips), Livingstone, Edinburgh, Chap. XVI.
10. Strachan, G.I. (1954) Radiography in obstetrics and gynaecology, in *Historical Review of British Obstetrics and Gynaecology, 1800–1950* (eds J.M. Munro Kerr, R.W. Johnstone and M.H. Phillips), Livingstone, Edinburgh, Chap. XXVIII.
11. Salmond, R.W.A. (1937) The uses and value of radiology in obstetrics, in *Antenatal and Postnatal Care* 2nd edn (ed. F.J. Browne), Churchill, London, p. 497.
12. Stewart, A., Webb, J., Giles, D. and Hewitt, D. (1956) Malignant disease in childhood and diagnostic irradiation in utero. *Lancet*, **ii**, 447.
13. McIlroy, A.L. (1954) Pregnancy and associated disease, in *Historical Review of British Obstetrics and Gynaecology, 1800–1950* (eds J.M. Munro Kerr, R.W. Johnstone and M.H. Phillips), Livingstone, Edinburgh, Chap. XXIV.
14. Gregg, N.M. (1941) *Trans. Ophthalmol. Soc. Aust.*, **4**, 119.
15. Browne, F.J. (1934) Are we satisfied with the results of antenatal care? *Br. Med. J.*, **2**, 194–7.
16. Campbell, J. (1924) *Maternal Mortality: Reports on Public Health and Medical Subjects*, No. 25, HMSO, London, p. 74.
17. Medical Officer of the Local Government Board (1915) *Memorandum on Health Visiting and on Maternity and Child Welfare Centres*, HMSO, London.
18. Wertz, R.W. and Wertz, D.C. (1977) *Lying-in: A History of Childbirth in America*, The Free Press, New York.
19. Chief Medical Officer of the Ministry of Health (1934) *Annual Report for 1933*, HMSO, London, pp. 75–6.
20. Logan, D. (1934) The general practitioner and midwifery. *Lancet*, **ii**, 141–3.
21. Dick-Read, G. (1933) *Natural Childbirth*, Heinemann, London.
22. Dick-Read, G. (1942) *Childbirth Without Fear*, Heinemann, London.

23. Williams, M. and Booth, D. (1980) *Antenatal Education*, 2nd edn, Churchill Livingstone, London.
24. Randall, M. (1949) *Training for Childbirth*, 4th edn, Churchill, London, p. 45.
25. Wrigley, A.J. (1934) A criticism of antenatal work. *Br. Med. J.*, **1**, 891–4.
26. Kerr, M.J.M. (1933) *Maternal Mortality and Morbidity: A Study of their Problems*, Livingstone, Edinburgh.
27. Oakley, *Captured Womb* (Quoting Lady Rhys-Williams) (1936) Malnutrition as a cause of maternal mortality. *Public Health*, **50**, 11–19.
28. Butler, N.R. and Bonham, D.G. (1963) *Perinatal Mortality*, Churchill Livingstone, Edinburgh.
29. Chamberlain, G., Philipp, E., Howlett, B. and Masters, K. (1978) *British Births, 1970 Vol. 2, Obstetric Care*, Heinemann, London.
30. Department of Health and Social Security: Central Health Services Council Standing Midwifery and Maternity Committee (1961) *Human Relations in Obstetrics*, HMSO, London.
31. House of Commons Social Services Committee Second Report (The Short Report) (1980) *Perinatal and Neonatal Mortality*, HMSO, London.
32. Royal College of Obstetricians and Gynaecologists (1982) *Report of the RCOG Working Party on Antenatal and Intrapartum Care*, HMSO, London.
33. Association of Community Health Councils for England and Wales (1987) *Antenatal Care: Still Waiting for Action*. ASCHC, London.
34. House of Commons Health Committee (Chairman Nicholas Winterton) (1992) *Maternity Services. Report*, vol. I, paras i–xciii (The Winterton Report), HMSO, London.
35. Flint, C. and Poulengeris, P. (1987) *The 'Know Your Midwife' Report*, 34 Elm Quay Court, London SW8 5DE.
36. Marsh, G. (1985) Introduction, in *Modern Obstetrics in General Practice*, (ed. G. Marsh), Oxford University Press, Oxford.
37. Reynolds, J., Yudkin, P. and Bull, M. (1988) General practitioner obstetrics: does risk prediction work? *J. R. Coll. Gen. Pract.*, **38**, 307–10.
38. House of Commons Health Committee (Chairman Nicholas Winterton) (1991) *Maternity Services: Preconception, vol. III, Appendices to the Minutes of Evidence*, HMSO, London, pp. 293–336.
39. Reid, M. and Garcia, J. (1989) Women's views of antenatal care, in *Effective Care in Pregnancy and Childbirth* (eds I. Chalmers, M. Enkin and M. Keirse), Oxford University Press, Oxford, Chap. 8.
40. Hall, M., MacIntyre, S. and Porter, M. (1985) *Antenatal Care Assessed*, Aberdeen University Press, Aberdeen, Chap. 7.
41. McKee, I. (1984) Community antenatal care: the Sighthill community antenatal clinic, in *Pregnancy Care for the 1980s* (eds L. Zander and G. Chamberlain), Royal Society of Medicine and Macmillan, London, Chap. 5.
42. Taylor, R. (1984) The interface between hospital and community-based care, in *Pregnancy Care for the 1980s* (eds L. Zander and G. Chamberlain), Royal Society of Medicine and Macmillan, London, Chap. 4.
43. Reid, I. and McIlwaine, G. (1981) Consumer opinion of hospital antenatal clinics. *Soc. Sci. Med.*, **14A**, 363–8.
44. House of Commons Health Committee (Chairman Nicholas Winterton)

(1992) *Maternity Services, vol. III, Appendices to the Minutes of Evidence,* HMSO, London, pp. 651–922.

45. Association of Radical Midwives (1986) *The Vision. Proposals for the Future of Maternity Service,* ARM, Ormskirk.

46. National Childbirth Trust, Alexander House, Oldham Terrace, Acton, London W3 6NH.

47. Korte, D. and Scaer, R. (1993) *A Good Birth, A Safe Birth,* Harvard Common Press, Boston, Massachusetts, p. 297.

48. Department of Health (1990) *Health and Personal Social Services Statistics for England,* HMSO, London, Table 8.1.

49. Jacoby, A. (1988) Mother's views about information and advice in pregnancy and childbirth: findings from a national study. *Midwifery,* **4,** 103–110.

50. Buxton, C. (1962) *A Study of Psychophysical Methods for Relief of Pain in Childbirth,* W.B. Saunders, Philadelphia.

51. Simkin, P. and Enkin, M. (1989) Antenatal classes, in *Effective Care in Pregnancy and Childbirth* (eds I. Chalmers, M. Enkin and M. Keirse), Oxford University Press, Oxford, Chap. 20.

52. Odent, M. (1984) How to help women in labour, in *Pregnancy Care for the 1980s* (eds L. Zander and G. Chamberlain), Royal Society of Medicine and Macmillan, London, Chap. 10.

53. Chamberlain, G. (1990) What is modern antenatal care of the fetus?, in *Modern Antenatal Care of the Fetus* (ed. G. Chamberlain), Blackwell, Oxford, Chap. 1, pp. 1–12.

54. Godfrey, K. (1985) A critical evaluation of modern techniques for fetal assessment during pregnancy, in *Modern Obstetrics in General Practice* (ed. G. Marsh), Oxford University Press, Oxford, Chap. 11.

55. McParland, P. and Pearce, J. (1990) Uteroplacental and fetal blood flow, in *Modern Antenatal Care of the Fetus* (ed. G. Chamberlain), Blackwell, Oxford, Chap. 6, pp. 89–126.

56. Kerr, M. (1980) The influence of information on clinical practice, in *Perinatal Audit and Surveillance* (ed. I. Chalmers), RCOG, London, pp. 319–26.

57. Chalmers, I., Enkin, M. and Keirse, M. (1989) *Effective Care in Pregnancy and Childbirth, vol. I, Pregnancy,* Oxford University Press, Oxford, Chaps 1–47.

58. Thomas, P., Golding, J. and Peters, T. (1991) Delayed antenatal care; does it effect (sic) pregnancy outcome? *Soc. Sci. Med.,* **32,** 715–23.

59. Hall, M. (1989) Critique of antenatal care, in *Obstetrics* (eds A. Turnbull and G. Chamberlain), Churchill Livingstone, Edinburgh, pp. 225–33.

60. Hall, M., Chng, P. and MacGillivray, I. (1980) Is routine antenatal care worth while? *Lancet,* **ii,** 78–80.

61. Wallenburg, H. (1989) Detecting hypertensive disorders of pregnancy, in *Effective Care in Pregnancy and Childbirth* (eds I. Chalmers, M. Enkin and M. Keirse), Oxford University Press, Oxford, Chap. 24, pp. 382–402.

62. Cartwright, W., Dalton, K. *et al.* (1992) Objective measurement of anxiety in hypertensive pregnant women managed in hospital and the community. *Br. J. Obstet. Gynaecol.,* **99,** 182–5.

63. Perry, I., Wilkinson, L. *et al.* (1991) Conflicting views on the measurement of blood pressure in pregnancy. *Br. J. Obstet Gynaecol.,* **98,** 241–3.

64. Collins, R. and Wallenburg, H. (1989) Pharmacological prevention and treatment of hypertensive disorders in pregnancy, in *Effective Care in Pregnancy and Childbirth* (eds I. Chalmers, M. Enkin and M. Keirse), Oxford University Press, Oxford, Chap. 33.

65. Blake, S. and Macdonald, D. (1991) The prevention of maternal manifestation of pre-eclampsia by intensive antihypertensive treatment. *Br. J. Obstet. Gynaecol.*, **98**, 244.

66. Hutton, J. and James, D. (1992) Management of severe pre-eclampsia and eclampsia by UK consultants. *Br. J. Obstet. Gynaecol.*, **99**, 554–6.

67. Bisson, D., MacGillivray, I. *et al.* (1991) Assessment and management of hypertension disorders by health professionals in the Avon district. *Br. J. Gen. Practit.*, **41**, 342, 23–5.

68. Wallenburg, H. and Rotmans, N. (1987) Prevention of recurrent idiopathic fetal growth retardation by low-dose aspirin and dipyridamole. *Am. J. Obstet. Gynecol.*, **157**, 1230–5.

69. Wallenburg, H. and Rotmans, N. (1988) Prophylactic low-dose aspirin and dypyridamole in pregnancy. *Lancet*, **i**, 939.

70. McParland, P., Pearce, J. and Chamberlain, G. (1990) Doppler ultrasound and aspirin in recognition and prevention of pregnancy induced hypertension. *Lancet*, **335**, 1552–7.

71. Uzar, S. *et al.* (1991) Prevention of fetal growth retardation with low dose aspirin: findings of the EPREDA trial. *Lancet*, **337**, 1427–31.

72. Douglas, K. and Redman, C. (1992) Eclampsia in the United Kingdom. The 'Best' way forward. *Br. J. Obstet. Gynaecol.*, **99**, 335–9.

73. Green, J. (1989) Diet and the prevention of pre-eclampsia, in *Effective Care in Pregnancy and Childbirth* (eds I. Chalmers, M. Enkin and M. Keirse), Oxford University Press, Oxford, Chap. 18, pp. 281–300.

74. Andersen, H., Andersen, L. and Fuchs, A. (1989) Diet, pre-eclampsia and intrauterine growth retardation. *Lancet*, **334**, 1146.

75. Secher, N. and Olsen, S. (1990) Fish-oil and pre-eclampsia. *Br. J. Obstet. Gynaecol.*, **97**, 1077–9.

76. CLASP (Collaborative Low-dose Aspirin Study in Pregnancy) Collaborative Group (1994) *Lancet*, **343**, 619–29.

77. Office of Population Censuses and Surveys (1990) *Perinatal and Infant Mortality: Social and Biological Factors, England & Wales*, DH3 no. 24, HMSO, London, Table 22.

78. Newton, R. and Hunt, L. (1984) Psychosocial stress in pregnancy and its relation to low birth weight. *Br. Med. J.*, **288**, 1191–4.

79. Mutale, T., Creed, F. *et al.* (1991) Life events and low birth weight – analysis by infants preterm and small for gestational age. *Br. J. Obstet. Gynaecol.*, **98**, 166–72.

80. Goldstein, P., Sacks, H. and Chalmers, T. (1989) Hormone administration for the maintenance of pregnancy, in *Effective Care in Pregnancy and Childbirth* (eds I. Chalmers, M. Enkin and M. Keirse), Oxford University Press, Oxford, Chap. 38, pp. 612–23.

81. Interim Report of the Medical Research Council/Royal College of Obstetricians and Gynaecologists (1988) Multicentre randomized trial of cervical

cerclage, MRC/RCOG working party on cervical cerclage. *Br. J. Obstet. Gynaecol.*, **95**, 437–45.

82. Crowther, C., Bouwmeester, A. and Ashurst, H. (1992) Does admission to hospital for bed rest prevent disease progression or improve fetal outcome in pregnancy complicated by non-proteinuric hypertension? *Br. J. Obstet. Gynaecol.*, **99**, 13–17.

83. Editorial (1992) Bed rest. *Br. J. Obstet. Gynaecol.*, 13–17.

84. MacLennan, A., Green, R. *et al.* (1990) Routine hospital admission in twin pregnancy between 26 and 30 weeks' gestation. *Lancet*, **335**, 267–9.

85. Department of Health and Social Security/Office of Population Censuses and Surveys (1980) *Hospital Inpatient Enquiry Maternity Tables 1973–6*, Series MB4 No. 8, HMSO, London, Table 7.

86. Department of Health and Social Security/Office of Population Censuses and Surveys (1988) *Hospital Inpatient Enquiry Maternity Tables 1982–5*, Series MB4 No. 28, HMSO, London, Table 2.2.

87. House of Commons Health Committee (Chairman Nicholas Winterton) (1992) *Maternity Services Report*, vol. II, HMSO, London, pp. 338–650.

88. Tuffnell, D. and Lilford, R. (1992) Randomised controlled trial of day care for hypertension in pregnancy. *Lancet*, **399**, 224–7.

89. McDonald, H., O'Loughlin, J. *et al.* (1992) Prenatal microbiological risk factors associated with preterm birth. *Br. J. Obstet. Gynaecol.*, **99**, 190.

90. McDonald, H., O'Loughlin, J. *et al.* (1992) Vaginal infection and preterm labour. *Br. J. Obstet. Gynaecol.*, **98**, 427–35.

91. Maclean, A. (1991) Infection and preterm labour. *Curr. Obstet. Gynaecol.*, **1** (2), 67–71.

92. Schultz, R., Read, A. *et al.* (1991) Genito-urinary tract infections in pregnancy and low birthweight: case controlled study in Australian Aboriginal women. *Br. Med. J.*, **303**, 1369–73.

93. Crowley, P., Chalmers, I. and Keirse, M. (1990) The effects of corticosteroid administration before preterm delivery; an overview of the evidence from controlled trials. *Br. J. Obstet. Gynaecol.*, **97**, 11–25.

94. Mugford, M., Piercy, J. and Chalmers, I. (1991) Cost implications of different approaches to the prevention of respiratory distress syndrome. *Arch. Dis. Childhood*, **66**, 757–64.

95. Davies, J. (1991) The Newcastle community care project, the project in action, in *Midwives, Research & Childbirth*, vol. 2 (eds S. Robinson and A. Thomson), Chapman and Hall, London.

96. Evans, F. (1991) The Newcastle community care project, the evaluation of the project, in *Midwives, Research & Childbirth*, vol. 2 (eds S. Robinson and A. Thomson), Chapman and Hall, London.

97. Durand, A. (1992) The safety of homebirth: the Farm study. *Am. J. Pub. Health*, **82**, 3, 450–2.

98. Oakley, A. (1985) Social support in pregnancy: the 'soft' way to increase birthweight? *Soc. Sci. Med.*, **11**, 1259–68.

99. Oakley, A., Rajan, L. and Grant, A. (1990) Social support and pregnancy outcome. *Br. J. Obstet Gynaecol.*, **99**, 182–5.

100. Bryce, R., Stanley, F. and Garner, J. (1991) Randomized controlled trial of

antenatal social support to prevent pre-term birth. *Br. J. Obstet. Gynaecol.*, **99**, 182–5.

101. Heins, H., Nance, N. *et al.* (1990) A randomized trial of nurse-midwifery prenatal care to reduce low birthweight. *Obstet. Gynecol.*, **75**, 341–5.

102. Pagel, M., Smilkstein, G. *et al.* (1990) Psycho-social influences on new born outcome: a controlled prospective study. *Soc. Sci. Med.*, **30**, 597–604.

103. Blondel, B., Breart, G. *et al.* (1990) Evaluation of the home-visiting system for women with threatened preterm labour: results of a randomized controlled trial. *Eur. J. Obstet. Gynaecol. Reprod. Biol.*, **34**, 47–58.

104. Dawson, A., Middlemiss, C. *et al.* (1989) A randomised controlled study of a domiciliary antenatal care scheme: the effect on hospital admissions. *Br. J. Obstet. Gynaecol.*, **96**, 1319–22.

105. James, D. (1990) Diagnosis and management of fetal growth retardation. *Arch. Dis. Childhood*, **65**, 390–4.

106. House of Commons Health Committee (Chairman Nicholas Winterton) (1992) *Maternity Services: Preconception*, vol. II, HMSO, London, pp. 1–291.

107. Doyle, W., Crawford, M. *et al.* (1989) Maternal nutrient intake and birth-weight. *J. Hum. Nutr. Dietet.*, **2**, 415–22.

108. Mahomed, K. and Hytten, F. (1989) Iron and folate supplementation in pregnancy, in *Effective Care in Pregnancy and Childbirth* (eds. I. Chalmers, M. Enkin and M. Keirse), Oxford University Press, Oxford, Chap. 19, pp. 301–17.

109. Medical Research Council Vitamin Study Research Group (1991) Prevention of neural tube defects: results of the MRC Vitamin Study. *Lancet*, **338**, 131–6.

110. Altman, D. and Hytten, F. (1989) Assessment of fetal size and growth, in *Effective Care in Pregnancy and Childbirth* (eds I. Chalmers, M. Enkin and M. Keirse), Oxford University Press, Oxford, Chap. 26.

111. Pearce, J. and Campbell, S. (1987) A comparison of symphysis-fundal height and ultrasound as screening tests for light-for-gestational-age infants. *Br. J. Obstet. Gynaecol.*, **94**, 100–4.

112. Spencer, J. (1990) Antepartum cardiotocography, in *Modern Antenatal Care of the Fetus* (ed. G. Chamberlain), Blackwell, Oxford, Chap. 9, pp. 163–88.

113. Lumley, J., Lester, A. *et al.* (1983) A randomized trial of weekly cardiotocography in high-risk obstetric patients. *Br. J. Obstet. Gynaecol.*, **90**, 1018–26.

114. Newnham, J., O'Dea, M. *et al.* (1991) Doppler flow velocity waveform analysis in high risk pregnancies: a randomized controlled trial. *Br. J. Obstet. Gynaecol.*, **98**, 956–63.

115. McIntosh, N. (1988) Clinical issues. *Br. Med. Bull.*, **44**(4), 1119–32.

116. McIlwaine, G., Mutch, L. *et al.* (1992) The Scottish Low Birthweight Study. *Arch. Dis. Childhood*, **67**, 6, 675–708.

117. Daker, M. and Bobrow, M. (1989) Screening for genetic disease, in *A Guide to Effective Care in Pregnancy and Childbirth* (eds M. Enkin, M. Keirse and I. Chalmers), Oxford University Press, Oxford, Chap. 8.

118. Medical Research Council European Trial of Chorionic Villus Sampling (1991) *Lancet*, **337**, 1491–9.

119. Firth, H., Boyd, P. *et al.* (1991) Severe limb abnormalities after chorion villus sampling at 55–66 days' gestation. *Lancet*, **337**, 762–3.

120. Cuckle, H., Wald, N. and Lindenbaum, R. (1984) Maternal serum alphafe-toprotein measurements: a screening test for Down's syndrome. *Lancet*, **i**, 926–7.

121. Wald, N., Kennard, A. *et al.* (1992) Antenatal maternal serum screening for Down's syndrome: results of a demonstration project. *Br. Med. J.*, **305**, 391–4.

122. Bryndorf, T., Christensen, B. *et al.* (1992) New rapid test for prenatal detection of trisomy 21 (Down's syndrome): preliminary report. *Br. Med. J.*, **304**, 1536–9.

123. Neilson, J. and Grant, A. (1989) Ultrasound in pregnancy, in *A Guide to Effective Care in Pregnancy and Childbirth* (eds M. Enkin, M. Keirse and I. Chalmers), Oxford University Press, Oxford, Chap. 12.

124. Proud, J. (1989) Placental grading as a test of fetal well-being, in *Midwives, Research and Childbirth*, vol. 1 (eds S. Robinson and A. Thomson), Chapman and Hall, London.

125. Marsh, G. (1985) 'New style' obstetric care, in *Modern Obstetrics in General Practice* (ed. G. Marsh), Oxford University Press, Oxford, Chap. 31.

126. Thacker, S. and Berkelman (1986) Assessing the diagnostic accuracy and efficacy of selected antepartum surveillance techniques. *Obstet. Gynecol. Surv.*, **41**, 121–41.

127. Bucher, H. and Schmidt, J. (1993) Does routine ultrasound scanning improve outcome in pregnancy? Meta-analysis of various outcome measures. *Br. Med. J.*, **307**, 13–17.

128. Lorenz, R., Comstock, C. *et al.* (1990) Randomized prospective trial comparing ultrasonography and pelvic examination for preterm labour surveillance. *Am. J. Obstet. Gynecol.*, **162**, 1603–10.

129. Larsen, T., Larsen, J. *et al.* (1992) Detection of small-for-gestational-age fetuses by ultrasound screening in a high risk population: a randomized controlled study. *Br. J. Obstet. Gynaecol.*, **99**, 469–74.

130. Beech, B. and Robinson, J. (1993) Ultrasound unsound? *AIMS J.*, **5**, 1.

131. Cartwright, R., McKinney, P. and Hopton, P. (1984) Ultrasound examinations in pregnancy and childhood cancer. *Lancet*, **ii**, 999–1000.

132. Kinnear Wilson, L. and Waterhouse, J. (1984) Obstetric ultrasound and childhood malignancies. *Lancet*, **ii**, 997–8.

133. Royal College of Obstetricians and Gynaecologists (1984) *Report of the RCOG Working Party on Routine Ultrasound Examination in Pregnancy*, RCOG, London.

134. Newnham, J., Evans, S. *et al.* (1993) Effects of frequent ultrasound during pregnancy: a randomized controlled trial. *Lancet*, **342**, 987–91.

135. Meire, H. (1987) The safety of diagnostic ultrasound. *Br. J. Obstet. Gynaecol.*, **94**, 1121–2.

136. Green, J. (1990) Prenatal screening and diagnosis: some psychological and social issues. *Br. J. Obstet. Gynaecol.*, **97**, 1172.

137. Romito, P. (1990) *Women's Paid and Unpaid Work During Pregnancy: A Psycho-social Analysis*. Thomas Coram Research Unit, London.

138. House of Commons Health Committee (Chairman Nicholas Winterton) (1991) *Maternity Services: Preconception, Report*, vol. I, paras 1–143, HMSO, London.

<table>
<tr><td>

4

</td><td>

The practices of attendants around the time of birth

</td></tr>
</table>

PRACTICES BEFORE 1900

Although the human mother, like other female mammals, is biologically endowed with instinctive behaviour to ensure the safe delivery of her offspring and so the survival of the species, civilization has taught her to distrust her instincts and rely on assistance of some kind from a birth attendant. The practices of attendants have varied according to culture and historical period. Presumably they have always been intended to improve welfare and reduce suffering and danger. Whether they were able to achieve this with little or much intervention has depended on the attitudes, beliefs and knowledge of the attendants and the place of birth. But however successful they may appear to have been in particular cases, regular observations were not made to confirm that they were so in most cases and current practices persisted for long periods before being rejected or displaced by others of equally unproven efficacy, a pattern as characteristic of recent as of earlier history.

Posture for birth

English manuals of midwifery in the 17th and 18th centuries [1] gave sensible advice about the need to reassure the mother and to maintain her confidence with supportive behaviour and her physical strength with suitable nourishment. As labour developed, the mother was to be encouraged to vary periods of activity with periods of rest and when delivery was imminent to adopt her own comfortable position, which could be standing, sitting on a suitable stool or kneeling. Midwives were told to 'notice that all women do not keep the same posture in their delivery; some lye in their beds being very weak, some sit on a stool or chair, or rest upon the side of the bed, held by other women that come to the labour' [2, p. 95].

All upright positions facilitate birth of the infant and the placenta if the process is to be assisted by gravity, but they are very inconvenient if the process is to be assisted by human intervention, manual or instrumental. In such a circumstance, the French surgeon-midwife of the 16th century, Ambroise Paré, advised delivering the woman on a bed [1, p. 52] and his advice was increasingly followed by his medical successors. Their well-to-do clients set the fashion and the phrase 'brought to bed' was recognized in 18th century literature as signifying the onset of labour, 'accoucheur' being a fitting title for the attendant doctor.

The woman's recumbent position implies weakness, inferiority and submission to the strong, superior 'obstetrician', the male attendant who stands before her to complete the process which her body finds it too difficult to do unaided. She did not realize that her recumbency itself contributed to her difficulty and she allowed the promptings of her instinct to be swept aside by medical persuasion. Naturally, recumbency was enforced by doctors who worked and taught in hospitals and it became accepted as the normal birth position also by midwives who were trained there. By the end of the 19th century it had become the general practice in Western medicine.

Midwives' intrapartum practices

The midwifery manuals advised midwives to apply lubricating ointments 'to the places concerned with travail', to administer herbal preparations reputed to relieve pain and stop bleeding and other complications, and to ensure frequent emptying of the bladder and bowels, by enema if necessary, for 'otherwise a full bowel and bladder could impede descent and contribute to uterine inertia' [3, p. 74]. The intention of such advice was to facilitate the natural process, not to interfere with it. But the natural process can be slow, tedious and frustrating for the mother and her attendants alike and it takes a very patient attendant to resist the temptation and pressure to speed things up, especially if the mother is in great pain. The good midwife has this patience and can communicate her (or his) confidence to the mother that eventually all will be well. But this virtue is not possessed by all females and is even less characteristic of males.

There is a long history of pharmaceutical and mechanical practices designed to induce or accelerate labour. Various herbal concoctions, such as quinine, have been used to encourage uterine contractions.

More vigorous was the use of emetics to cause vomiting, or strong snuff or pepper to cause sneezing in the hope of initiating reflex uterine reactions or contractions strong enough to shift a fetus whose passage appeared to be obstructed. The naturally occurring drug, ergot, was used for a long time in many countries, despite the danger that if its administration was mistimed and the fetus was not ready to move, the uterus could rupture with fatal consequences. For this reason, it had only a brief period of popularity in Britain [4] and the USA [5, pp. 65–6] in the early 19th century for the purpose of expediting labour, although it continued to be used to control postpartum haemorrhage.

The positive advice of the midwifery manuals was accompanied by warnings against certain mechanical practices which had become prevalent. Midwives were enjoined 'not to induce labour by tearing the membranes with their nails or scissors, a practice connected with the frequent occurrence of prolapsed limbs and dry labours' nor 'to pull on the prolapsed arms, nor to push on the fundament, nor to hasten birth by stretching the passages with fingers and hands' [3, pp. 73–4]. This advice notwithstanding, the practice of 'tearing' (or sweeping or stripping) the membranes to encourage the onset of labour persisted: it was still common throughout the 20th century, and often achieved its purpose (page 155). The painful accelerating process was sometimes tackled by 'tying the reluctant woman to the obstetric chair and in more obstinate cases by tossing her in a blanket, rolling and rocking her, or by other violent measures' [6, p. 11], which may not have been quite as barbaric as they may now sound, for they could indeed encourage relaxation of the cervix or achieve a more favourable lie for the fetus, and so a quicker birth [7].

Unorthodox fetal presentations seem to have been common enough for some midwives to become skilled at internal podalic version (page 43). Perhaps more gently than 'pushing on the fundament', the 17th century midwife was reminded of the previous century's advice 'to stroke down the birth from above the navel easily with her hand' [2, p. 95]. This technique is reminiscent of the widespread 20th century practice among traditional attendants in less developed countries of massaging the mother's abdomen to position the fetus before birth [8].

Doctors' intrapartum practices

Medical midwifery fell partly in the province of surgeons, who tended to favour intervention, and partly in the province of physicians, who had more faith in the sufficiency of the physiological process and accepted more willingly that interventions could be harmful. The guiding rule of the celebrated English physician of the 17th century,

William Harvey, 'was to wait on nature and only intervene when it was absolutely necessary' [1, p. 72]. His precept was still followed by a 19th century American Professor of Obstetrics who taught that 'Dame Nature is the best midwife in the world. . . . Meddlesome midwifery is fraught with evil. . . . The less done generally the better. Non-intervention is the cornerstone of midwifery' [5, p. 65]. In Britain, until well into the 20th century the physicians' influence was the stronger and medical students were taught the virtues of 'masterly inactivity'. 'The greatest attribute of a man who intends to practise midwifery is to know when to leave patients alone' [9, p. 733].

Despite these precepts, many of the births attended by doctors, either through initial choice of the mother or emergency call from the midwife, were accomplished with the help of instruments. The obstetric forceps invented in England in the 16th century (page 41) were followed by many more sophisticated and effective designs [10]. They were used in cases of apparent obstruction, but doctors, who retained the monopoly of their use and the cachet that went with this right, were always tempted to overdiagnose obstruction and the failure of the natural process, as they had done in Margaret Stephen's day (page 44).

The feasibility and incidence of instrumental delivery was increased after chloroform, which was first used in 1847 by Dr James Simpson of Edinburgh, became generally available [11]. Chloroform, together with increased awareness of the necessity for asepsis, increased the feasibility of the ultimate instrumental delivery, caesarean section, but the operation was still very dangerous and very uncommon before 1900.

Doctors as readily resorted to blood-letting as a remedy for problems of labour as of pregnancy (page 87). It was thought to accelerate the birth by relaxing a rigid cervix and to forestall postpartum haemorrhage! It was used also to relieve labour pains, effectively by eventually rendering the mother unconscious. Its popularity for most uses was waning towards the end of the 19th century – chloroform offered an alternative means of producing unconsciousness – but it continued for many more years to be a favoured treatment for puerperal convulsions in women who developed eclampsia or toxaemia of pregnancy, on the hypothesis that toxaemia was literally 'poisoned blood' and would be mitigated by removing some of the poisoned substance [12].

Although chloroform could be used to produce unconsciousness, or at least to reduce the awareness of pain, it became obvious that its safe administration required skill. Many doctors doubted that they had the necessary skill and preferred to continue to use opium, belladonna and ether [11]. These were apparently more respectable analgesics than the gin dispensed by the less reputable midwives or handywomen.

Managing the third stage of labour

The importance of completely evacuating the placenta was always realized. If it was not expelled naturally with the aid of gravity, herbal remedies, including ergot, to be taken by mouth or applied as a poultice, could be tried. Sneezing could be provoked and the abdomen massaged. All else failing and despite the dangers, manipulation of the umbilical cord and manual removal were undertaken by midwives as well as doctors [1, p. 122].

Treatment for puerperal sepsis

Also lacking were effective treatments for postpartum complications. The most dangerous of these was puerperal fever, the scourge of maternity hospitals in the 18th and 19th centuries. It is caused by infection of the genital and urinary systems: the uterus, with its large raw area where the placenta has detached, and the tissues of the vagina and external genitalia which have been stretched, torn or damaged by instruments are extremely vulnerable to invading organisms.

That such infection was the cause of the fever and that the principal vector was actually the obstetrician whose unclean hands and instruments carried the bacteria from affected to unaffected patients, was suspected at least as early as 1841, when the Registrar General's annual report included a discussion of the subject [13], and was supported by evidence accumulated and presented in 1843 by the American anatomist, Oliver Wendell Holmes [14]. It was convincingly demonstrated when Ignaz Semmelweis made known the results of his study in the Vienna Maternity Hospital in 1846 [5, p. 121]. Effective as he showed ruthless hygiene to be as a preventive measure, its absolute necessity was not widely accepted or practised, so that puerperal sepsis remained a major cause of maternal death right up until the 1940s.

The nature of the harmful substance which the birth attendants were unwittingly transmitting remained a mystery, further confused because there were cases of infection where the birth attendant could not have been the vector. It was not until the later 19th century that the mystery began to be solved by the discoveries of the great European microbiologists, notably the German Robert Koch and the Frenchman Louis Pasteur, who were able to identify streptococci in the blood of infected patients. Research was pursued by microbiologists of many nationalities and led over the next fifty years to the identification of additional micro-organisms which could cause puerperal fever and explain the variety of its incidence (pages 284–5).

In view of the ignorance about the disease and its causes, it is not surprising that the treatments offered, even by doctors of high repute, now sound bizarre. They included blood-letting and keeping the patients in bed sedated with strong opiates [1, p. 156] and copious and repeated draughts of wine and spirits, while cheaper, though even more noxious folk-remedies like turpentine were also prescribed [6, p. 17].

Lying-in

Up to the 18th century, it was customary for the mother to be allowed three to five days to rest and recover from the birth even when delivery had been complicated [1, p. 77]. As the 19th century progressed and doctors became involved in more confinements of the richer patients, the accepted lying-in period was stretched to twelve to fourteen days, although 'the midwives were keen to get the patient up early, within 24 hours, to help drain the lochia from the uterus thereby preventing its stagnation' [1, p. 156]. The early risers seemed none the worse for their activity and indeed escaped dangerous circulatory complications, like 'white leg' (*phlegmasia alba dolens*) which became increasingly common among the rested mothers.

CHANGING PRACTICES BETWEEN 1900 AND 1950

Posture for birth

A midwifery textbook of 1908 [1, p. 197] showed the influence of doctors on the instruction of midwives. They were now taught to manage delivery by allowing the woman to move around as she wished in the first stage of labour but putting her to bed for the second stage; and how to fix up contraptions for her to pull on and push her feet against to assist her to bear down during contractions, a pathetic compensation for depriving her of her choice of delivering upright. A Handbook of Midwifery published twenty-four years later in 1932 [1, p. 222] confirmed that the mother was to deliver in bed, lying on her left side, with the same contraptions for pulling and pushing on. Even so, the mothers who gave birth at home with midwives as attendants enjoyed the better option.

By the 1930s, appreciable numbers of deliveries were taking place in medical institutions under the supervision of doctors who might consider instrumental assistance necessary. It was much more convenient for them if the delivery bed was in effect an operating table with the mother fixed in the lithotomy position, lying on her back with her legs spread apart and strapped high in the air in 'stirrups' and perhaps with arms strapped down. This position may be advantageous if the operation is, as its name signifies, to cut out stones (from the bladder), but it is most disadvantageous for the labouring woman and her child. Being held in a fixed position throughout the pain of muscular contractions increases her awareness of their painfulness and so her need of pain relief; without the help of gravity, greater force is required to push the burden uphill through an opening now prevented from stretching to accommodate the descending head, which increases the incidence of lumbar strains and perineal tears and creates the need for episiotomy and forceps assistance; impeding the process in this way adds to its duration, while the dorsal position exposes the important blood vessel, the vena cava, to the pressure of the heavy uterus, impairing the mother's blood circulation and the oxygen supply to the fetus [15, pp. 117–18]. The unnatural posture in fact made an important contribution to the complications which obstetric management was imposed to relieve. This was the fate of increasing numbers of women as the trend moved towards birth in hospital.

The intrapartum practices of trained midwives

In 1908 [1, p. 197] midwives were instructed to limit vaginal examinations because of the danger of infection, to ease the patient's pain by rubbing her back and to safeguard the perineum by delivering the head slowly between contractions, a technique of proven efficiency which, however, was later to become neglected in favour of episiotomy (page 150). Only minor changes in management were described in the 1932 handbook. By then [1, p. 222] the unsophisticated method of induction, the castor oil, hot bath and enema regimen, was being recommended and shaving the pubic hair had been adopted as a routine precaution against infection. Despite repeated research evidence that it is ineffective and despite client disapproval, the practice was still widely observed by midwives and doctors in the 1980s [15, pp. 43–5].

Relieving pain

Beyond moral support and back-rubbing, the only pain relief the midwife was allowed to give was mild sedatives. However, from 1936 the small minority who had been trained to use it, and could transport the necessary apparatus, could offer inhalational analgesia, gas and air, and from 1950 they were allowed to give pethidine (page 56). The general practitioner's previous monopoly of these methods of pain relief encouraged one domiciliary patient in four to book his attendance [16]. When he was called in by the midwife to deal with complications he was naturally expected to intervene with drugs or instruments, to cope with problems by methods similar to those used in hospital, except that caesarean section would not be carried out in the home.

Effective anaesthesia was, however, more easily and less dangerously provided in the hospital. Early in the 20th century a new type of anaesthesia, described as 'twilight sleep', was developed in Germany.

This technique involved injecting the woman with morphine at the beginning of labour and then giving her a dose of an amnesiac drug, scopolamine, which caused her to forget what was happening; once the fetus entered the birth canal, the doctor gave ether or chloroform to relieve the pain caused by the birth of the head. Altogether, the procedure dulled awareness of pain and, perhaps more important, removed the memory of it [5, p. 150].

On regaining consciousness the mother could be left with the feeling that birth had been a good experience.

The offer of such a prospect made twilight sleep very attractive to women and for thirty years it was used extensively in the USA and rather less so in Britain. Its satisfactory usage seemed to depend on adjusting the dosage of the different drugs to suit the patients' needs, which varied from one individual to another, and other adjuvant drugs, such as barbiturates, were tried. Where a correct balance was not achieved, there were undesirable side-effects, including prolongation of labour, troublesome restlessness and depressed respiration of the infant [11]. The adverse side-effects of gas and air were far fewer.

Means of avoiding the dangers of general anaesthesia were found from the late 1920s in the application to obstetrics of local anaesthesia, particularly in performing episiotomies and repairing all perineal tears. Spinal anaesthesia, which allowed a woman to remain conscious while feeling nothing from the waist down, but which required the continuous attendance of a skilled anaesthetist to cope with dangerous complications, was frequently used in the 1940s in American hospitals [5, p. 181], but it never gained popularity in British hospitals [11].

The possibility of remaining conscious while avoiding or coping with pain was offered by Dick-Read's training in relaxation and deep breathing techniques, but the method was used in relatively few deliveries in Britain before 1950 (page 96).

Doctors' instrumental deliveries: the use of forceps

The intervention of doctors was sought when uterine contractions were failing to deliver the child and the assistance of traction by forceps was called for. A frequent reason for obstructed labour was malpresentation of the fetus and, depending on the nature of the malpresentation, different designs of forceps were appropriate. A modification, primarily for rectifying malpositions of the fetal head by means of rotation, was devised by Kielland in 1913 and became widely used [4].

Many malpresentations were forestalled by external version (pages 87,

150, 171), but attempts to correct faulty positions and attitudes of the fetal head antenatally were less successful. For these and oblique presentations encountered during labour, internal version continued to be used, although for placenta praevia and contracted pelvis it came to be superseded by caesarean section. Antenatal external version reduced the incidence of breech deliveries, but where they did occur, prevention of damage to the after-coming head was a perpetual source of concern [4].

Episiotomy

Since instrumental deliveries, but some unassisted births also, often resulted in perineal tears because the perineal opening failed to stretch sufficiently, the theory was developed that widening it by an anticipatory incision would both ease the baby's passage and prevent the tears. In 1920, an eminent Chicago obstetrician, Dr Joseph DeLee, recommended combining this episiotomy with forceps rotation as routine practice. His procedure [5, p. 141]

> involved sedating the woman and allowing her cervix to dilate, giving ether when the fetus entered the birth canal, making a cut of several inches through the skin and muscles of the perineum, the area between the vagina and the anus, applying forceps to lift the fetus's head over the perineum while monitoring the fetal heart via stethoscope, using ergot or one of its derivatives to contract the uterus, and then extracting the expelled placenta with a 'shoehorn maneuver'. Finally the doctor should stitch up the perineal cut.

By the 1930s, episiotomy and outlet forceps had indeed become accepted as routine procedure in many American hospitals, although it was less popular in other countries. In Britain, episiotomy to enlarge the birth canal became a routine procedure in the breech delivery of first-time mothers, but otherwise it is rarely referred to in the history of British obstetrics up to 1950, which suggests that the operation was not by then as widespread as it was to become in the following decades [4].

Caesarean section

Aseptic practice and general anaesthesia having reduced the extremely high maternal mortality formerly associated with caesarean section, this had become a feasible treatment for the most intractable mechanical complications. American and British obstetricians in the early years of the 20th century followed the example of the German surgeon, Max Sänger, who from 1882 used this method to deliver women with deformed pelves with a fair measure of success, and they achieved even greater success. There was at first considerable experimentation to develop a sound technique and to decide when best to operate. Better results were judged to come from lower segment incisions, which reduced the chance of later uterine rupture, and from operations done before or early in labour [4, p. 125, 5, p. 139]. As confidence grew, the use of caesarean section was extended to other complications. Nevertheless, by 1950 it was still too dangerous to be frequently undertaken.

Caesarean section and blood transfusions were the treatments believed to have been responsible for the great decline in maternal mortality associated with the fairly uncommon condition, placenta praevia, in the first half of the 20th century. The outcome for the infant was only slightly improved, but more hopeful possibilities were suggested by the good results reported in 1946 of expectant treatment, keeping the mother resting in hospital, with blood transfusions if necessary and protected from infection, so as to prolong the pregnancy as far as possible [17].

Technical advances

Improvements in blood transfusion techniques in the 1930s and 1940s used in conjunction with the new knowledge about anaemia in pregnancy and rhesus blood groups opened the way to much more effective obstetric treatments. For the mother it became possible not only to reduce the direct dangers of blood loss following surgical interventions or postpartum haemorrhage, but also to fortify her resistance to infection through maintaining her strength. For the baby, blood transfusion could reduce the mortal risk of haemolytic disease resulting from incompatible parental rhesus blood groups.

Intranatal obstetrics also profited from the dramatic pharmacological advances of the period. The antibiotic drugs proved as effective against puerperal fever as against other infections (pages 92, 284). The effectiveness of antiseptic agents was being improved.

Less successful were the early efforts to reproduce oxytocin, the secretion of the maternal pituitary gland which stimulates the uterus to contract, for the purpose of inducing and augmenting or accelerating labour. Experimental work continued, however, and by 1948 a more efficient method of administering oxytocin by the slow intravenous infusion of a very dilute solution was developed, although this too brought its own dangers (page 155) [15, p. 148]. Until then, artificial rupture of the membranes was found to be a more reliable method of induction and from the 1930s became widely used in British hospitals [4, p. 81].

However painful and distressing mothers found the natural birth process, obstetric intervention made it even more so. The upsetting experience was shared by the attendants and could only be compensated by more effective artificial pain relief and/or by shortening the duration of labour. Moreover, higher perinatal mortality was often observed to be associated with long labour, although probably the real danger came from the factors which caused the labour to be long. Although shortening the process is certainly not the same as making it safer, the powers of accelerating labour promised by the new drugs encouraged obstetricians to set arbitrary time limits for each stage of labour, after which intervention, pharmacological, instrumental or surgical, should be accepted practice. The risks of intervention were considered, without evidence, to be less than the risks of delay (pages 158–9).

Updating management of the third stage of labour

In 1908 the midwife was instructed to leave the umbilical cord untied until it had stopped pulsating [1, p. 197]. The placenta would be forced by uterine contractions into the upper part of the vagina within an hour of the birth but, denied the help of gravity, it would probably need the midwife's intervention to complete the expulsion. Following the 19th century practice, she was to wrap a tight binder round the mother's abdomen, which it was believed would maintain intra-abdominal pressure and stimulate the uterus to contract, so promoting separation of the placenta and preventing haemorrhage. By 1932, if fundal pressure had failed to expel the placenta, midwives were permitted, like doctors, to administer liquid extract of ergot or its newly synthesized equivalent, ergometrine [1, p. 224]. From 1933, doctors found it more effective to give ergometrine by intramuscular injection than by mouth to control postpartum haemorrhage. From 1947, the routine was to administer the injection just after the baby's head was born, with the intention of hastening expulsion of the placenta and reducing the risk of haemorrhage [4, p. 111].

Changed needs for lying-in care

From the mid-1930s, sepsis was rapidly ceasing to be the predominant and intractable puerperal complication and dangerous postpartum haemorrhages were also declining. Heroic efforts by obstetricians were less in demand.

The suggestive association between prolonged bed-rest and circulatory complications was not picked up and the fashion for the longer lying-in period spread to all classes who could afford it. At first, 20th century midwives were trained to nurse the mother and baby for ten days and from 1937 for fourteen days, tending the mother like a bed-bound patient needing an invalid diet, in marked contrast to the robust expectations of earlier times [1, p. 267].

As well as monitoring the involution of the uterus and the healing of perineal damage, the midwife had to supervise the satisfactory establishment (or suppression) of lactation. Every other newborn mammal knows instinctively how to find and in its own time make use of its mother's milk-providing nipple and the mother knows instinctively how to facilitate this process. These instincts, essential to survival, are assumed to be inactive in the human baby and mother and to need relearning under professional guidance. This may be so for frail compromised babies and sick exhausted mothers, but it is an extraordinary indictment of the induced attitudes of civilization that the guidance (or interference) should be considered a routine necessity for most births. Breast-feeding problems have, however, been recognized at least since the 18th century.

Babies born in hospital were quickly removed to the nursery where they were looked after exclusively by midwives, being brought to their mothers only at set times for feeding. Babies born at home were not so deprived of intimate contact, but even there the fashion set by popular paediatricians, like Dr Truby King, and encouraged by midwives, was to handle the child as little as possible. Discipline could not start too early.

THE CHANGED PICTURE BY 1950

Thus the first steps along the road towards the scientific management of labour had been taken in Britain by 1950, although there was less unanimity that scientific management was the correct objective for good maternity care than there was in the USA and other countries where obstetricians had greater influence and where greater progress along the road had already been made. The doctrine of 'masterly inactivity', although still widely favoured, was becoming outmoded and adhered to with ever diminishing conviction by a growing body of doctors. The training of midwives was surely understood as meaning that they were intended to practise such interventive techniques as they learned. It was being ever more thoroughly impressed on mothers that professional attendants knew best and that instinctive reactions were to be mistrusted and overridden.

THE FLOURISHING OF INTERVENTIVE PRACTICES AFTER 1950

Conversion to the philosophy that obstetric interventions improved the efficiency of the natural birth process, and hence its safety, was not achieved by factual evidence, for accumulating results indicated the reverse (Chapters 7 and 8). No attention was paid to the sound biological reasons why obstetric practices, such as the lithotomy position for delivery, made the natural process less efficient and less safe.

In cases of extreme pathology, when the natural process had broken down, certain interventions may well have been life-saving, but claims to this effect have to be taken on trust, for there is a disturbing lack of evaluated evidence that they were so more often than not. Certainly, the assumed benefits of treatment in hospital never counteracted all the pathological dangers, for mortality there was always significantly higher than when delivery took place at home, no matter how poor or overcrowded the homes [18, p. 63]. Many of the overall benefits from antibiotic therapy, blood transfusion and even the prevention of rhesus factor sensitization were absorbed in compensating for the damage inflicted by other aspects of obstetric treatment.

In cases where the natural process was functioning normally or where it had not broken down seriously, there was no evidence that it was improved by interventive birth practices. But no-one seemed to think such evidence essential. Their rigorous training courses had the objective of fitting obstetricians to perform interventions competently, not to prove that the interventions made birth safer. Their enthusiastic self-confidence was infectious. They became most effective masters of the arts of propaganda. In this spirit they encouraged everyone to believe that women should deliver their babies in suitably equipped hospitals, staffed by specialist doctors, and they encouraged health authorities to provide more maternity beds there. They pressed on towards a goal of perfecting interventive technology and widening its application.

As long as doctors and midwives had been commercial rivals for the same clients, doctors were concerned to guard for themselves the instruments and skills of intervention. After the National Health Service finally ended the competition and obstetricians gained domination of the maternity service, implementing their policy needed the collaboration, not of practitioners of a different conception of midwifery, but of technically competent obstetric nurses. So midwives had to be trained how to use the equipment. Moreover, they had to be trained to believe that it was right to use it, although this conflicted with their traditional ethos. The distinction between the practices of midwives and the practices of doctors became increasingly blurred.

The obstetricians' aims were to identify the maternal characteristics and conditions likely to lead to perinatal problems and to develop procedures which would forestall adverse outcomes. Forestalling frequently meant shortening pregnancy or labour on the hypothesis, usually untested, that this would benefit either the mother or the baby or both.

Interventions to induce labour

By 1958, 13% of births in Britain were being induced [19, p. 183]; the indications for 77% of these were maternal toxaemia and postmaturity, with other indications accounting for less than 4% each. The unsophisticated method of induction, castor oil, hot bath and enema, which did not require the facilities of a hospital, was often not effective, even when used in conjunction with gentle digital sweeping of the membranes away from the lower segment of the uterus, a method thought to stimulate uterine activity through encouraging the release of maternal prostaglandins [15, p. 58].

The surgical procedure, amniotomy or artificial rupture of the membranes (ARM), was found to be more effective and was used alone in 48% of the inductions (6.2% of births). When the cervix has already become 'favourable', ready to dilate, it may be further stimulated by the pressure of the baby's head once the cushion of amniotic fluid has been released, so that labour, which would probably have happened spontaneously quite soon, is precipitated and starts within twenty-four hours in 70–80% of cases after amniotomy alone [15, p. 57]. Releasing the amniotic fluid before the baby's head has descended to occupy the whole outlet passage can occasionally allow a loop of umbilical cord to slip past and become trapped between the fetus and uterus, so creating the grave danger of cutting off the vital supply of oxygen and nourishment; otherwise, amniotomy does not directly increase the risk to the baby's life, but it does increase the force and frequency of uterine contractions and so the mother's discomfort.

The simplicity (for the attendant) and apparent safety of this method of induction encouraged its more frequent use – to 11.4% of births by 1970 [20, p. 165]. But in cases where spontaneous labour was not imminent, induction by amniotomy alone was unsuccessful and, without the protection of the aseptic amniotic fluid, a high risk of intrauterine infection was created, a risk aggravated by the antepartum pelvic examinations thought necessary at this stage. A complementary method of induction was called for and this was provided by advances in pharmacology.

It had become possible to synthesize natural oxytocin and by 1955 the product, Syntocinon, was commercially available. At first its administration by intravenous infusion caused serious side-effects, but in the 1960s an instrument, the Cardiff pump, was developed to titrate the dose accurately so as to achieve the rate of contractions desired by the obstetricians and avoid overdosing, which could lead to uterine tetany or rupture, with fetal death. Control was improved after 1979, when a more refined instrument for administration became available [15, pp. 59–60]. A respected textbook pronounced 'Oxytocin has revolutionised the management of labour by providing the obstetrician with a means of stimulating, but at the same time controlling, uterine activity [21, p. 460]. The risk of failed induction was virtually eliminated. Oxytocin was used in 23% of inductions (3.1% of births) in 1958 [19, p. 185], but in 39% of inductions (10.2% of births) in 1970 [20, p. 177].

The induction rate was 13% in 1958 and 13.4% in 1964, but doubled to 26% by 1970 and trebled to 39.4% in 1974 [22]. It varied widely between centres: it was negligible for births at home and low in general practitioner units; in obstetric hospitals it could be as low as 8% [23] or higher than 50%, 'and reached 75 per cent among some individual consultants' [24, p. 19]. The increased rate did not correspond to an increased incidence of the mortal dangers which induction was claimed to avert. As early as 1970, it was carried out in 23% of births at the lowest predicted risk [20] and during the 1970s in nearly the same proportion of births without as with 'complication or anomaly' [22].

For obstetricians had quickly persuaded themselves and mothers that they could remove the irritating uncertainty about the date and time of delivery without offsetting disadvantage. It had hitherto been accepted as 'a truism that more babies are born between 7 p.m. and 7 a.m. than during the rest of the 24 hours' [9, p. 731]. The indication for most of the additional inductions was social convenience, to some extent for the mother, but probably to a greater extent for the obstetrician.

> . . . in some hospitals it was surmised that the quality of obstetric care was better in the day-time than at night. From this it was a short step to consider that the care provided might also be better on weekdays than at weekends when facilities were likely to be less adequately staffed. [20, p. 164]

That these views became practical policy is confirmed by the lower incidence, in 1970, of births in obstetric hospitals (27%) than at home (35%) between 01.00 and 08.00 hours, the period when perinatal mortality was found in the 1958 survey to be lowest, and by the lower incidence in the 1970s of birth at weekends and public holidays [25]. The pattern still obtained in the 1980s.

However, in reality induction with oxytocin does have offsetting disadvantages. The contractions it produces start suddenly, giving the mother's mind and body less time to adjust to them, occur in quicker succession and cause more pain than natural contractions. The intravenous drip usually confines the mother to bed and restricts her ability to find a more comfortable position and distraction from the pain [15, pp. 63–4]. Many mothers found this an unwelcome price to be paid for the promised convenience and widespread public protests were made. The induction rate fell back to around 37% until 1978 and then more than halved to 17.3% by 1984 and dropped further to an estimated 12% (4% surgical amniotomy, 8% using oxytocin) by 1989–90 [26, p. 376].

This last figure is an estimate by the Department of Health, the routine collection, collation and publication of hospital maternity statistics having broken down since 1985, but it is much lower than the figure suggested by an unofficial postal enquiry of a national sample, methodologically validated, of recently delivered mothers in 1989. This found that 26% of births were induced by drugs and 46% by amniotomy (the amount of overlap was unstated). The proportion of amniotomies had more than doubled since a corresponding enquiry in 1984, which suggests that the official figure for inductions in that year also was a considerable underestimate. The wide variation found between different areas indicates a wide variation in individual obstetricians' policies, rather than a wide variation in the need for induction [27].

How much these recorded reductions were in deference to public opinion or to obstetricians' own appreciation of the disadvantages cannot be gleaned from the literature, which contains many studies comparing different methods of inducing labour but conspicuously few comparing the value of intervening to end pregnancy with awaiting the spontaneous onset of labour [28]. The former comparisons illustrate obstetricians' conviction that intervention improves the process of childbearing and also their failure to pursue deeper understanding of the immensely complicated natural biochemistry and endocrinology which govern human reproduction. The latter comparisons are more important if promoting the welfare of mothers and babies is the criterion.

Though many labours were eventually induced, this was often achieved after failed attempts. The intention could be thwarted by a cervix not ready to relax and give up its function as a retaining sphincter, a sign that the fetal systems were not yet ready for independent existence. The decline in the induction rate happened to coincide with the increase in knowledge about and availability of prostaglandins. These are a complex group of chemicals made by the body's tissues as part of its defence against injury and were found also to activate muscular control of the uterus and to make the cervix softer and readier to stretch – indeed they are an essential element in the body's preparation for labour. In due course, a synthetic version in the form of a vaginal pessary was developed which has the welcome advantages of being non-invasive and non-restrictive to the mother's mobility, with few adverse side-effects. By themselves, prostaglandins have been fairly effective in inducing labour – further amniotomy or oxytocin infusion was found to be unnecessary in over 70% of cases [29] – and in decreasing the incidence of prolonged labour and instrumental deliveries, though these benefits may rather be the favourable side-effect of facilitating greater mobility in labour [28].

It is not known how widely prostaglandins became used in the 1980s. It is probable that their use spread considerably and probable also that labours officially recorded as induced did not include all, or indeed any, of those where prostaglandins alone were used. In so far as these were omitted from the records, this would account for at least part of the apparent decline in the induction rate and for its variation between hospitals. Where prostaglandins were not by themselves sufficient to encourage labour to start, amniotomy with or without oxytocin infusion remained the induction methods of choice.

Duration of labour

Induction, by definition, shortens the period of gestation. While its effect of intensifying pain was acknowledged, it was widely believed to shorten labour also. This belief was eventually discredited by a randomized controlled trial which did not find early amniotomy to be an effective method of reducing the duration of labour [30].

A long natural labour ending in spontaneous delivery is not necessarily painful or distressing for the mother, or dangerous for the baby [20, p. 132], but pain and fear can inhibit progress and make labour long and distressing. The mother's exhaustion is increased if, as is often the practice, she is denied food as a precaution in case general anaesthesia is eventually used. Her risk of infection is increased the longer the interval after the membranes ruptured or the more frequent the pelvic examinations. The more exhausted and distressed she becomes, the more likely is her labour to end in operative delivery.

Long labours are tedious and distressing for birth attendants also, as well as disrupting patient flow through the hospital accommodation. Man-midwives and their obstetrician successors have always wanted to hasten the natural process. It would be supportive of their predilections if long labour were known to endanger the infant also.

There has, in fact, never been any evidence that labour will run into danger if it does not keep within a specified time limit. Records from one London teaching hospital show that the neonatal mortality rate between 1939 and 1946 was actually substantially lower for labours lasting over, rather than under, forty-eight hours, while in a second one the perinatal mortality rate between 1946 and 1951 was substantially lower for labours lasting over, rather than under twenty-four hours [31].

Given that the onset of labour cannot be precisely timed, the 1958 perinatal survey showed that the mortality rate rose above average only when labours were very short (under three hours) or very long (over forty-eight hours); mortality was lowest when the first stage lasted between twelve and twenty-four hours for first births and between three and twenty-four hours for later births [19, p. 157]. Obstetricians felt justified in intervening to prevent exceeding the 'optimal' duration, but their criterion of 'optimal' was quite unjustified, for according to the report of the 1970 survey the critical limits were set arbitrarily at eighteen hours for first births and twelve hours for later births. Even tighter schedules have been advocated [32].

By 1970 the percentage of first births with a first stage of under twelve hours had been raised to 57%, compared with 46% in 1958, and the percentage lasting between twelve and twenty-four hours, the optimal period in 1958, had been reduced to 27% from 34% [20]. Similarly among later births the percentage with first stages under six hours had risen to 48% from 41% and between six and twelve hours, the optimal period in 1958, had fallen to 31% from 34% [20]. This degree of shortened labour was not likely to have resulted from natural causes. The presumption must be that it resulted from obstetric intervention. It was hardly likely to make birth safer.

Nor did the results of the 1958 survey support the view that shortening the second stage of labour was advantageous for the baby. In first births perinatal mortality was only above average when the second stage lasted under thirty minutes or over four hours, which happened in 16% and 1% of deliveries respectively, so that it was unnecessary to shorten the second stage in nearly all cases and positively dangerous to shorten it to under thirty minutes, the interval associated with more than twice average mortality. For later births a short second stage was not dangerous; perinatal mortality rose above average only for the very few (2%) which lasted over two hours.

A study analysing 4403 first births in an American hospital in the 1970s found no significant increase in perinatal or neonatal mortality or neonatal morbidity with increasing length of the second stage of labour up to three hours; on the contrary it was to the unwarranted surgical interventions to end labour that any dangers of increased postpartum haemorrhage and maternal feverishness were due [33].

In a third London teaching hospital a study of first babies in 1983–4 found that poor condition, as assessed five minutes after birth, occurred by far the most frequently when labour lasted under four hours and least frequently when it lasted twenty-four hours or more [31].

Their increasing power to control the length of labour has encouraged obstetricians to disregard evidence of lowest mortality and morbidity and impose standards which better suit their convenience, to substitute treatments which carry definite dangers as remedies for conditions which rarely carry danger. In so far as midwives and general practitioners were persuaded or obliged to act in accordance with these standards, many women who would have completed their labour safely in their own time, were transferred to hospital for interventions which carried higher risk (pages 339–41). Midwifery textbooks favoured the shorter intervals: 'it is common to expect the active stage of the first stage of labour to be completed within 12 hours. Primigravidae [first time mothers] will take most of the 12 hours, multigravidae [other mothers] less' [34]. However, in 1958 in more than half the first births and one-fifth of the later births the first stage took over twelve hours [19].

The records quoted should be as valid measurements of present as of past experience, for evolution would not be expected to bring about changes in the timing of the natural processes of human reproduction within a few years. The actual evidence notwithstanding, an eminent obstetrician wrote in 1988:

> . . . it has become traditional for obstetricians to remain concerned about the effects of long labour, and this has led to dramatic changes in practice, with increasing use of caesarean section to shorten labour or alternatively the augmentation of labour with oxytocin in up to 55% of primigravidae. [31]

Neither are later births immune from such interventions.

The 'traditional concern' of obstetricians was finally discredited by the findings of a retrospective analysis of 25 069 singleton term births, vertex (head first) presentation, in an English Health Region in 1988. Like the American findings of the 1970s, long second stages were associated with postpartum haemorrhage and maternal infection and probably for the same reasons – the consequences of surgical interventions to end labour – since long second stages were even more strongly associated with operative deliveries and maternal pyrexia in labour, as they were also with the heaviest babies and with first births as might be expected for physiological reasons. Second stages lasting even as long as three hours were not found to carry undue risk for the fetus; the babies were not born in poor condition nor in need of special care [35]. In short, the advantages for the baby of routine shortening of labour have never been demonstrated.

Accelerating labour

In shortening the period of gestation, induction brings the serious risk that, since the interval from conception is seldom known exactly, it may lead to the birth of immature infants, with all the attendant dangers. In the 1970 survey, 21% of births before thirty-nine weeks of gestation had been induced, many probably as a result of miscalculation. This particular risk can be avoided, while obstetric control is maintained, if intervention is delayed until the spontaneous onset of labour and is directed at accelerating its progress.

The first stage can be accelerated by the artificial rupture of membranes and the intravenous infusion of oxytocin, with the same disadvantage as in induction. This type of intervention was not common before 1970. It was used in only 1.4% of the 1970 survey births and could have accounted for very little of the observed trend towards shorter labours. It became more widely practised as more became known about the timing of the successive stages of normal labour.

The length of the first phase, when the cervix dilates to about 3 cm, may vary, but thereafter dilatation progresses fairly regularly and rapidly by at least 1 cm per hour in first births and faster in later births, until at 10 cm the presenting part is ready to descend and the mother is ready to push, so assisting rotation and descent into position for final expulsion. Based on expectations of normal progress, a method was developed of assessing progress in individual cases by means of a partogram, a graph on which the hourly state of dilatation is recorded and compared with the desired standard [36]. When dilatation is slower than this, intervention is advocated to speed it up. Indeed, amniotomy at 3 or 4 cm dilatation is often advocated and adopted as routine practice in many hospitals. It is frequently described by those who practise it at this stage as not really interfering with the normality of labour. Decisions are based on what the partogram shows, not on how the mother feels. The mother is discounted as a reliable witness of her current state.

Besides accelerating progress through intensifying contractions and increasing pressure on the cervix, amniotomy enables the fetus's wellbeing to be assessed first by observing the quantity and quality of the amniotic fluid, then by monitoring its heart rate via an electronic device clipped to its scalp and by determining the oxygen concentration in its blood by analysing samples drawn from its scalp. Further acceleration is achieved by the administration of oxytocin, high doses of which bring the risk of acute complications, calling for emergency treatment [37].

As the rate of induction stabilized after 1974 and decreased after 1978, the frequency of acceleration increased. The official recorded rate for England rose to 10.5% in 1979 [21] and 12.1% in 1985]38], the last year for which statistics were published, but it is doubtful that all cases were reported. Certainly in some hospitals the rate was very much higher. In the obstetric section of one large teaching hospital between 1981 and 1984 it was used in 30% of 13 394 labours, though in only 8.0% of the 2295 of labours in its integrated general practitioner unit [39]. The unofficial postal enquiries found that in 46% of births amniotomy was carried out after the onset of labour in 1989, hardly changed since 1984, suggesting a much wider practice of acceleration than that officially recorded [27].

The physical reason for slow progress in labour is that the uterine muscles fail to contract efficiently. Uterine contractility is regulated by hormones which the body produces in reaction to its emotional state. The early muscle changes are involuntary, slow and gradual; they need the mother's body to produce only small amounts of oxytocin to initiate them and larger amounts of prostaglandins to keep them going. This is best accomplished when the mother feels relaxed. If the changes are obstructed, they will cause more pain and the body will produce more of its own pain-relieving hormone, beta-endorphin, which has the effect also of slowing down labour. In turn, oxytocin and prostaglandins need the co-operation of another hormone, oestrogen, if labour is to be started and kept going.

Later the mood and hormonal balance change. As the baby inches its way down the widening cervix, it sends a message for much more oxytocin. If fear does not inhibit responses to the order, the assistance of the voluntary muscles is powerfully enlisted and with a wonderful co-ordination of hormonal and nervous signals and much effort, the baby is born [40].

Perpetuation of the species depends on a mother bringing her baby to birth in a safe environment, one which she finds reassuring, where she is allowed to follow her instincts and behave in a familiar, reassuring way. Many women do not find adequate reassurance in a hospital setting under obstetric management or, indeed, in any setting after constant indoctrination about the dangers of childbirth. The hormone messages sent to her uterine muscles are not strong enough completely to overcome her apprehension, so labour proceeds at a reluctant pace. It is frequently observed that contractions stop when the mother arrives at hospital and, unless she is soon reassured, her professional attendants may intervene to restart the process artificially. She is likely to be reassured more quickly if she is free to respond to the stimulus of pain, the useful function of which is to prompt her to adopt pain-relieving positions, or simply walk around, which activity not only distracts her, but helps her fetus to move to the optimum starting position for the delivery journey [40]. She is reassured also if she can eat and drink, as she feels the need, and if she can receive continuous moral and social support from a comforting companion or attendant.

There is abundant evidence that, when empathetic midwives have provided this service, labours have progressed smoothly without undue delay (Chapters 7 and 8). But there is now evidence that the successful companion need not be an expensively trained, professional midwife. A randomized controlled trial in a busy austere American obstetric hospital showed much better results over a range of outcomes – shorter labours, fewer interventions, less morbidity for both mother and baby – for the mothers who had the continuous companionship throughout labour of a 'doula', a labour support woman, herself a mother, briefly and inexpensively trained in the arts of soothing behaviour and encouraging conversation [41]. In situations where midwives cannot be provided to carry out their simple original function of being 'with woman', the employment of 'doulas' would greatly reduce the maternity service's high financial cost associated with technological interventions, as well as the human costs of its policies.

Assisted vaginal delivery: forceps and vacuum extraction

The second stage of labour may be shortened by instrumental interventions by doctors at different phases, the risk to the baby being least the nearer it has already reached unassisted delivery. Forceps may be used in the last minutes to lift out a baby, who may be distressed, from a tired or oversedated mother. At an earlier phase, if progress is slow, forceps may be used to correct the position of the fetus and assist its rotation, especially when the natural process has been impeded by previous interventions, such as induction of labour or epidural anaesthesia. Forceps may also be used to assist the delivery of the after-coming head in a breech presentation.

In the 1958 survey forceps were applied to 4.7% of all deliveries [19, p. 147]; they were used in 40% of all deliveries by hospital doctors and 20% of all deliveries by general practitioners, these deliveries making up 9.3% and 4.4% respectively of the total [19, pp. 151, 175]. The forceps rate increased quickly and was officially recorded as 8% in 1962 and 13% in 1977 [22], though it was only 7.8% in the 1970 survey – 43% of all deliveries by hospital doctors and 23% of all deliveries by GPs [20, p. 181]. After 1978 the official rate fell back to 9.1% in 1985 and this was the rate officially estimated for all instrumental deliveries in 1988–9 [26, p. 375].

The forceps rate obviously depends on the proportion of deliveries in which a doctor, not a midwife, is in control of the delivery and on the rate of certain preceding interventions. But it must also depend on the incidence of other precipitating factors, for though the risk of a forceps delivery was much higher after an induced than a spontaneous labour (1.76 times in 1979–82), most actual cases followed spontaneous labour [42].

It depends also on the alternative modes of delivery practised. Until 1978 the rising forceps rate reflected the increases in hospitalization, in epidural anaesthesia and induction, slightly modified by the rising rate of caesarean section. After 1978, despite the continued upward trend in hospitalization and epidural anaesthesia, the forceps rate declined, reflecting the falling rates of induction and the rising rate of caesarean section and perhaps also a lower incidence of other precipitating factors. Between 1958 and 1982, the rate for low outlet forceps rose from 3.6% to 5.7%, relatively less than the rate for rotational forceps, which rose from 1.0% to 4.6%. This reflects the greater use of inhibiting interventions, particularly epidural anaesthesia [43]. By 1985, the rates had fallen to 5.3% and 3.8% respectively [38]; in 1989–90 the rate for all instrumental deliveries in England was estimated at 9% [26, p. 375].

The association between the forceps rate and the dominance of doctors in intranatal care was well illustrated by contrasting rates in the 1960s quoted for Chicago, 66%, Sydney, 11%, and Kuala Lumpur 3.5%; and in the 1980s in American and Australian teaching hospitals, 70% and 25% respectively [44, p. 340]. In America by the 1990s, instruments were still used in 25% of deliveries in all obstetric hospitals, in marked contrast to less than 1% in freestanding birth centres [45, p. 129].

Vacuum extraction, which was introduced in the 1950s and was used in 0.7% of the British births in the 1970 survey [20, p. 181], had not increased further in popularity in England by the 1990s. In contrast, obstetricians in other European countries prefer this intervention to forceps delivery. It has the merits of requiring less complex forms of analgesia or anaesthesia, as well as resulting in less severe maternal injury and, except for cephalhaematoma, fewer injuries to the baby's head and face. The conclusion from randomized trials is that vacuum extraction is the better treatment [46].

Episiotomy

A further intervention to expedite delivery in episiotomy – cutting the perineum to enlarge the vaginal opening (page 150). The need for this is increased when induction and acceleration of labour have prevented the gradual thinning and stretching of the perineal muscles to allow the head to be born and when the birth position, especially the lithotomy position, further restricts such stretching [15, pp. 130–44]. It nearly always has to be used when forceps are used. As part of obstetric management, the American example was followed and the procedure became popular in Britain after 1950. By 1958 it was carried out in 16% of deliveries, in 21% of those in obstetric hospitals, 14% of those in general practitioner units and 2.7% of those at home. It was used in 34% of first births but in only 6% of later ones [19, p. 161].

Besides the alleged advantages to mother and baby of shortening labour, episiotomy was supposed to prevent severe perineal tears and minimize damage to the pelvic floor, so reducing the risks of future urinary incontinence and uterine prolapse. None of these advantages for the mother have been substantiated by later experience, while perineal tears are found to heal just as quickly as surgical cuts [47]. Episiotomy certainly increases the field for postpartum infection. Wide ranging reviews of the evidence have suggested also that it actually predisposes to third and fourth degree lacerations and is associated with greater postpartum pain and discomfort and with serious complications including maternal death [48–50].

Whatever its merits and demerits, obstetricians in Britain favoured the procedure, but carrying it out was time-consuming and so the right to perform it routinely was extended to midwives, after 1967 using local anaesthesia. Learning how and when to do it has since become a standard part of midwives' training. Their traditional training was to prevent tears by asking the mother to breathe the head out gently between contractions (page 148), but working under obstetricians they came to distrust their conservative skills and accept that episiotomy was the treatment of choice; by performing it routinely, inflicting deliberate damage, they hoped to escape the risk of tears, incidental damage, which to the midwife are the mark of professional failure [15, pp. 133–41].

The practice of episiotomy in England rose on average from 48% in 1973 to reach 52% in 1980 [51]. It varied considerably between regions – from 40% to 56% in 1973 and from 47% to 58% in 1980. In certain hospitals it was known to be much higher, up to 90% by 1980 [15, pp. 140–1], and it was commoner for first births – inflicted on 50–90% of them – than for later births [52, p. 231]. But perhaps prompted by evaluated results, enthusiasm waned somewhat, so that by 1985 the average rate had fallen to 37%, with regional variations from 31% to 44% [38, p. 34]. This downward trend was confirmed by the unofficial postal enquiry, which noted a decline from 43% in 1984 to 36% in 1989 [27]. In view of the evaluated results, it could be further reduced without disadvantage, certainly if other interventive or restrictive intranatal practices were discontinued.

Caesarean section – its increased use

The ultimate operative intervention to shorten gestation or labour is caesarean section, the safety of which was greatly increased from the 1940s onwards by advances in surgical, nursing, anaesthetic, aseptic and transfusion techniques. Nevertheless, delivery by caesarean section has always carried such a higher risk to the life and health of both mother and baby, that it is likely to be advantageous only in cases of serious complication.

In Britain in 1958 the proportion of births delivered by this method was only 2.7% – 1.3% as election before labour and 1.4% as emergency during labour [19, p. 148]. Increasing confidence pushed up the rate, so that by 1972 in England it had doubled to 5.3% [22] and by 1985 doubled again to 10.5%, 4.9% being elective [38]. Then the pace of increase slowed. By 1989–90 the rate, as officially estimated, had risen only to 12% (5% elective), with regional variation from 11% to 14% [26, p. 375], and the estimate from the unofficial postal enquiry was only slightly higher at 13%, up from 10% in the corresponding enquiry in 1984 [27]. By 1993 the official rate had risen to 14%, with 19.5% in one London hospital.

In the United States the caesarean rate, 3% in the 1960s, rose eightfold in two decades, from 5.5% in 1970 to 24.7% in 1988, nearly one birth in four. But there too the upward trend faltered; the rate fell back to 23.5% in 1990 and stayed the same in 1991. By the late 1980s between other countries where the statistic was recorded, rates ranged widely, with around 7% in Ireland, the Netherlands and Japan, 17.5% in Italy and nearer 20% in Canada. Such figures reflect neither relative degrees of prenatal risk nor postnatal results. They reflect the wide disagreement between obstetricians on when the operation is appropriate; some find a rate of under 5% adequate, many others prefer a rate over 20%. Even higher rates have become common in hospitals in countries with a well-organized obstetric profession with payment guaranteed by a co-operative insurance system, as in North America and Australia, where the upward trend started to gather momentum in the 1960s, earlier than in Britain [45, 53, 54].

Disagreement about the conditions which caesarean section would benefit reflects the paucity of evaluated results from alternative treatments. It may also reflect differences in motivation and attitudes of individual obstetricians and indeed mothers: the eagerness of the former to take over and the willingness of the latter to surrender the responsibility of bringing the child into the world. It may reflect that obstetricians find the surgical technique easier to master, and for them quicker to carry out, than the arts of collaborative midwifery. It may simply reflect attitudes formed by their training, or an increasingly generous ratio of obstetricians to deliveries, obstetricians seeking to justify their training and employment by performing a task which they alone can do and which they do very competently, while the taxpayer or the insurance contributor pays the higher bills involved. Higher section rates in teaching hospitals can be explained at least as much by the practice requirements of trainees as by the morbidity of the patients, and the more practitioners are trained, the more often the practice will have to be carried out to keep their skill in good order.

It must have some significance that in many countries the incidence of caesarean section, for which obstetricians are paid most, is highest among private, fee-paying patients – women whose standard of living is associated with the highest standards of health, which makes them fittest to reproduce, women who are least likely to develop the complications whose dangers caesarean section is thought to reduce [55]. In a cohort of 245 854 singleton births in California in the 1980s, the caesarean rate was much higher for rich white women than for poor Mexicans. It was 10.9% in the lowest income group compared with 17.4% in the highest. The rates were related to the socio-economic status of the subject, not to complications of delivery. In Southern Brazil half the private patients have a caesarean section; the intervention is related to the patient's income and inversely related to her degree of physical risk [56]. Private patients in Britain too are more likely to have caesarean sections than NHS patients. The average perinatal mortality rate after caesarean section will be the lower, the more the babies of these healthy mothers are included.

The experience of caesarean section among a large group of such healthy mothers, delivered in an American hospital, was found to vary, from 19% to 42%, according to which of the eleven obstetricians was in charge. This variance could not be explained by any predelivery risk factor present in the patients, nor did better neonatal outcomes justify retrospectively the higher section rates. It could only be explained by the personal preferences of the obstetricians concerned, which did not appear to be based on actual clinical or legal experiences [57].

However, defence against possible litigation on the grounds that they did not take every available measure to prevent a disastrous outcome was offered by 53% of American and 20% of British obstetricians as justification for their ultimate intervention, 84% of the Americans and 42% of the Britons attributing the upward trend in their national rate to this cause [55]. This means that in a substantial proportion of cases any medical indication for the operation was of secondary importance.

Unequivocal evidence identifying conditions where caesarean section is indeed the best measure for preventing disaster is extremely hard to find, but this fact notwithstanding, the obstetric profession of the 20th century has managed to convince the legal profession (page 244) of the rightness of the view of the 18th century midwife, already quoted above in Chapter 2, '. . . there is no appeal from what a doctor does, being granted he did all he could on the occasion' (page 44).

American official statistics show that the risk of having a caesarean section is greater for women who, besides having higher socio-economic status, are giving birth for the first time or are in older age groups. 'A woman in her early twenties has one chance in eight of having a primary cesarean; a woman thirty-five years old or older has one chance in four.' [45, p. 141] The older women are more likely to include those who have already had a section; the first-time mothers are more likely to have long labours, medically diagnosed as failure to progress or dystocia (page 158). Repeat section and dystocia are the indications in both America and Britain which together account for around two-thirds of all caesarean sections – repeat sections made up 30% of all sections done in a large English teaching hospital between 1978 and

1983 [58]. Fetal distress and breech presentations each made up another 10%.

Repeat caesarean sections

In 1916 an American obstetrician pronounced the dictum 'Once a section, always a section' [5, p. 139]. The surgical technique then used created the real danger of rupture of the uterine scar in a subsequent vaginal delivery, but improved methods have now made this danger very small. Moreover, the reasons for the primary caesarean section are usually not repeated in a later pregnancy, so that a second section should often not be necessary.

Nevertheless, it needed the agitation of vigorous consumer groups, notably in America (page 240), who, rebelling against being barred from ever giving birth in the normal way, persuaded some obstetricians to let them try. They soon demonstrated that vaginal birth after cesarean (VBAC) could be safely accomplished. Although the results of elective operation and trial of labour have not been compared in properly controlled trials, prospective comparative studies have shown that about 80% of the women allowed to try vaginal delivery did succeed and they and their babies had fewer complications than the women who underwent a repair section [59, p. 248]. Despite these results, some obstetricians stick to the long-standing precept; 'in 1990 four out of five United States women who had cesareans and gave birth again had repeat cesareans' [45, p. 143] and even under the more open-minded obstetricians the rate for repeat section tends to exceed 50%. To this extent, caesarean section is a self-perpetuating intervention and a high rate of primary section will maintain a high overall section rate.

Caesarean section and poor progress in labour

Dystocia, literally *bad birth*, should describe conditions where the normal process is obstructed for some physical reason and so prolonged, but it has come to be used to describe any labour which is taking longer than the arbitrarily set standard. In the days when deformed maternal pelves were common, a frequent reason for obstruction was cephalopelvic disproportion, but since the 1950s true disproportion has become rare. However, if the mother is kept immobile and in such a position that her pelvis cannot expand as it should to accommodate the passage of the baby's head, disproportion will be diagnosed. The obstetric management of labour in recent decades has itself been a fertile contributor to the increased frequency of diagnosed disproportion, which in turn has contributed greatly to the increased frequency of caesarean section.

American researchers have found that the early administration of medications and regional, especially epidural, anaesthesia often prolong labour. In particular, they found that epidural anaesthesia in first labours is associated with an increased risk of caesarean section for dystocia, the risk being increased the more, the earlier the epidural is administered [45, p. 145]. Poor progress in labour is often attributed to uterine inertia, a state associated with emotional tension (page 158), also often generated by the obstetric management of labour, including the feeling of urgency created by trying to keep within the arbitrary time limits which inhibits rather than encourages progress. Away from such constraints, dystocia was strikingly absent among the evacuated mothers in war-time Britain (page 287). It occurs more often after induced labours, but whether this happens because of the induction or the reasons for induction is uncertain.

Caesarean section and fetal distress

Fetal distress has been more frequently, but not more reliably, diag-nosed from what are interpreted as abnormal heart rate patterns recorded by continuous electronic monitoring (page 178). The fact that many babies, born by emergency caesarean section, show no signs of recent distress indicates that many obstetricians do not correctly distin-guish abnormal from normal patterns of stress, for the process of phy-siological birth exposes the fetus to many stresses, as it finds its way from the safe environment of the uterus to the world outside. These natural stresses are not harmful, but are necessary preparations for vital systems to make the adaptations necessary for healthy independent existence. Stress hormones are generated which actually slow down the fetus's heart rate and enable its organs to withstand the variations in blood (and oxygen) supply caused by uterine contractions, though the efficiency of the adaptation process may be prejudiced by the more violent contractions of drug-induced labours. These normal variations in the fetal heart rate caused by *stress* are often misinterpreted as signals of fetal *distress*, calling for prompt intervention to relieve the lack of oxygen. Although misinterpretations may be corrected by analysis of blood samples taken from the fetal scalp, facilities for carrying out this test may not be available or used to prevent unnecessary caesarean sections [53].

Caesarean section and breech presentation

Elective caesarean section has become increasingly preferred for breech presentations. Most of those diagnosed antenatally will have turned, naturally or assisted by external version (page 150) to the vertex (head first) position before labour starts. Many of the minority which do not turn are malformed or undeveloped with little chance of survival, but even the normally developed babies who come breech first are more likely to die than those who come head first. Although there has been no randomized trial of the two methods of delivery, certain studies have found lower mortality and morbidity for the infant following abdominal than vaginal delivery [53]. To some extent the apparently superior results are achieved because caesarean section is only undertaken when there is a fair prospect of rescuing a potentially viable fetus, leaving the ill-fated ones to swell the mortality rate for vaginal delivery. These results, though inconclusive, persuaded more obstetricians to favour abdominal delivery: their training gave them more skill and confidence to perform the surgical operation than to supervise and assist natural delivery in the breech position, though good outcomes for healthy fetuses carefully delivered vaginally by the breech have also been reported [60].

In a Norwegian hospital between 1972 and 1975, 8.1% of the breech births were delivered by caesarean section, but between 1976 and 1979 this rate rose to 32.6%. There was, however, 'no definite improvement in mortality in spite of the fourfold increase in caesarean sections. . . . It therefore appears difficult to defend without reservation the sharp increase in the use of caesarean section in breech delivery, as reported from a number of countries' [61].

A prospective randomized trial might eliminate the bias in predelivery viability and establish which method is the safer. In the absence of such decisive information, a retrospective analysis was made of the 3447 singleton breech deliveries at term which represented 3.6% of all the singleton term births in a London Health district over the three years 1988–90; of the breeches, 28% were delivered vaginally and 72% by caesarean section, 30% emergency and 42% elective. For the vaginal breech births the neonatal death rate was 0.83%, twenty-eight times higher than the 0.03% for those delivered abdominally but, more surprisingly, about ten times higher than the 0.08% (77 deaths/93 062 births) for the mature singleton vertex births delivered vaginally [62]. This study was unique in finding caesarean breech birth actually safer than vaginal birth for most term singletons, which suggests that the accuracy of the computer database might be questioned and hence the validity of the conclusions obtained from the analysis.

This finding of the greater safety of caesarean section for the baby was not repeated in a study, based on births in Cape Town between 1975 and 1986, to measure the relative safety of caesarean and vaginal birth for the mother, 'the effects of medical disorders and other acute pre-existing physiological disturbances' having been excluded. For all cases so defined, the maternal death rate was 0.04%, but there were five deaths following caesarean for every one death following vaginal delivery. The relative risk as between emergency and elective sections was 1.5 : 1 [63].

The need for operative delivery for breech presentations would obviously be reduced if there were in the event fewer breech presentations. Randomized trials have now shown that this can be safely achieved by the more frequent practice of external version, which, if performed at term rather than earlier in the pregnancy as used to be done and if appropriate drugs are used to relax the uterus, significantly reduces the incidence of breech presentations at birth and so the call for caesarean sections. Version may even be delayed until after the onset of labour, particularly if birth is to take place in a hospital with facilities to carry out an emergency section, should a dangerous complication arise in the few cases where version is unsuccessful [64] (pages 87, 91, 150).

Other reasons for elective caesarean section

Caesarean section is carried out electively in the interest of the mother and/or the baby to terminate pregnancy in cases of maternal pre-eclampsia or suspected retarded fetal growth. Disturbingly often, suspicion proves to have been ill-founded. Gestation can be seriously over-estimated and intervention result in the birth of a premature, but not growth-retarded, infant [65]. Such iatrogenic immaturity partly accounts for the higher mortality and morbidity associated with caesarean section. Moreover, it has not yet been demonstrated that the truly growth-retarded babies thrive better in the neonatal intensive care unit than in the unsatisfactory uterus. For this indication, as for breech births, the confidence of some obstetricians is being disturbed by the results achieved. 'In view of the maternal morbidity associated with a caesarean section and the poor neonatal outcomes at birthweights <1500 grams, the use of operative delivery for very low birthweight infants deserves further scrutiny' [66]. Various other conditions, including placenta praevia, for which an elective operation may well be life-saving if the condition is correctly diagnosed, are each fairly uncommon and together account for around 10% of all sections [58].

Operative delivery has become increasingly favoured by obstetricians as the safest method for solving potential problems in multiple births, certainly those of higher order. These births have a much greater than average chance of being born preterm, but whether their chances of survival are improved by elective preterm delivery has not been demonstrated.

The rapid increase in the overall caesarean section rate coincided with the rapid decrease in the overall perinatal mortality rate and led, particularly in North America, to the familiar, mistaken hypothesis that the former trend was the cause of the latter. But the hypothesis could not be supported: the perinatal mortality rate decreased as much in series where the caesarean section rate did not increase [67, 68]. Nor have recent trends towards lower or stable section rates been reflected in corresponding increases in perinatal mortality rates.

NEW TREATMENTS FOR PAIN RELIEF

The degree of pain in childbirth perceived by a woman depends not only on the physical stimulus but also on her emotional state and her cultural expectations. Her perceived pain is less when she feels relaxed, unafraid and reassured by the continuous, comforting support of her birth attendant. Not all doctors or midwives can inspire peaceful confidence and this is rarely the atmosphere in a large obstetric hospital where the obstetric practices themselves have the effect of intensifying physical pain.

Women from cultures which believe that all pain should and can be relieved by medical means come to expect relief at low levels of suffering. Belief that other medical means are available in itself undermines the woman's willingness to endure or to rely on the prophylaxis of emotional support. Unfortunately the medical remedies have the effect of making the birth slower and less efficient, which in turn prompts further obstetric interventions with further pain. It is not, therefore, surprising that the increase in hospitalization and obstetric management in the pain-averse Western cultures of the later 20th century has coincided with, indeed been facilitated by, a tremendous increase in the amount of medical pain relief asked for and given at the time of delivery. In Britain in 1946, 51% of mothers received neither anaesthetics, analgesics nor sedatives [18, p. 86]. By 1958 this rate had shrunk to less than 22% [19, p. 167], and by 1970 to 3% [20, pp. 193–4], around which low level it subsequently continued [15, p. 93]. By 1990 when the National Birthday Trust conducted its Confidential Enquiry into Pain Relief in Labour and when 99.5% of women delivered in an obstetric hospital or other medical institution, its questionnaires were designed on the assumption that all labouring women would ask for and be given some kind of medical pain relief at some stage. In the event too few questionnaires were correctly completed for the sample surveyed to be sufficiently representative of all births. This deficiency limits the generalizations which can confidently be made from the aggregated data [69].

The demand for and supply of medical means of pain relief is high in cultures accustomed to obstetric interventions in labour. In the United States drugs are used to relieve pain in most deliveries, 80–98% of those in high-tech. hospitals but much less for those in low-tech. birth centres. In contrast, attitudes are more resilient in the Netherlands and Japan where mothers, especially those under midwives' care, get by very successfully with far fewer pain-relieving drugs or none at all.

In Britain in 1946 18% of mothers had general anaesthesia, but because of the obvious risks, especially to the mother, and the advent of alternatives, general anaesthesia became less favoured. By 1958 it was given to only 5.7% of mothers and in 1970 to 5.3%. Over this period its use was maintained at 95–97% for caesarean sections, but was reduced from 59% to 10% of the forceps deliveries and from 17% to 5% of the vaginal breech deliveries. By 1990 it had even been replaced by epidural anaesthesia for 51% of the increased number of caesarean sections then performed [69].

For the instrumental vaginal deliveries, as well as for episiotomies and perineal repairs, it became more popular to numb the pudendal nerves, which supply most of the perineum, vulva, vagina and pelvic muscles, by the injection of an anaesthetic agent such as lignocaine, because this local anaesthesia gave effective pain relief without the dangerous drawbacks of general anaesthesia [15, pp. 107–8]. Infrequent in 1946, the use of pudendal blocks or local infiltration increased between 1958 and 1970 from 36% to 64% of the forceps and from 24% to 52% of the vaginal breech deliveries. General practitioners were slower to adopt the new techniques and though they used forceps far less often than hospital doctors, they used general anaesthesia in relatively more of their assisted deliveries. These modes of regional anaesthesia also had some adverse side-effects on fetus and mother and in the 1970s gave way to more attractive alternatives.

As the availability increased of equipment for administering inhalational analgesia, by midwives as well as by doctors, so did its use: from 16% of mothers in 1946 to 78% in 1958. Holding the face-mask by herself, the mother can breathe in enough of the mixture of gas (nitrous oxide or trichloroethylene) and air (later oxygen) to ease her awareness of pain without overdosing and losing consciousness and without the compound entering, or lingering in, her or her baby's blood circulation. Most women found it of some help, but apparently it did not satisfy the needs of all women, or perhaps the needs of their birth attendants, whose health might suffer from continued exposure to the gases, for its use declined to 61% by 1970, but increased again to an estimated 75% by 1990. The use of trichloroethylene continued to diminish but another inhalational analgesic, methoxyfluorine, became popular and was found helpful by 90% of women [70]. Although more effective in pain relief, it has other adverse side-effects and is probably more useful in short but painful labours where delivery is imminent [71].

After 1950 there was a great increase also in the use of narcotic drugs which, like the others, brought both advantages and disadvantages. One of these, pethidine (Demerol in America), a synthetic narcotic, administered usually by intramuscular injection, was introduced in 1940. After 1950 midwives were allowed to administer it on their own authority and many became eager to do so, having more faith in this pharmacological method of relieving pain than in their traditional prophylaxis of psychological support, on which their training had come to lay less stress [15, pp. 102–5]. By 1958 it was being given to 56% of mothers [19, p. 163].

By making the mother drowsy, pethidine reduces her awareness of pain but also her active control of labour and slows down the process [72]. It may make her nauseous, but more dangerously it crosses the placenta and until the baby's body can eliminate its share, which may take hours or days to complete, it depresses the baby's instincts to breathe and suck [15, pp. 102–5]. Despite its disadvantages, its use was extended to 69% of mothers by 1970 and it continued to be commonly prescribed in the 1980s, alternative drugs, intended to produce fewer adverse effects on the baby, not having gained widespread acceptance [71]. By 1990 it was still being used for about half of all labours, but only 30% if epidurals were also being used.

For seriously sedated babies a narcotic antagonist drug, such as naloxone, may have to be injected intravenously or intramuscularly. Babies whose breathing is not quickly and satisfactorily established have to have the immediate assistance of a mechanical ventilator and run the risk of future respiratory problems. Babies whose sucking reflex is impaired likewise need the assistance of artificial methods of feeding. The Special Care Baby Unit became a necessary adjunct to the liberal use of analgesia in childbirth. Such units were introduced in British obstetric hospitals in the 1960s and were later followed by Neonatal Intensive Care Units in the larger hospitals, both bringing dangers of their own [73] (pages 206, 363).

Many of the dangers and drawbacks associated with general anaesthesia and narcotic drugs are avoided by lumbar epidural anaesthesia which became increasingly popular from the 1970s. Birth attendants had no hesitation in recommending it because of its undoubted advantages, on the one hand giving the mother complete relief of pain while she remains conscious, and on the other hand giving them a compliant, undistressed and undistressing patient. These advantages obtained in both vaginal and abdominal deliveries. They find support in a long list of research reports in journals read by anaesthetists [74].

The disadvantages were considered of less importance and were often not mentioned, even after research had confirmed them. Because impaired function of the uterine muscles obstructs the natural rotation and descent of the fetus and prevents the mother's urge to push, labour is prolonged and the need for forceps assistance, with its attendant dangers to the child, is greatly increased [43]. Likewise the problem of slow progress often has to be resolved by caesarean section. Like most others, the drug used crosses the placenta and has a depressing effect on the fetus which it may take weeks, or possibly longer, to outgrow [75].

Acute, and sometimes very serious, consequences for the mother are fortunately rare. Less serious but chronic consequences were overlooked until research, prompted by complaints made to the consumer body, AIMS (page 236) [26, p. 491], established a significant association between back pain and epidural anaesthesia [76]. Further research found associations between intranatal drug usage and several maternal illnesses of body and mind [77] (page 303).

The technical difficulties of administration are such that, though specially trained midwives are permitted to 'top up' the anaesthetic dose, the constant supervision of a skilled anaesthetist and the availability of equipment to deal with emergency complications are essential. It is, therefore, a method of pain relief feasible only in the well-equipped obstetric hospital, with anaesthetist staffing for twenty-four hours a day seven days a week. The argument that the option of epidural anaesthesia should be given to all childbearing women requires that all births should take place in such hospitals [78, 79] whatever other disadvantages enforcing this may bring (Chapters 7 and 8).

Because a naturally occurring state of relaxation bodes well for a smooth labour, birth attendants are apt to assume that drug-induced relaxation will be equally felicitous. It will certainly make the mother easier to manage, but it is liable to be followed by adverse side-effects for the mother and infant, similar to those resulting from anaesthetic and narcotic drugs. In most countries where Western style obstetrics reign, the use of opiates, sedatives and tranquillizers has become ever more liberal. In Britain they were given to 7% of mothers in 1946, 25% in 1958 and the widening range available was extensively prescribed in the 1980s [71]. The use of sedatives and tranquillizers was not reported in the 1990 Enquiry. Instead of being a treatment of last resort needed by the few, they are dispensed as first-line therapy, not only as the necessary antidote to the adverse consequences of intranatal intervention, but as early prophylaxis to blunt the labouring woman's awareness of impending troubles.

The long-term consequences of any event are intrinsically hard to trace and determine reliably, taking into account the possible influence of many later events. Irrespective of other circumstances, there seems to be for the mother an increased risk of lasting postnatal depression after certain drugs used to relieve pain in labour. For the child there may be an increased risk that the opiate drugs he has absorbed as a fetus from his mother may predispose him to opiate addiction as an adult. Research data supporting this hypothesis has been published [80]. If the association is real and holds for other drugs which may impair the natural ability of human beings to withstand the provocations of life, then the liberal use of drugs to relieve the pain of childbirth, much of which is aggravated by obstetric interventions ostensibly undertaken to improve outcome, is an appalling potential danger.

Dependence on artificial pain relief originates from a misinterpretation of the physiological role of pain, which tells the sufferer that the present situation is not right and prompts him to change it. Pain in the various stages of labour prompts the mother to move and change her position. Freedom to move as her body dictates helps to relieve her pain and, more importantly, helps the fetus, whose efforts to be born initiate the painful stimuli, to move to the correct place in its journey.

> Freedom from pain depends on allowing uterine contractions to do their work without interference from the mind and the external environment. Painful contractions are an indication that labour is becoming less efficient. Pain slows labour by increasing β-endorphin secretion. β-endorphin is the biochemical cause of prolonged labour, also known as uterine inertia and dystocia. Prolonged labour is caused by physical and mental stress. If we can teach women how to reduce their stress levels then they can have pain-free contractions. [40, p. 111]

Experience already referred to is that women have found mental stress eased, simply but effectively, by the comforting presence of chosen companions, by their reassuring physical contacts, stroking and rubbing; by applying hot or cold compresses or physical pressure to sensitive places; by enjoying warm showers and relaxing in warm baths – all without harm. Immersion in a warm bath has been advocated by the French surgeon turned obstetrician, Michel Odent, as helping women to re-discover their instinctive behaviour. His advocacy has even encouraged converts to persuade several local hospitals to install birthing tubs in which many women have been allowed to labour at length and some to give birth, despite reservations from orthodox obstetricians about the difficulties of carrying out monitoring procedures which this poses. Water birth has not been scientifically evaluated, but very few adverse outcomes have been reported.

Other less simple and not yet evaluated methods of relieving pain without recourse to drugs include acupuncture and TENS (transcutaneous electrical nerve stimulation, whereby a low-voltage electric current is transmitted from a battery-powered generator to the skin producing a tingling sensation and distracting attention from pain from other sources). TENS seems to be effective in early labour but needs supplementation to deal with more intense later pain and it was used in relatively few labours in 1990.

As in the case of other mammals, nature has evolved a balanced set of behaviours which enable the human mother to co-operate with and advance the physiological changes that will result in the efficient birth of offspring. These pain-avoiding, pain-relieving behaviours may not be powerful enough to overcome the ingrained fears and expectations of women, brought up in cultures where excruciating pain is accepted as an inevitable part of childbirth, an ordeal which is intensified by the pain-creating interventions organized by the professional managers of childbirth and from which they are encouraged to believe that only drugs can offer an escape.

INTRANATAL ELECTRONIC FETAL MONITORING (EFM)

Interventions to shorten gestation or labour cannot hope to improve the baby's safety unless the natural birth process is deviating from normality and the fetus is becoming distressed. Obstetricians believe that fetal distress can be detected through abnormal patterns in the fetal heart rate. Traditionally, since Pinard invented his stethoscope for this purpose in the 19th century, the birth attendant has monitored the heart rate by non-invasive auscultation, which, being intermittent, runs the risk of missing significant indications of deterioration.

In the 1960s obstetricians harnessed new knowledge from the science of electronics to invent instruments whereby the reactions of the fetal heart could be monitored continuously over periods in labour, as in pregnancy, long enough to reveal useful warnings of fetal distress. The fetal heart rate reflects the adequacy of its oxygen supply. Knowing when this is insufficient should, in theory, make possible timely interventions, intended to prevent fetal death or damage, particularly neurological damage, by hastening the end of unsatisfactory uterine life and starting extra-uterine resuscitation.

Electronic fetal monitors, even models using telemetry, the 1980s' technological advance, restrict the labouring mother's mobility, completely or partly and the internal devices necessitate artificial rupture of membranes, to the detriment of the natural process. Like partograms (page 161), they downgrade the mother as a less reliable witness to progress than the impersonal instruments and reduce the amount of personal attention and support she receives from her attendants. Fixing a monitoring electrode to the presenting part of the fetus after amniotomy is not without danger and may well cause it pain [15, pp. 88–9].

The monitor should record whether the fetal heart accelerates and decelerates appropriately in response to increases and decreases in fetal activity or uterine contractions. Correct interpretation of the traces recorded in pregnancy or in labour is, however, notoriously difficult, for there is a wide overlap between the recorded responses of healthy and distressed fetuses. While a normal trace is very likely to indicate a healthy fetus, an abnormal trace has only a 50–70% chance of indicating a distressed fetus. Moreover, there has been wide variation between the interpretations of different observers and variations also between the interpretations of the same trace by the same observer on different occasions [81]. Obstetricians' attempts to err on the safe side led to a great increase first in the diagnosis of fetal distress and then in obstetric interventions, with their attendant and often unnecessary dangers. Overdiagnosis and interventions were somewhat reduced when greater credence was given to the complementary analysis of oxygen concentration (pH level) of blood samples taken intermittently from the baby's scalp which often contradicted the interpretation of the monitor's traces [82].

The introduction and increased application of electronic fetal monitors coincided with the decline in perinatal mortality and obstetricians again fell into the trap of illogically inferring a cause and effect relationship between the variables [83]. Their mistaken belief encouraged the wider use of the method, to the point where not to have used it might be judged professional negligence in cases of litigation (pages 244–5). But whatever benefit the information provided by electronic monitoring in pregnancy or labour may have been in individual cases, no one has yet been able to show that it contributed to the general decline in perinatal mortality or morbidity [84, 85] or indeed to any improvement in outcome for either mother or child [86]. A prospective comparison of selective and universal EFM in 34 995 pregnant women in Texas found that the only significant difference in outcomes was the higher rate of caesarean section associated with universal monitoring. This led to the conclusion that all pregnant women, particularly those at low risk, do not need continuous EFM [87].

But action prompted by the warnings of fetal distress from continuous monitoring failed to benefit births at high risk also. A randomized controlled trial found better neurological outcomes up to eighteen months after birth – better mental and psychomotor development and less cerebral palsy – for the preterm babies weighing less than 1750 grams whose heart rate had been monitored by periodic auscultation than by electronic monitoring [88].

These findings are consistent with those of the earlier large scale randomized controlled trial in Dublin [89] where the lower rate of neonatal neurological damage which followed continuous as opposed to intermittent monitoring was found to have disappeared by early childhood. The neonatal seizures which were prevented were not those associated with long-term problems; the incidence of cerebral palsy was not reduced in the group randomized to electronic monitoring [90].

Faced with the mounting evidence, leading obstetricians have eventually had to concede that no greater benefit has been found from the routine use of the high technology electronic monitoring than of low technology intermittent auscultation, not only for low-risk births but for high-risk births also. The American College of Obstetricians and Gynecologists has made specific recommendations for using auscultation [45, p. 112]. In 1993, the *British Journal of Obstetrics and Gynaecology* brought out a special supplement volume devoted to 'Cardiotocography Technology', which includes fetal monitoring. One of the eminent obstetrician contributors in his paper, 'Clinical overview of cardiotocography' (CTG) repeated the verdict that 'the use of CTG has been associated with an increase in interventions in labour, particularly caesarean section, without clear evidence of benefit'. He went on to admit that the relationship between fetal heart rate, fetal blood pH (oxygenization) changes and long-term outcome remains obscure [91]. Their imperfect understanding of the subject was emphasized by another contributor who pointed out that 'arguments between experts reveal lack of agreed standards in cardiotocography' [92].

It will probably take some time longer before maternity services, which have invested heavily in the necessary capital equipment and the training of doctors and midwives to operate it, revise their practices in the light of evidence and the belated admission by experts of their fallibility.

PRECAUTIONARY STARVATION

Obstetricians have been increasingly disposed to deal with unforeseen complications by carrying out operative deliveries for which general anaesthesia may be required. Maternal death may occur if an anaesthetized woman vomits and inhales the contents of her stomach. To guard against this danger, obstetricians have made it standard practice in recent years to withhold (or drastically ration) food and drink from all labouring women, although even in 1988–9 only a small minority of them (7% in England) [26] were delivered by an unplanned caesarean section and despite the more frequent use of regional anaesthesia.

For a woman whose labour lasts longer than her normal fasting time between meals this is a weakening deprivation at a time when considerable physical and emotional exertions are being demanded of her body, often in a hotter atmosphere than usual. The longer her starvation, the more likely it is to upset the woman's normal blood chemistry and reduce the efficiency of her muscles. The chemical imbalance may have to be corrected by intravenous feeding, which imposes a further restriction on her mobility [15, pp. 52–4], while the infusion of glucose and fluid may lead to hyperinsulinism in the fetus and hypoglycaemia in the neonate [93], calling for intervention and special care to avoid potential damage to the infant brain.

Deprivation of nourishment and refreshment may well aggravate the complications which then have to be treated by operative delivery. Likewise, it probably weakens the fetus and contributes to the diagnosed distress which triggers the intervention. And so a vicious circle is set up. Avoiding one danger which could affect a small minority is achieved by courting other dangers which affect a large majority. No study has yet confirmed that the advantage of pursuing the former objective outweighs the disadvantages of suffering the consequences.

DEVELOPMENTS IN THIRD-STAGE MANAGEMENT

The female reproductive system has evolved to complete the process of birth by detaching the placenta from the uterine wall, sealing off the blood vessels and expelling the placenta with minimal loss of blood. Retained placentae and postpartum haemorrhages are reportedly rare when the mother gives birth in an upright position and without interference [15, pp. 145–6], but this simplicity became less assured with the 'civilizing' influence of medical management and the manifest dangers of the complications were worrying. In the 1930s, interest was revived in the natural drug, ergot, which produced speedy and strong contractions of uterine muscle but was shunned because of its other damaging effects. Chemical derivatives of it suitable for intravenous or intramuscular injection, in Britain ergometrine, were developed. These avoided most of the offsetting dangers but not the risk that mistimed administration would trap an undelivered placenta in a firmly contracted uterus [15, p. 147].

It had also been discovered that natural oxytocin would cause similarly rapid uterine contractions and a synthetic form, Syntocinon, was produced in 1954. Experimental work in the early 1960s established that a mixture of Syntocinon and ergometrine, Syntometrine, injected intramuscularly with the birth of the first shoulder and followed by controlled traction of the cord, gave time for the placenta to be delivered before the uterus contracted enough to prevent haemorrhage.

With this apparent solution of the problem, within the competence of midwives as well as doctors, management of the third stage in this way soon became routine prophylaxis for all women, since there is no sure way of identifying in advance the minority of mothers who would otherwise suffer a retained placenta or postpartum haemorrhage. For the majority who would not, the treatment cannot be beneficial. It brings new risks to the mother, of unfavourable reactions in muscles, heart and blood vessels: it may raise her blood pressure to a dangerous level [94, 95] and go towards explaining the occurrence of late onset pre-eclampsia already noted in the Aberdeen study (page 115). It brings new risks also to the baby: it either deprives it of its final quota of blood if the cord is clamped immediately or subjects it to a violent overdose of drug-contaminated blood forced from the placenta by the strong uterine contractions as long as the cord is left unclamped. The drugs react adversely on the baby's tissues and may go towards explaining the higher incidence of neonatal jaundice in managed deliveries [15, pp. 148–52].

Traction of the cord may not always deliver the placenta successfully. The two may separate completely or partially, leaving all or a portion of the placenta behind, or if the placenta is not ready to detach, traction may invert the uterus. In these contingencies the mother is likely to suffer haemorrhage, severe shock and the manual removal of the placenta under general anaesthesia.

Various methods of assisting expulsion of the placenta by external manipulation have been practised by birth attendants. Assistance from the production of natural oxytocin, stimulated simply by the infant sucking the breast, was long neglected. Though this potentiality was increasingly acknowledged in the 1980s, there was no sign of reliance on it to usurp routine administration of Syntometrine as preferred therapy.

The preventive use of ergometrine and Syntocinon made an important contribution to reducing the incidence of, and mortality from, postpartum haemorrhage, but in so far as this third stage complication results from earlier obstetric management, from induction, from oversedation of the mother or inflicted damage of tissues, the drug therapy may only serve to mitigate unnecessary risks unnaturally created [95–97].

However, a large randomized controlled trial, conducted within an English obstetric hospital by staff accustomed to obstetric methods, compared postpartum blood loss in two groups of women: one having the routine preventive drug injection and the other only being encouraged to adopt all the 'natural' practices said to protect against postpartum haemorrhage. The results showed that in this setting, blood loss was significantly greater in the 'natural' group as assigned by randomization [98]. In the event, only 47% of the women assigned to the 'natural' group actually received 'natural' postpartum treatment: 20% had prophylactic oxytocin drugs, 49% adopted postures where descent of the placenta could not be helped by gravity, 40% had cord traction and 49% had the cord clamped before delivery of the placenta, while preventive drug treatment was not given to a few of those assigned to receive it. In an attempt to overcome one of the weaknesses of the methodology of the randomized controlled trial where results ought to be assessed in the groups as randomized, a secondary analysis was carried out to compare outcomes in the smaller groups which actually had the treatment allocated. The preventive drug treatment again led to significantly fewer postpartum haemorrhages and other serious third-stage problems. However, the 'natural' group had not been assured of 'natural' treatment throughout the earlier stages of labour, which may be a fair prerequisite for their effectiveness.

A later randomized controlled trial in Dublin of 1429 women at low risk of haemorrhage compared outcomes after 'active', using preventive ergometrine as was the normal routine, and 'natural' postpartum management. Although physiological practices were followed far more often in the 'natural' group, there were deviations from the proposed protocol; ergometrine, which could be used if necessary as treatment, was so used in 14% of 'natural' cases. Even so, primary blood loss was significantly higher in the 'natural' group, with two of the 724 women (0.3%) needing blood transfusion, but for most women any complications were not severe and were short-lived. In contrast, the incidence of various more serious postpartum complications, including secondary haemorrhage, was significantly higher in the 'active' group. The broader findings of this study indicate that for healthy women, which most childbearers now are, the loss of up to 750 ml of blood does not present a serious problem. It is possible that at this stage women's bodies are reversing the physiological increase in blood volume necessary in pregnancy. This suggests that the conventional criterion of dangerous postpartum blood loss of over 500 ml is inappropriate and invites a style of routine management likely in the end to do more harm than good [99].

REVISED ATTITUDES TO LYING-IN

In war-time Britain, speedy mobilization after delivery became a necessary air-raid precaution. Birth attendants were surprised that mothers seemed the better for it, but it was not until after 1950 that it came to be understood why, for physiological reasons, recumbent inactivity is dangerous. From the 1960s other changes in the maternity service were making it convenient to give effect to this new knowledge by shortening the lying-in period. Propaganda advocating hospitalization, coinciding with the rise in the birth rate, overtook the supply of hospital beds, which could most easily be augmented by cutting short the in-patient stay. In selected cases discharge in forty-eight or thirty-six hours or even less was dared, so that the average postnatal stay was steadily whittled down to reach 5.7 days in 1977 [22] and 5.2 in 1985 [38], the rest of the postpartum care being carried out by community midwives visiting mothers in their homes. Obstetricians, having little to contribute to an uncomplicated puerperium, are willing to relinquish control. Following vaginal delivery the stay in bed was progressively reduced from days to hours, so the postpartum period ceased to be the invalid experience of lying-in and mothers were quickly able to attend to their own hygiene.

Early discharge from hospital was appreciated by those mothers who, with the co-operation of community midwives, were able to make satisfactory arrangements for domestic care and assistance, but others, who could not enlist the help of relations or friends and without access to a generous community service, would have welcomed hospital care for longer if this had been available [100, p. 103, 101].

But despite earlier mobilization, the 1970 survey [20, pp. 235, 237] found venous complications in 5.1% of mothers in the first postpartum week, as well as genito-urinary tract infections in 4.4%. Both disorders occurred more frequently among women delivered in hospital and after intranatal interventions, yet other evidence of disadvantage following obstetric management. The survey of postpartum morbidity in 1987 [77] did not ask about these causes of illness.

CARE OF THE NEWBORN

Mothers were increasingly allowed to take some part in looking after their babies, whose cots from the 1970s were most likely to be next to their mothers' beds. It ceased to be the practice to banish normal babies to the nursery to be looked after exclusively by midwives; a greater proportion of babies, however, were judged to need nursing in special or intensive care units under the care of neonatal paediatricians, because they were premature or of low weight or had suffered intranatal intervention which always, to a greater or lesser degree, has adverse consequences for the baby [102]. By the 1980s many babies who had formerly been thought to need special care were also being left with their mothers in the postnatal ward, for paediatricians were realizing that they throve better there.

Nature obviously intended that the umbilical cord should briefly continue its life support function while the neonate's respiratory and circulatory systems adapt to their new role. Medically oriented midwifery early adopted the tidier practice of promptly clamping the cord, with the disadvantage for the baby of abruptly withdrawing its natural support and interrupting the ordered process of transition. At the same time, it endangered the mother by interfering with the physiological process of placental separation and encouraging postpartum haemorrhage. The healthy baby is remarkably resilient and obviously withstands deviations from its physiological expectations, but the more frail, more immature babies are probably more dependent on all the natural support they can obtain, yet these are the ones most likely to be immediately deprived of it, so that they can be rapidly transferred to the technological equipment for resuscitation in the intensive care ward. A randomized control trial showed that delay of only thirty seconds in severing the cord of preterm infants led to a milder form of respiratory distress with a much shorter period of oxygen dependence [103].

Nature also intended that an infant's air passages should be able to clear themselves and be ready to take over their respiratory function immediately on arrival. This would be the experience of healthy, mature infants, unless they were sedated and depressed through sharing the anaesthetic or analgesic drugs given to the mother (page 174). So many hospital-born infants have had to share their mothers' drugs that artificial suctioning of airways has become a routine hospital practice, regardless of individual need and of the potential damage to the infant's respiratory and cardiac systems [15, p. 179]. Less healthy and immature infants are at even greater danger from secondary sedation. Analysis of the results of the 1970 survey showed that breathing difficulties were much more often suffered by, and proved fatal to, babies born in hospital, despite the fact that a much greater proportion of them were transferred to special care units [104].

For such babies whose breathing reflex has been damaged by intranatal care, postnatal resuscitation is essential. Since 1970 technological advances, at high financial cost, have made possible a manifold increase in the numbers receiving ventilatory support and in their chances of survival. By the late 1980s data from the Northern Health Region of England show that just over 1% of live births were so treated for non-surgical reasons, with about three-quarters of all those ventilated surviving until fit for hospital discharge [105]. The more babies who survive but need this treatment, the higher is the total cost of neonatal care. But that is not the end of the cost, for the methods of resuscitation can themselves inflict further damage and leave the ventilated babies at increased risk of other respiratory disorders needing treatment in infancy and childhood [106–108].

Mature infants are born with the instinct to suck and a digestive system to process the intake. Their involuntary infusion of drugs can impair both these functions. Their feeding problems have to be overcome with artificial assistance, as have those of the infants born too immature for the sucking instinct and digestive system to have adequately developed.

For the proliferation of more radical interventions obstetricians were dependent on advances in anaesthetic and surgical techniques, in asepsis and pharmacology. But they came to be no less dependent on advances in neonatology for rescuing infants who emerged from the labour wards with impaired chances of survival. Yet the scale of this dependence may have become exaggerated, for a survey in an English Health Region in 1990 found that as many as 40% of the admissions to a neonatal unit were unnecessary [26, p. 450] and this prompted the health authority concerned to ask the purchasers of the service to review admission criteria with the providers [26, p. 369].

Life in the neonatal unit is far from restful. Constant monitoring indicates the need for frequent treatments, painful enough for the baby to resent and fear. It is difficult to believe that there will be no lasting psychological damage from this troubled early experience. The psychological damage may be aggravated by the early separation from the mother which intensive care necessitates, and to the mother who is more likely to suffer psychological damage after intranatal interventions, early separation may be the last straw [109, 110].

OBSTETRICIANS' CONCESSIONS TO CLIENTS' DEMANDS

Social surveys of women's attitudes to the maternity service invariably uncover satisfaction with some aspects of it but also widespread and serious dissatisfaction with others. The complaints have been felt keenly enough for reforming associations to be formed (pages 234–40). These submitted well-researched evidence to the House of Commons Health Committee's Inquiry in 1990–2 and several individual mothers felt strongly enough to submit personal accounts of their experiences. The Committee's Report [111], followed by *Changing Childbirth* [101], left no doubt that the existing service still did not nearly meet women's genuine needs, although obstetricians have not been utterly impervious to the mounting criticism and since the late 1970s have thought it prudent to agree to palliative changes. American obstetricians on the whole have been less accommodating.

Humanizing hospitals

To keep abreast of rising standards of home comfort and patients' expectations, all hospitals in recent decades have softened the austerity of their surroundings. Maternity hospitals also have tried to give labour wards more home-like furnishings and a few have gone so far as to provide alternative birth rooms, in which they discreetly conceal the apparatus for technological interventions with a view to reducing the apprehension these inspire, while having them available for immediate use as required. Obstetricians have considered it politic to provide as far as possible the reassuring environment valued by the proponents of home birth, so that they can claim to offer the best of both worlds.

Offering the best of both worlds was hospital obstetricians' expressed justification for their policy of replacing 'isolated' general practitioner maternity units on separate sites with 'integrated' units on the same site. Results in Britain and other countries (pages 220, 339) have consistently shown that such integration facilitates the infiltration of the stronger influence of hospital-trained obstetricians and midwives, with more frequent diagnosis of complications, wider use of interventions and worse outcomes for mother and child. The same is true of 'integrated' birth rooms.

In the home setting without interventions and without equipment at hand, complications which need such equipment do not often actually arise. If all the essentials of the home setting were faithfully replicated in hospital – and the intimacy of home is difficult to recreate in the large hospitals now recommended – the equipment would be little needed and little used. The need for obstetricians would be much reduced, so would be the need for new obstetricians and the opportunity to train them. It is only too plausible that they would find excuses to justify using the equipment and installing further sophisticated innovations, by diagnosing, as they have so often done in the past, complications that do not exist. If obstetric interventions were only used for the few complications where they really do reduce the risk (and which these are has still to be unequivocally demonstrated), hospitals could indeed justify their claim of offering the best of both worlds, but such restraint has not been observed in the past, and indeed is completely contrary to obstetricians' philosophy and self-destructive to their profession.

Suspicion that this would be their reaction is fuelled by their tactics when the Royal College of Obstetricians and Gynaecologists, in collaboration with the National Birthday Trust, carried out a national survey of the facilities – staff and equipment – available at all the places of birth in 1984, without at the same time collecting information measuring outcome in any way, so that the effectiveness of the facilities, individually or as a whole, could not be evaluated [79]. This omission could be interpreted as betraying (well-grounded) fear, that results would show that the facilities do not make birth safer. Without such frank contradiction, the impression could be left unchallenged that the facilities enumerated improve outcome, that birth is safest in the places where there are the most technological equipment and specialist staff, which would of course be the large obstetric hospitals. This is the unshaken but unsubstantiated belief reiterated in their submissions to the House of Commons Health Inquiry by individual obstetricians and their organized body, the RCOG [111]. Obstetricians are naturally as unwilling as any other occupational group to hasten their own redundancy.

Changing attitudes to posture for birth

Until the 1970s it was hardly questioned wherever modern obstetrics held sway that a woman would give birth lying on her back or side. This is what medical students were taught [20, p. 221], despite the known physiological reasons why an upright position is more efficient in maximizing the pelvic outlet, assisting the descent of the fetus and placenta, in avoiding unnatural strains on the mother's back and abdominal muscles and perineal tissues, and in avoiding the risk of a heavy uterus pressing on a major vein interrupting her venous blood supply.

A randomized trial of low-risk mothers in South America reporting in 1979 found that the group giving birth upright had easier, shorter labours and less pain [15, pp. 50–1]. In the 1970s, Michel Odent, was developing his philosophy that the natural physiology of labour should not be disturbed and devising a suitable setting in his hospital at Pithiviers near Paris where this could happen, where women were not confined in bed but could move around and find the positions which best suited them. Although his system was not scientifically evaluated, his publicized message created great interest [112].

At the same time some women, rebelling against the increased medicalization and regimentation of birth, were informing themselves about physiological facts and realizing that many obstetric birth practices promoted neither greater safety nor greater satisfaction. In particular they latched on to the advantages of free choice of posture, in fact reverting to the accepted practice of earlier centuries when women could walk around and stand, sit, kneel, squat or lie to give birth, as nature prompted. In the late 1970s a group of these women attempted to give birth in upright positions in a London hospital. One obstetrician was sympathetic, but others so strongly disapproved that the practice was banned. This provoked the foundation of the Active Birth Movement in 1982 and the writing of the Active Birth Manifesto, which set down the physiological disadvantages of a recumbent posture and the physiological advantages of upright postures, especially supported squatting, which mothers could adopt to suit their individual feelings. Also provoked was a public protest rally, where some 6000 women demanded the right to vary their posture when giving birth [113]. In face of their demands, some obstetricians relaxed hospital regimens, invested in bean bags and birth chairs, though the benefit of these had not been proven, and accepted the greater inconvenience for the birth attendant, usually the midwife, so long as their requirements for electronic fetal monitoring and intravenous medication had priority and the women were in bed for the examinations in which the obstetricians were involved.

The 1980s saw a gradual extension of this concession on posture, but often the concession is only a compromise, to a semi-recumbent or semi-sitting position, which gains only slightly more assistance from gravity and still leaves the weight of the body resting on the sacrum (the second lowest bone of the spinal column), thus restricting by up to 30% the maximum widening of the pelvic outlet. In this way obstetricians sought to pacify critics and accommodate this potential threat to their professional domination. American obstetricians have so far been less responsive to the proponents of Active Birth. The lithotomy position is still in frequent use there [45].

Making good the lack of moral support

The historic function of the midwife had been to give the labouring woman not only physical help but also continuous companionship and support, the latter service being no less important than the former. When birth took place at home support could also be given by members of the family and friends, usually female. As hospitalization increased and hospital staffs concentrated on the physical aspects of birth, the mother's emotional needs were neglected. Attention to instruments took precedence over attention to women; midwives, far less doctors, had not time to attend to both. Women complained bitterly of their emotional isolation. Lay antenatal teachers at the classes organized by, for example, the National Childbirth Trust appreciated the need and began to infiltrate the hospital system and gained permission to sit with the labouring woman they had 'prepared' (page 235). Gradually hospitals acquiesced, indeed welcomed, the presence of lay companions who thus eased their work load. The role of participating companion/helper has been extended to any friend of the mother and especially to willing fathers, who were formerly excluded and left to pace the corridors outside. Most readily tolerated are fathers who, like their partners, have been 'prepared' in antenatal classes. In environments where women cannot be given continuous support by midwives or chosen companions, outcomes would be greatly improved by the provision of a 'doula' (pages 162–3).

Something for nothing

The obstetricians' modest concessions all have the obvious merit of making the procedures more pleasant for the mother, and in addition have the underlying merit of making the outcome safer. Thus doctor/ patient relationships are smoothed, immediately and ultimately. These modest changes represent sheer gain for the obstetrician for, while reducing the workload on staff, they involve no sacrifice of his clinical dominance, no threat to the supremacy of his profession, with its philosophy of the ultimate superiority of the medical management of childbirth. Nor is this threatened by the lesser frequency in the 1980s of induction, forceps deliveries and episiotomies, for these interventions are still undertaken often enough to impress everyone that they are necessary instruments for dealing with the ever possible obstetric emergencies against which, as obstetricians continue to assert, obstetric management in obstetric hospitals is the only safe insurance [111].

On present showing, it is unlikely that obstetricians would be prepared to trade something for something, if the concession required an appreciable surrender of power.

REFERENCES

1. Towler, J. and Bramall, J. (1986) *Midwives in History and Society*, Croom Helm, London.
2. Towler, J. and Bramall, J. *Midwives in History* (Quoting J. Sharp (1671) *The Midwives Book*, London).
3. Towler, J. and Bramall, J., *Midwives in History* (Quoting P. Willoughby (c 1650) *Observations on Midwifery. A Country Midwife's Opusculum*, University of Manchester. Radford Collection).
4. Munro Kerr, J.M. (1954) Obstetric operations, in *Historical Review of British Obstetrics and Gynaecology, 1800–1950* (eds J.M. Munro Kerr, R.W. Johnstone and M.H. Phillips), Livingstone, Edinburgh, Chaps VI (1800–50), XII (1850–1900) and XX (1900–50).
5. Wertz, R.W. and Wertz, D.C. (1977) *Lying-in: A History of Childbirth in America*, The Free Press, New York.
6. Donnison, J. (1977) *Midwives and Medical Men*, Heinemann, London.
7. Gaskin, I.-M. (1992) Head Midwife, The Farm, Tennessee, personal communication.
8. Mangay-Maglacas, A. and Pizurki, H. (eds) (1981) *The Traditional Birth Attendant in Seven Countries: Case Studies in Utilisation and Training*, Public Health Papers 75, World Health Organisation, Geneva.
9. Berkeley, C. (1929) The teaching of midwifery. *J. Obstet. Gynaecol. Br. Emp.*, **37**, 701–55.
10. Llewellyn Jones, D. (1982) *Fundamentals of Obstetrics and Gynaecology Vol. 1, Obstetrics*, 3rd edn, Faber & Faber, London, Chap. 50.
11. Claye, A.M. (1954) Obstetric anaesthesia and analgesia, in *Historical Review of British Obstetrics and Gynaecology, 1800–1950* (eds J.M. Munro Kerr, R.W. Johnstone and M.H. Phillips), Livingstone, Edinburgh, chap. XXVII.
12. Siddall, A.C. (1980) Blood-letting in American obstetric practice 1800–1945. *Bull. Hist. Med.*, **54**, 101–10.
13. General Register Office (1843) *Fifth Annual Report of the Registrar General*, HMSO, London, pp. 380–93.
14. Holmes, O. Wendell (1843) The contagiousness of puerperal fever. *New Engl. Q. J. Med.*, April, 503–3.

15. Inch, S. (1982) *Birthrights*, Hutchinson, London.
16. Cookson, I. (1967) The past and future of the maternity services. *J. Coll. Gen. Pract.*, **13**, 143–62.
17. Johnstone, R.W. (1954) The haemorrhages, in *Historical Review of British Obstetrics 1800–1950* (eds J. Munro Kerr, R. Johnston and M. Phillips), Livingstone, Edinburgh, chap. XVII.
18. *Maternity in Great Britain* (1946) (Survey undertaken by a Joint Committee of the Royal College of Obstetricians and Gynaecologists and the Population Investigation Committee), Oxford University Press, Oxford, p. 63.
19. Butler, N.R. and Bonham, D.G. (1963) *Perinatal Mortality*, Churchill Livingstone, Edinburgh.
20. Chamberlain, G., Philipp, E., Howlett, B. and Masters, K. (1978) *British Births 1970, Vol. 2, Obstetric Care*, Heinemann, London.
21. Tomkinson, J.S. (ed.) (1970) *The Queen Charlotte's Textbook of Obstetrics*, 12th edn, Churchill, London.
22. Office of Population Censuses and Surveys Monitors (1981, 1984) *Maternity Statistics MB4*, HMSO, London.
23. Williams R. and Studd, J. (1980) Induction of labour. *J. Matern. Child Health*, **5.1**, 16–21.
24. Stirrat, G.M. (1985) Overall trends in obstetrics, in *Modern Obstetrics in General Practice*, (ed. G. Marsh), Oxford University Press, Oxford, p. 19.
25. Macfarlane, A. (1978) Variations in numbers of births and perinatal mortality by day of week in England and Wales. *Br. Med. J.*, **2**, 167.
26. House of Commons Health Committee (1992) *Maternity Services*, vol. II, HMSO, London, pp. 338–650.
27. Fleissig, A. (1993) Prevalence of procedures in childbirth. *Br. Med. J.*, **306**, 494–5.
28. Chalmers, I. and Keirse, M. (1989) Evaluating elective delivery, in *Effective Care in Pregnancy and Childbirth* (eds I. Chalmers, M. Enkin and M. Keirse), Oxford University Press, Oxford, chap. 60, pp. 981–7.
29. Gordon-Wright, A. and Elder, M. (1979) Prostaglandin E_2 tablets used intravaginally for the induction of labour. *Br. J. Obstet. Gynaecol.*, **86**, 32–6.
30. Fraser, W., Sauve, R. *et al.* (1991) A randomized controlled trial of early amniotomy. *Br. J. Obstet. Gynaecol.*, **98**, 84–91.
31. Steer, P. (1988) Risks of labour, in *Pregnancy and Risk* (eds D. James and G. Stirrat), John Wiley, Chichester.
32. O'Driscoll, K. (1975) An obstetrician's view of pain. *Br. J. Anaesth.*, **47**, 1053–9.
33. Cohen, W.R. (1977) Influence of the duration of second stage labor on perinatal outcome and puerperal morbidity. *Obstet. Gynecol.*, **49**, 266–9.
34. Bennett, R. and Brown, L. (eds) (1989) *Myles Text Book for Midwives*, 11th edn, Churchill Livingstone, Edinburgh.
35. Saunders, N., Paterson, C. *et al.* (1992) Neonatal and maternal morbidity in relation to the length of the second stage of labour. *Br. J. Obstet. Gynaecol.*, **99**, 381–5.
36. Bull, M.J.V. (1985) Intervention in labour: acceleration, induction and other

'active' procedures, in *Modern Obstetrics in General Practice* (ed. G. Marsh), Oxford University Press, Oxford, pp. 300–9.

37. Keirse, M. (1989) Augmentation of labour, in *Effective Care in Pregnancy and Childbirth* (eds I. Chalmers, M. Enkin and M. Keirse), Oxford University Press, Oxford, chap. 58.

38. Department of Health and Social Security/Office of Population Censuses and Surveys (1988) *Hospital Inpatient Enquiry (England) Maternity Tables 1982–1985, Series MB4 no. 28*, HMSO, London, Tables 2.2, 4.5.

39. Reynolds, J.L., Yudkin, P. and Bull, M. (1988) General practitioner obstetrics: does risk prediction work? *J. R. Coll. Gen. Pract.*, **38**, 307–10.

40. Jowitt, M. (1993) *Childbirth Unmasked: (The Science, Art and Humanity of Childbirth)*, Peter Wooller, Craven Arms, Shropshire.

41. Kennell, J., Klaus, M. *et al.* (1991) Continuous emotional support during labor in a US hospital: a randomized controlled trial. *J. Am. Med. Assoc.*, **265**, 2197–2201.

42. Tew, M. (1986) Do obstetric intranatal interventions make birth safer? *Br. J. Obstet. Gynaecol.*, **93**, 659–74.

43. Hoult, I.J., Maclennan, A.H. and Carrie, L.E.S. (1977) Lumbar epidural analgesia in labour: relation to fetal malposition and instrumental delivery. *Br. Med. J.*, **1**, 14–16.

44. Llewellyn Jones, D. (1971) *Fundamentals of Obstetrics and Gynaecology. Vol. 1. Obstetrics*, 1st edn, Faber and Faber, London, p. 340.

45. Korte, D. and Scaer, R. (1993) *A Good Birth: A Safe Birth*, Harvard Common Press, Harvard, Massachusetts.

46. Chalmers, J. and Chalmers, I. (1989) The obstetric vacuum extractor is the instrument of first choice for operative vaginal delivery. *Br. J. Obstet. Gynaecol.*, **96**, 505–6.

47. Sleep, J. (1991) Perineal care: a series of five randomised controlled trials, in *Midwives Research and Childbirth*, vol. 2 (eds S. Robinson and A. Thomson), Chapman and Hall, London, pp. 199–251.

48. Simpson, D. (1988) Examining the episiotomy argument. *Midwife, Health Visitor and Community Nurse*, **24**, 6–17.

49. Thacker, S. (1987) The efficacy of intrapartum fetal monitoring. *Am. J. Obstet. Gynecol.*, **156**, 24–30.

50. Thorpe, J. and Bowes, W. (1989) Episiotomy: can its routine use be defended? *Am. J. Obstet. Gynecol.*, **160**, 1027–30.

51. Department of Health and Social Security/Office of Population Censuses and Surveys (1986) *Hospital Inpatient Enquiry Maternity Tables 1977–1981, Series MB4, no. 19*, Table 4.5, HMSO, London.

52. Sleep, J., Roberts, J. and Chalmers, I. (1989) The second stage of labour, in *A Guide to Effective Care in Pregnancy and Childbirth* (eds M. Enkin, M. Keirse and I. Chalmers), Oxford University Press, Oxford, p. 231.

53. Kennedy, R. and Patel, N. (1986) The significance of increasing caesarean section rates. *Br. J. Hosp. Med.*, November, 336–4.

54. Savage, W. and Francome, C. (1993) British caesarean section rates: have we reached a plateau? *Br. J. Obstet. Gynaecol.*, **100**, 493–6.

55. King, J. (1993) Obstetric interventions and economic imperatives. *Br. J. Obstet. Gynaecol.*, **100**, 303–4.
56. Gould, J., Davey, B. and Stafford, R. (1989) Socio-economic differences in rates of caesarean section. *N. Engl. J. Med.*, **321**, 233–9.
57. Goyert, G., Bottoms, S. *et al.* (1989) The physician factor in caesarean birth rates. *N. Engl. J. Med.*, **320**, 706–9.
58. Yudkin, P. and Redman, C.W.G. (1986) Caesarean section dissected, 1978–1983. *Br. J. Obstet. Gynaecol.*, **93**, 135–44.
59. Enkin, M. (1989) Labour and delivery after previous caesarean section, in *A Guide to Effective Care in Pregnancy and Childbirth* (eds M. Enkin, M. Keirse and I. Chalmers), Oxford University Press, Oxford.
60. Mann, L.I. and Gallant, J.M. (1979) Modern management of the breech delivery. *Am. J. Obstet. Gynaecol.*, **134**, 611–14.
61. Oian, P., Skramm, I. *et al.* (1988) Breech delivery. An obstetric analysis. *Acta Obstet. Scand.*, **67**, 75–9.
62. Thorpe-Beeston, J., Banfield, P. and Saunders, N. (1992) Outcome of breech delivery at term. *Br. Med. J.*, **305**, 746–7.
63. Lilford, R., De Groot, H. *et al.* (1990) The relative risks of caesarean section (intrapartum and elective) and vaginal delivery: a detailed analysis to exclude the effects of medical disorders and other acute pre-existing physiological disturbances. *Br. J. Obstet. Gynaecol.*, **97**, 883–92.
64. Hofmeyr, G. (1989) Suspected fetopelvic disproportion and abnormal lie, in *A Guide to Effective Care in Pregnancy and Childbirth* (eds M. Enkin, M. Keirse and I. Chalmers), Oxford University Press, Oxford.
65. Hall, M., Chng, P. and Macgillivray, I. (1980) Is routine antenatal care worth while? *Lancet*, **ii**, 78–80.
66. Pinion, S. and Mowat, J. (1988) Pre-term caesarean section. *Br. J. Obstet. Gynaecol.*, **95**, 277–80.
67. Harley, J.M.G. (1980) Caesarean section. *Clin. Obstet. Gynaecol.*, **7**, 529–57.
68. O'Driscoll, K. and Foley, M. (1983) Correlation of decrease in perinatal mortality and increase in caesarean section rates. *Obstet. Gynaecol.*, **61**, 1–5.
69. Chamberlain, G., Wraight, A. and Steer, P. (1993) *Pain and its Relief in Childbirth*, Churchill Livingstone, Edinburgh.
70. Rosen, M. (1975) Survey of current methods of pain relief in labour, in *The Management of Labour* (eds R. Beard, M. Bradwell, P. Dunn and D. Fairweather), Proceedings of the Third Study Group of the Royal College of Obstetricians and Gynaecologists, London, pp. 140–8.
71. Lim, K.B. and Hawkins, D. F. (1985) Intervention in labour: drugs in normal labour, in *Modern Obstetrics in General Practice* (ed. G. Marsh), Oxford University Press, Oxford, p. 295.
72. Thomson, A. and Hillier, V. (1994) A re-evaluation of the effect of pethidine on the length of labour. *Journal of Advanced Nursing*, **19**, 448–56.
73. Richards, M. (1978) A place of safety? An examination of the risks of hospital delivery, in *The Place of Birth* (eds S. Kitzinger and J. Davis), Oxford University Press, Oxford, chap. 5, pp. 66–84.
74. Reynolds, F. (1989) Epidural analgesia in obstetrics. *Br. Med. J.*, **299**, 751–2.
75. Rosenblatt, D., Belsey, E. *et al.* (1981) The influence of maternal analgesia

on neonatal behaviour: epidural bupivacaine. *Br. J. Obstet. Gynaecol.*, **88**, 407–13.

76. MacArthur, C. (1990) Epidural anaesthesia and long term backache after childbirth. *Br. Med. J.*, **301**, 9–12.

77. MacArthur, C., Lewis, M. and Knox, E. (1991) *Health After Childbirth*, University of Birmingham, HMSO, London.

78. Association of Anaesthetists of Great Britain and Ireland (1987) *Anaesthetic Services for Obstetrics – A Plan for the Future*, London.

79. Chamberlain, G. and Gunn, P. (1987) *Birthplace: The Report of the Confidential Enquiry into Facilities Available at the Place of Birth*, John Wiley, Chichester.

80. Jacobson, B., Nyberg, K. *et al.* (1990) Opiate addiction in adult offspring through possible imprinting after obstetric treatment. *Br. Med. J.*, **301**, 1067–70.

81. Lotgering, F., Wallenburg, H. and Schouten, H. (1982) Interobserver and intraobserver variation in the assessment of antepartum cardiotocograms. *Am. J. Obstet. Gynecol.*, **144**, 701–5.

82. Godfrey, K.A. (1985) Interventions in labour: machines in labour, in *Modern Obstetrics in General Practice* (ed. G. Marsh), Oxford University Press, Oxford, chap. 23, p. 313.

83. Edington, P., Sibanda, J. and Beard, R.W. (1975) Influence on clinical practice of routine intrapartum fetal monitoring. *Br. Med. J.*, **3**, 341–3.

84. Prentice, A. and Lind, T. (1987) Fetal heart rate monitoring during labour – too frequent intervention, too little benefit? *Lancet*, **ii**, 1375–7.

85. Banta, D. and Thacker, S. (1979) Assessing the costs and benefits of electronic fetal monitoring. *Obstet. Gynaecol. Surv.*, **34**, 627–42.

86. Friedman, E. (1986) The obstetrician's dilemma. *N. Engl. J. Med.*, **315**, 611–13.

87. Leveno, K., Cunningham, F. *et al.* (1986) A prospective comparison of selective and universal electronic fetal monitoring in 34 995 pregnancies. *N. Engl. J. Med.*, **315**, 615–19.

88. Shy, K., Luthy, D. *et al.* (1990) Effects of fetal-heart-rate monitoring as compared with periodic auscultation on the neurological development of premature infants. *N. Engl. J. Med.*, **322**, 588–93.

89. MacDonald, D., Grant, A. *et al.* (1985) The Dublin randomised controlled trial of intrapartum fetal heart rate monitoring. *Am. J. Obstet. Gynecol.*, **152**, 524–39.

90. Grant, A., O'Brien, N. *et al.* (1989) Cerebral palsy among children born during the Dublin randomized controlled trial of interpartum monitoring. *Lancet*, **ii**, 1233–6.

91. Spencer, J. (1993) Clinical overview of cardiotocography. *Br. J. Obstet. Gynaecol.*, **100** (Suppl. Cardiotocograph Technology), 6–7.

92. Symonds, E. (1993) Litigation and the cardiotocogram. *Br. J. Obstet. Gynaecol.*, **100** (Suppl. Cardiotocograph Technology), 8–9.

93. Johnson, C., Keirse, M. *et al.* (1989) Malnutrition and position in labour, in *A Guide to Effective Care in Pregnancy and Childbirth* (eds M. Enkin, M. Keirse and I. Chalmers). Oxford University Press, Oxford, chap. 31, pp. 183–9.

94. Turnbull, A.C. (1976) Traditional uses of ergot compounds. *Postgrad. Med. J.*, **5** (Suppl.), 15–16.
95. Browning, D.J. (1974) Serious side-effects of ergometrine and its use in routine obstetric practice. *Med. J. Aust.*, **1**, 957–8.
96. Gilbert, L., Porter, W. and Brown, A. (1987) Postpartum haemorrhage – a continuing problem. *Br. J. Obstet. Gynaecol.*, **94**, 67–71.
97. Hall, M., Halliwell, R. and Carr-Hill, R. (1985) Concomitant and repeated happenings of complications of the third stage of labour. *Br. J. Obstet. Gynaecol.*, **92**, 732–8.
98. Prendiville, W., Harding, J. *et al.* (1988) The Bristol third stage trial: active versus physiological management of third stage of labour. *Br. Med. J.*, **297**, 1295–1300.
99. Begley, C. (1990) A comparison of 'active' and 'physiological' management of the third stage of labour. *Midwifery*, **6**, 3–17.
100. House of Commons Health Committee (1991) *Maternity Services: Preconception*, vol. II, HMSO, London, pp. 1–291.
101. Department of Health (1993) *Changing Childbirth Part I: Report of the Expert Maternity Group*, HMSO, London.
102. Chamberlain, R., Chamberlain, G., Howlett, B. *et al.* (1975) *British Births 1970. Vol. 1. The First Week of Life*, Heinemann, London, chap. 6.
103. Kinmond, S., Aitchison, T. *et al.* (1993) Umbilical cord clamping and preterm infants: a randomized trial. *Br. Med. J.*, **306**, 172–4.
104. Tew, M. (1980) Facts not assertions of belief. *Health Soc. Serv. J.*, 12 September, 1194–7.
105. NRHA (Northern Regional Health Authority) (1989) *Collaborative Survey of Perinatal, Late Neonatal and Infant Deaths in the Northern Region*, NRHA.
106. Skeoch, C., Rosenberg, K. *et al.* (1987) Very low birthweight survivors: illness and readmission to hospital in the first 15 months of life. *Br. Med. J.*, **2**, 579–80.
107. Powell, T.G., Pharoah, P.O.D. and Cooke, R.W.I. (1986) Survival and morbidity in a geographically defined population of low birthweight infants. *Lancet*, **i**, 539–43.
108. Steiner, E., Sanders, E. *et al.* (1980) Very low birthweight children at school: comparison of neonatal management methods. *Br. Med. J.*, **281**, 1237–40.
109. Gordon, B. (1978) The vulnerable mother and her child, in *The Place of Birth* (eds. S. Kitzinger and J. Davies), Oxford University Press, Oxford, chap. 13, pp. 201–15.
110. Klaus, M. and Kennell, J. (1972) Maternal attachment – importance of the first postpartum days. *N. Engl. J. Med.*, **285**, 460–3.
111. House of Commons Health Committee (1992) *Maternity Services*, vol. I, HMSO, London, paras 1–458, pp. i–xciii.
112. Odent, M. (1984) *Birth Reborn*, Souvenir Press, London.
113. Balaskas, J. (1989) *New Active Birth*, Unwin, London.

5

Maternity care: a public concern

AWAKENING TO THE NEED

Until the foundation in the later 18th century of the charitable lying-in hospitals and dispensaries for the relief of the sick poor, maternity care, like medical care in general in Britain, was a matter only of personal concern. The concept of public health began to develop in the 19th century when the important influence on it of the physical environment, particularly in the rapidly growing towns, was coming to be realized. Enlightened policies were implemented by sanitary engineers for the provision of uncontaminated water supplies and the safe removal of sewage. These ambitious reforms were soon rewarded by striking reductions in deaths from cholera, typhoid and other infections. The extent of these reductions could be measured, for since 1837 in England and Wales and 1855 in Scotland the State had made the registration of deaths compulsory.

In the treatment of disease there was a recognized need to protect people from the activities of unqualified practitioners and in this the public interest coincided with the interest of the established medical profession. After much political agitation, the State intervened to pass in 1886 an Act of Parliament, the *Medical Registration Act*, restricting the practice of medicine to those doctors who showed an understanding of medicine, surgery and midwifery, to a standard considered satisfactory by the relevant professional bodies. This State intervention was followed in 1902 by the *Midwives Act*, which similarly restricted midwifery practitioners and set up machinery for regulating the training of midwives (as discussed in Chapter 2). Thus by the 20th century, the State had sanctioned the professional monopolies of birth attendants. It took more time for the framework in which they were to function to develop.

The recruitment of soldiers for the Boer War had drawn public attention to the poor physical condition of young men. Concern was such that the government set up an Interdepartmental Committee on the Physical Deterioration of the Population which reported in 1904 [1]. Its recommendations emphasized the need for improving the social conditions of the poor, the education of mothers and the welfare of infants and young children, particularly their nutrition. Legislation towards this end followed and some financial assistance was given through the Local Government Board to local authorities to set up milk depots, schools for mothers and to employ health visitors (discussed in Chapter 3). The *National Insurance Act* of 1911, which instituted compulsory medical insurance for low-paid workers, allowed the men's wives and women workers a cash maternity benefit, which for most was equal to at least half their weekly wage.

By 1914, the Local Government Board's flow of advisory circulars were referring to the need for medical advice and treatment for expectant mothers [2–8]. From this tender beginning was to grow the general provision of municipal antenatal clinics, which, like their provisions of subsidized milk supplements and their employment of salaried midwives for necessitous mothers, local authorities were empowered to fund under the *Maternity and Child Welfare Act* of 1918. They also had to reimburse doctors whom under the second *Midwives Act* of 1918 midwives were compelled to call in cases of emergency.

THE CREATION OF THE MINISTRY OF HEALTH

The nation's health was becoming accepted as a proper subject for public involvement and to deal with the issues of concern the government set up, in 1919, the Ministry of Health, with a separate department for maternity and child welfare to which was appointed a very able and highly motivated Senior Medical Officer, Dr Janet Campbell. She promptly set in train a series of investigations into the teaching of obstetrics in medical schools, into the training of midwives and into maternal and infant mortality, leading to influential reports which appeared between 1923 and 1932 [9–14].

From her sample enquiry [14] she concluded that 'avoidable maternal deaths are a matter of every-day occurrence' and, although her methodology of examining only deaths and not survivors prevented her from making 'trustworthy comparisons' between outcome and contributory factors, she felt able 'with some confidence (to) assign responsibility primarily to *the adequacy or otherwise of the professional attention during pregnancy and at the time of birth*' [14, p. 55]. She found, with some surprise, that puerperal infection, the chief cause of maternal death, was not associated with the insanitary surroundings found in many homes, but that 'manual interference of any kind (including the use of forceps) inevitably increases risk of infection' and 'when the means of securing full surgical cleanliness and antisepsis are lacking . . . the risk is proportionately increased' [14, p. 90].

Her findings led her to recommend an improvement, through education, in the quality of professional attendants and the extension of social and educational measures – diet supplementation where necessary and widespread propaganda directed at the women themselves and the general public to convince everyone of the importance of attention to health throughout childbearing. The public was to be involved also through the local authorities which should provide preventive midwifery, antenatally and postnatally in maternity outpatient clinics and inpatient prenatal beds, as well as intranatally in more hospital beds and should subsidize 'a sufficient service of competent (domiciliary) midwives'. They should also finance 'investigation by the Medical Officer of Health of all maternal deaths due to childbirth and of all cases of puerperal infection, whether fatal or not.' For '. . . the establishment of a comprehensive and efficient Maternity Service designed steadily to improve the standard of midwifery and thus to eliminate the avoidable risks of childbearing is largely a matter of administration and finance' [14, pp. 90–3].

Dr Campbell's recommendations were soon followed by vigorous activity on the part of obstetricians through the setting up of their professional college to raise not only their own standards of technical competence but also those of their non-specialist colleagues (Chapter 2). They were able to extend their inadequate training facilities by persuading the local authorities to upgrade obstetric and gynaecology units in the former poor law hospitals which the Local Government Act of 1929 had transferred to municipal control [15, p. 84]. Likewise, the Central Midwives Board further upgraded the required qualifications for midwives (also discussed in Chapter 2). The scope of diet supplementation, with its potential benefits, was restricted by those local authorities which limited expenditure by imposing irksome and sometimes humiliating rules which applicants had to satisfy to prove their need, but the principle survived. Propaganda was certainly broadcast as recommended, but since it was not known in what way the maternity services offered would improve maternal health, the process of education had to be based on surmise and became heavily biased in favour of the most confident birth attendants, the obstetricians.

Official enquiries into maternal deaths were carried out and in due course became routine, but since they perpetuated Dr Campbell's methodology, being an audit of one aspect of the problem and not an evaluation of the total problem, they shed only limited light on the causative factors (pages 292–304). Reports in 1930 [16] and 1932 [17] attributed 33% of the avoidable deaths to the lack of antenatal care and a further 17% to the mother's own negligence. These were grounds for emphasizing the need to educate the mother, especially about the importance of attending for antenatal care, although they had no actual evidence that antenatal procedures improved the chance of survival (Chapter 3).

Financial uncertainties about providing 'a sufficient service of competent domiciliary midwives' were settled by the third *Midwives Act* of 1936, which charged the local authorities in England and Wales, as did the 1937 *Maternity Services Act* in Scotland, with paying midwives salaries either directly or through voluntary associations, so replacing the independent midwife. As employees of the local authority, all midwives could now count on a regular income, off-duty time and annual leave and could participate in the municipal antenatal clinics [18, p. 226].

The government in war-time Britain demonstrated its concern for childbearing women by arranging for the evacuation of those living in towns at risk from air raids to make-shift premises in safer locations in the country and by allowing them extra food rations and dietary supplements, both provisions being rewarded with unexpectedly favourable results (pages 287, 314).

THE 1946 SURVEY OF MATERNITY IN GREAT BRITAIN

Society had initially become concerned about the maternity service because it feared that a falling birth rate and a high infant mortality rate would lead to a decline in population and a loss of political power. The same concern was felt in the 1930s, despite the fall in infant mortality, and in 1936 a Population Investigation Committee was set up. In 1946, with the collaboration of the Royal College of Obstetricians and Gynaecologists (RCOG) – now the acknowledged experts in the field – it carried out an inquiry into pregnancy and childbirth, in an attempt to identify the reasons for a low birth rate and to provide base-line information for the impending restructuring of the health service.

The joint report bears the imprint of the obstetricians' influence, for the reasoning expressed and the relevant recommendations made were those on which obstetricians were thereafter to rely in pursuing their campaign to medicalize childbirth. The report admitted 'the complete lack of reliable statistics on the provision of antenatal care and the results it achieves' [19, p. 6], but naively interpreted as causal the apparent association between 'regular antenatal supervision, begun early in pregnancy' and 'the low incidence of prematurity and neonatal death and the increased likelihood of breastfeeding' [19, p. 202], disregarding the fact that the early regular attenders were most likely to come from social classes I and II and have these outcomes irrespective of antenatal care. On the basis of this optimistic misinterpretation, which favoured obstetricians' ambitions, the report recommended that 'Greater efforts should be made to publicise the antenatal services and stress the importance of early and regular supervision' [19, p. 210].

Although births at home included disproportionately more of those at higher risk on account of poor housing and high parity, they had much lower stillbirth and neonatal mortality rates than had births in hospital. But some 5% of births booked for home delivery developed complications for which they were transferred to hospital and their mortality was very high. Although in total the risk of booking for home (including the risk of transfer) was less than booking for hospital and although 'a large proportion of mothers would prefer a good domiciliary maternity service' [19, p. 203], the report considered that 'Until the incidence of such emergencies can be reduced, there is a good case for the encouragement of institutional delivery' [19, p. 203], for after all 'if a sufficiency of maternity beds is provided in suitable institutions . . . , there is little doubt that in England, as in America, the institutional habit would be established for the large majority of confinements' [19, p. 204]. However distasteful it was for the birth attendants to deliver women in overcrowded homes, the survey found no increased mortality for the baby, just as Dr Campbell's investigation in 1924 had shown no increased mortality for the mother in insanitary houses.

THE NATIONAL HEALTH SERVICE

The British electorate had become convinced that health was very much a public concern when Parliament passed the *National Health Service Act* in 1946 to transform the health services by making them all free to the user at time of need and paying for them out of general and local taxation and compulsory State health insurance. The Act, which came into force in July 1948, was to facilitate developments in the maternity service not planned by the social reformers.

Its operation added weight to the changing balance between the service users and the service providers and between the competing service providers. It appeared to give mothers more choice, but the new paths were to lead quite soon to ever-decreasing choice. At first they could book care, antenatal and intranatal, from a doctor as well as a midwife and propaganda was telling them that doctors were safer and specialists safest of all; after all they had long been preferred by clients who could afford them. So patronage of local authority antenatal clinics rapidly declined, making redundant the medical officers whose function had been limited to giving advice and leading to the professional downgrading of midwives by depriving them of a centre in which to practise their supervisory skills according to their own principles. Choosing to deliver in hospital with obstetric care was, in due course, to lead to the withdrawal of all other options.

Demand for maternity care from general practitioners immediately increased. Local obstetric committees were set up to prepare an 'obstetric list' of doctors with adequate qualifications and experience in midwifery and around 75% of them were included, but only around 30% were later found to be really interested in the work [20]. The authorized extra payments were sufficient to encourage many general practitioners to offer antenatal care, for they were required to perform only two examinations, but the extra fees encouraged fewer of them to offer intranatal care, for they did not compensate for the extra inconvenience involved. The process of discouragement was steadily to be intensified through the creation of further administrative and professional obstacles.

Obstetricians, like other specialist doctors, agreed to work in the Health Service only if control of hospitals was removed from local authorities and voluntary organizations and transferred to management bodies on which they were well represented and well placed to wield effective power. In this they found a new ally, for a new profession of Health Service administrators had to be created to manage the new structure with its disparate sections, hospitals, general practice and the variety of services provided by local authorities. Of these, hospitals were the tidiest units to comprehend; consultants and hospital doctors became salaried employees of the Hospital Management Committees appointed by the Regional Health Boards, unlike general practitioners who retained their financial autonomy. Hospitals were the places of ultimate treatment for the most serious disorders, which made it easy for the new administrators to accept the specialists' valuation that they were the most important providers of care and hospitals were the most important places of care. Certainly this was so in the maternity field, and administrators apparently did not question that obstetricians were right to claim domination.

THE REPORT OF THE GUILLEBAUD COMMITTEE 1956

Understandably, the new National Health Service soon encountered problems, in particular financial problems to investigate which an official Committee of Enquiry was set up under the chairmanship of C.W. Guillebaud. In the brief reference to the maternity service in its report in 1956 [21, para. 635], it noted

There was a general feeling among witnesses that in most areas 50 per cent would represent an adequate provision for hospital confinement – a view which is shared by the Ministry [of Health]. The Royal College of Obstetricians and Gynaecologists, on the other hand, recommended that 'institutional confinement' provides the maximum safety for mother and child, and therefore the ultimate aim should be to provide obstetric beds for all women who need or will accept institutional confinements.

Since the committee did not feel qualified to judge the medical issues and disagreements involved, it recommended an early review of the maternity services and another committee, under the chairmanship of Lord Cranbrook, was appointed to do this.

THE REPORT OF THE CRANBROOK COMMITTEE 1959

This committee proceeded to take 'evidence' from a wide range of persons representing directly or indirectly the providers and users of the service, 'evidence' comprising accounts of differing actual experience and differing, unevaluated opinions. The opinions which carried most weight, regardless of evaluation, were those of the most prestigious and politically most powerful providers – the hospital specialists. Providers identify the interest of the user with the services it best suits their profession to render. Medical instruction distinguished the users' physical interests from their emotional interests and the former as the more important, but other opinions disagreed.

The Royal College of Obstetricians and Gynaecologists reiterated its unsubstantiated opinion that hospital confinement offered maximum (physical) safety, referring also to the danger of occasional unforeseen complications in home births, while other witnesses canvassed the countervailing (emotional) advantages of home delivery. Epidemiological studies having established that certain maternal characteristics are associated with higher mortality rates, the committee accepted, without proof, the consensus that in such cases hospital confinement was safer, but considered that 'the advantages of home confinement for the apparently normal case probably outweigh the very slight risk of unforeseen complications' [22, para. 57]. Adding the numbers in the higher risk categories to the number of other women persuaded by propaganda to deliver in hospital, the committee estimated that providing hospital beds for 70% of births would generously meet all needs. It further estimated that 20–25% of expectant mothers would need antenatal inpatient care and beds should be provided accordingly [22, paras 70–1]. It rejected the option of increasing hospital accommodation by shortening the length of the postpartum stay from the then standard ten days [22, para. 81]. However, its grounds surely rested less on the supposed welfare of the mothers than on the need for captive subjects to meet the prescribed regulations for the training of midwives in post-natal nursing and to even out the workload for hospital midwives, of whom there was always a shortage because inferior status and working protocols made these appointments less attractive [22, paras 75, 77, 99].

Obstetricians' satisfaction at the recommended increase in hospital beds must have been somewhat alloyed by the rider that the extra lying-in beds should, where possible, be general practitioner beds, to be reserved for normal cases. However, these beds were preferably to be situated within or near obstetric hospitals and under the supervision of a consultant obstetrician [22, para. 258].

Thus, in proposing a framework for intranatal care, the committee sought a compromise which included something to please all the interested care providers. But although it stated that 'Nothing should be done to lessen the importance of the midwife' [22, para. 107], the recommended contraction of domiciliary midwifery did precisely that. The midwife's diminished authority was confirmed by the recommendation that 'a general practitioner obstetrician should, whenever possible, attend all domiciliary confinements, to safeguard the mother and baby against unforeseen emergencies. . . . The conduct of a normal confinement is the joint responsibility of the doctor and midwife' [22, para. 212]. Her unimportance was stressed by omitting the midwife from the participants at the proposed 'clinical meetings which could bring together for discussion of clinical cases all those persons responsible in a particular area for carrying out maternity care' [22, para. 314].

Nor did the committee's recommendations in the field of antenatal care redress this demotion, for in officially acknowledging the reduced role of medical care in the municipal clinic and the redundancy of the local authority medical officer whose work now overlapped with that of the hospital doctor and general practitioner, they tacitly accepted that midwives were being deprived of their best opportunity for responsibility in antenatal supervision (page 71). Whether carried out by midwife or general practitioner, adequate antenatal care had to be provided and the responsibility for ensuring this was placed on the doctor, although doing so would usually require more of him than his two statutory antenatal examinations. The work of the municipal antenatal clinic was henceforth to concentrate on health education and mothercraft instruction, a service given less satisfactorily in hospital and GP antenatal clinics, but not using the primary skills of midwives.

Opinions regarding the professed advantages of hospital confinement and disadvantages of home confinement were advanced by advocates of greater hospitalization, notably by organized obstetricians and the Regional Hospital Boards, while contrary opinions were advanced by its opponents, notably by organized midwives and municipal authorities. Some organizations representing consumers' interests shared the former opinions and some the latter, but always the critical consideration was the greater safety claimed, without evaluation, for hospital birth [22, para. 52]. The committee discerned inconsistency between the hospitals' admission policy and their practice which allowed women, predominantly from the better-off classes, who had been the first to be persuaded of the advantages of hospital care, to make such a large claim on available beds that accommodation was restricted for women in the higher risk categories, predominantly from the poorer classes [22, para. 224].

Did the recommendations by the Cranbrook Committee shape future events or did they at most endorse trends which would have happened without them? By the 1960s, the general consensus was that the first responsibility of the National Health Service was the treatment of disease; professional opinion was that the best method of dispensing treatment was to concentrate facilities in all specialities in a District General Hospital, serving a large enough population to justify the high costs of installing and using the new equipment required by the innovations of expanding technology. Disease was a physical condition to be treated by physical means; if this treatment conflicted with emotional or social factors involved, these were considered of much less importance. It was better to bring patients, even long distances, to centres of expertise than to maintain a scatter of small, poorly equipped, if geographically and socially more convenient, hospitals. A programme of erecting suitable buildings should be embarked on.

These arguments were considered to apply with equal validity to the speciality of obstetrics, although childbirth was not a disease and emotional and social factors were extremely important. Despite the increase in the birth rate, the recommended rate of 70% for hospital confinement was reached in 1965 and by 1968 had risen to 79%. This was achieved partly by an increase of 18% in maternity beds, but mostly by rejecting the Cranbrook recommendation and reducing the average postnatal stay to 6.6 days, leaving it to the community midwives to complete the postnatal care [23, p. 67]. At the same time, demand for their intranatal care was being reduced fast as, after 1964 when the number of births in total began to fall, community midwives were faced with a diminishing proportion of a diminishing number of clients for domiciliary delivery.

THE REPORT OF THE PEEL COMMITTEE 1970

To consider and advise on the related problems of the future of the domiciliary midwifery service and the bed needs of maternity patients (sic, for everyone had now been indoctrinated to accept the medical view that childbearing was an illness, to be treated like other illnesses by doctors), yet another committee, this time a sub-committee of the Minister of Health's Standing Maternity and Midwifery Advisory Committee, was set up in 1967 under the chairmanship of Sir John Peel, then President of the RCOG. It reported its recommendations in 1970 [23].

With the same methods of enquiry and the same disregard for the need to substantiate claims with evaluated results, the Peel Committee did no more than add its seal of approval to the trends that were being set up by the most powerful providers of care. Content to note the rise in institutional confinements and to opine that this made 'discussion of the advantages and disadvantages of home or hospital confinement in one sense academic' [23, para. 248], it recommended that 'sufficient facilities should be provided to allow for 100% hospital delivery' [23, para. 277]. It further recommended that 'Small isolated obstetric units should be replaced by larger combined consultant and general practitioner units in general hospitals' [23, para. 283].

It ignored the view of 59% of the general practitioners, who replied to a questionnaire sent out by local medical committees and who represented 34% of all general practitioners. This minority considered that domiciliary midwifery should continue, believing that 'the present trend towards hospital confinement is largely the result of a misleading pressure on the public, encouraging them to believe that hospital confinement is always better', and their preference for providing maternity services in separate general practitioner hospitals was likewise dismissed [23, Appendix F].

The recommendations regarding place of birth necessarily had implications for birth attendants. The delivery of care through obstetric teams was advocated, the team leaders of course being consultants. Although the number of consultant beds had increased between 1955 and 1968 by only 7%, the number of consultants had increased between 1959 and 1968 by 26%. (Not surprisingly, the rate of forceps deliveries increased by 50% and of caesarean sections by 61% between 1958 and 1966.) To meet the projected increase in workload, including at least two antenatal examinations of every pregnant woman, would require further substantial increases in the number of consultant obstetricians and obstetricians in training.

The increased involvement of general practitioner obstetricians in antenatal and postnatal care, replacing the few remaining local authority doctors, was encouraged and their reduced involvement in intranatal care, which must be restricted to normal cases, was certainly not deplored. Their need for further training in obstetrics was reiterated.

The committee's report confirmed the declining status of the midwifery profession. Midwives were even more rapidly to lose their opportunities for delivering mothers according to their ancient principles of facilitating, but not interfering with, the normal process and in exchange they were to gain opportunities for assisting obstetricians in the 'scientific' management of labour. And if non-interventive midwifery could not be practised, the techniques involved could not be observed and learned by students, either midwives or doctors. In partial compensation, more midwives working in the community were to be attached to general practices where they could build up reassuring relationships with women they would not be allowed to deliver and develop skills in the peripheral aspects of childbearing and childrearing, which doctors did not want to corner for themselves; they could also give reassuring postnatal care to women they had not delivered (pages 71–3).

As for the mothers, the report pointed to a future of less choice of where, and less control of how they could give birth. That there might be some objection to this restriction once the proposals were realized was foreseen by the committee, for its final recommendation was

The changes in professional thought and administrative action which, it is recommended in this report, should flow from it, must be associated with a change in community attitudes towards midwifery and maternity matters. . . . The obstetric team, which we have indicated as necessary for the service itself, should include amongst its responsibilities the education of the community to the desirability and benefits of the reorganisation. [23, para. 286]

Enough members of both the medical and midwifery professions, with greater or lesser enthusiasm, carried out this exhortation, so that community attitudes were effectively changed in the desired direction and opposition to the trends was muted.

Special care baby units

The upward trend in hospital confinements and the downward trend in home confinements continued apace. The Cranbrook report had recommended the setting up of special units to care for sick babies, whether premature or mature. The need for such facilities was accentuated as more babies were delivered by obstetric methods which, it was soon found, increased their chances of suffering morbidity, notably breathing difficulties and neonatal jaundice, although it was argued, without supporting evidence, that the complication for which the intervention was thought to be appropriate would have resulted in more morbidity, if not mortality. More facilities, to be sited in the larger and District General Hospitals, with specially equipped regional referral centres for the most serious cases, were recommended by a series of official committees [24–26].

As units were set up, they were rapidly filled. In 1970 12% of babies born in England and Wales were admitted to such a unit compared with 18.4% in 1975 [27, p. 77]. Mostly, the babies concerned had been delivered in the same hospital [24, para. 6.4], criteria of need where transfer was most convenient being readily adjusted to keep the facility fully used, criteria of need where transfer was less convenient being more strictly applied. Ironically, the stricter criteria seemed to be protective, for analysis of the results of the survey of British Births 1970 showed that babies had both a much smaller chance of suffering breathing difficulties and a much greater chance of surviving them if they were born at home or in a GP unit than in hospital, even though a much greater proportion of the affected babies born in hospital were transferred to special care units [28].

Many other studies found adverse psychological consequences from the imposed separation of mother and baby [27]. Official committees, persuaded by the theoretical arguments of current medical opinion that new diagnostic instruments ought to prevent the causes of most intranatal deaths, overlooked the facts that the need for special, and later neonatal intensive, care facilities was largely created by obstetric intranatal management and that these care facilities in turn introduced their own potential dangers. Recommendations were made as to the numbers of special cots and appropriate levels of staffing required, with even more generous ratios of attendants to cots and of experienced to less experienced attendants for intensive care [24, paras 7.1–7.17]. By the 1980s, medical opinion was realizing the disadvantages of separating the newborn from the mother. Stricter criteria for admission to the special care wards were applied and available cots were underused, but demand for intensive care grew at a level for which it was to prove difficult to provide trained nurses. The improving survival rate of babies of low birthweight was attributed, by the professionals concerned and hence generally, to the use of sophisticated technological equipment and so considered to justify the very high operating costs. However, a review of existing evaluative studies found 'no firm evidence that measures of the use of neonatal intensive care adequately reflect the desire, need or demand for these services. Indeed it is possible that the supply of neonatal intensive care determines its use rather than the converse' [29]. The importance of the supply side was emphasized by the 1988 report on medical care of the newborn, prepared by a working party of the Royal College of Physicians of London, a group almost entirely composed of neonatologists and allied clinicians and nurses with a direct interest. This report recommended more generous provision of intensive and special care cots in relation to births and more generous medical and nursing staffing ratios per cot [30].

THE REPORT OF THE SHORT COMMITTEE 1980

Although the recommendations of the Peel Report, especially with regard to place of birth, had been largely implemented, the House of Commons Social Services Committee under its chairwoman, Mrs Renee Short, felt the need to set up an enquiry into perinatal mortality 'because of mounting public concern that babies were unnecessarily dying or suffering permanent damage during the latter part of pregnancy and the earliest part of infancy' [31, para. 1]. Mortality rates in Britain had certainly fallen, but not as fast as in some other countries and experience still varied widely across social classes and geographic regions. The committee's investigations, which covered many aspects of the problem, and their interpretation of the material presented to them were guided by three expert advisers, respectively Professors of Obstetrics, Paediatrics and Clinical Epidemiology (formerly a paediatrician), whose loyalty to the claims of their professional specialities far outstripped their loyalty to academic ideals of requiring beliefs to be substantiated with factual evidence.

The committee expressed its awareness of the lack of convincing evidence on several issues. For example, it had to admit that 'While we unhesitatingly accept the often reiterated aim of antenatal care as a means of reducing perinatal and neonatal mortality, what antenatal care consists of and how it works has been less clear to us' [31, para. 46], for the committee could be shown no demonstration of the effectiveness of its various components [31, para. 48]. The benefits for women might be uncertain, but the benefits for obstetricians were certain. So the committee was persuaded to put aside its common sense reservations, in favour of the intended meaning of the professional view as put ambiguously by a Professor of Obstetrics from Nottingham, 'It is probably reasonable to assume that the level of antenatal and intrapartum care has some bearing on the subsequent outcome of pregnancy, and indeed our whole practice depends on this belief' [31, para. 47], and to recommend unequivocally that 'Every effort should be made to encourage women to attend as early as possible in their pregnancies for antenatal care' [31, para. 523.1].

Disregard of the evidence already published discrediting the professional view of the benefits of obstetric intranatal care was even less pardonable. The most important recommendation, from which many of the remainder follow, was that 'An increased number of mothers should be delivered in large units; selection of patients should be improved for smaller consultant units (CUs) and isolated GP units (GPUs); home delivery should be phased out further' [31, para. 523.10]. The committee deplored the paucity of informative statistics routinely collected and was obviously not made aware of analyses already in print (Chapter 2, references [28–31]) of the various publicly available statistics which did exist, all of which pointed to the conclusion that mortality was higher in obstetric hospitals at all identified levels of predicted and coincidental risk, a conclusion which obstetricians could find no evidence to refute (Chapters 7 and 8).

Furthermore, the committee was allowed to misuse the statistics, specially supplied by the Department of Health and Social Security (DHSS), of stillbirth rates (SBR) in 1978 in hospitals of different types and sizes (Table 5.1), in order to justify its recommendation of concentrating deliveries in the largest hospitals. It let itself be impressed that the SBR was fractionally lower in the 'largest and usually best equipped and staffed units' where it was told 'it is policy to deliver high risk mothers and one would expect to see the highest mortality'. It was led to reiterate obstetricians' judgement that 'It is therefore of some significance that the largest units, those delivering 4,000 or more babies a year, actually have lower stillbirth rates than units delivering between 1000 and 3999 babies a year. Either the selection process is not working as it should or the care offered in the largest units is so much better that it is compensating for high risk' [31, para. 395]. In contrast, it let itself be disturbed that CUs with 500–999 births, and according to policy fewer at high risk, had an SBR as high as 7.7/1000 [31, para. 396].

The largest hospitals are certainly the most exciting places for obstetricians and neonatal paediatricians to work in, but from the evidence

Table 5.1 Stillbirth rate per 1000 births in National Health Service hospitals, England, 1978

Number of deliveries	Units with		
	Obstetric beds only	Obstetric and GP maternity beds 'mixed'	GP maternity beds only
Less than 500	4.0	1.4	1.7
500–999	7.7	3.5	0.8
1000–1999	9.0	8.8	–
2000–2999	8.8	8.9	–
3000–3999	9.2	9.3	–
4000 and over	8.9	8.4	–
All units	8.8	8.7	1.6

Source: Perinatal and Neonatal Mortality, Second Report from the House of Commons Social Services Committee, 1980, Table 7.

they are far from being the safest places for babies to be born in, for the application of a simple, but mandatory, statistical test (page 266) would have revealed that the observed differences between the stillbirth rates in all units with obstetric beds having over 500 births and in all 'mixed' units (obstetric and GP maternity beds) having over 1000 births did not nearly reach the accepted minimum level of statistical significance, which means that they could have happened by chance far more than five times in a hundred ($p > 0.05$). Moreover, the average SBR per 1000 births in these larger units in 1978 (8.9) was very significantly higher than in the remaining smaller obstetric and mixed units (3.4) – this difference could have happened by chance less than once in a thousand times ($p < 0.001$). In turn, this average was very significantly higher ($p < 0.001$) than the average SBR in isolated GPUs (1.6), where mortality is consistently relatively low [28].

The explanation of these results, insistently repeated by the professionals and accepted uncritically by the committee, is said to be that births in the larger hospitals, and indeed in any obstetric hospital, include those at the highest predelivery risk. When tested against actual data, however, this always turns out to be a very insufficient explanation (Chapter 8). The converse arguments are offered, with the same invalidity, to explain why perinatal mortality rates are so low for planned births at home. The committee was persuaded by obstetricians' time-honoured but still unproven beliefs that immediate obstetric interventions always reduce the dangers from serious complications; since these can occasionally arise in deliveries outside hospital and are manifestly not reduced by transfer to hospital as always witnessed by the exceptionally high mortality rates for such cases (pages 338–41, 352–4), these occasional dangers would be avoided if all births took place close to emergency and resuscitation facilities, namely in the larger hospitals [31, para. 523.17]. The committee was shielded from the evidence that the serious complications are much more likely to arise under obstetric management and that cases when interventions are life-saving are far outnumbered by cases where they are not (pages 205–6, 324).

The committee regretted that 'some techniques in common use in perinatal medicine have never been properly evaluated' [31, para. 452]. Yet it made sweeping recommendations to ensure their continued and extended use. On electronic fetal monitoring, for example, the evidence given to them [31, para. 79] had certainly not been 'properly evaluated' and the committee was left unaware of valid evaluative studies then existing [32] which cast serious doubt, to be later confirmed (page 179) [33], on the net benefits to be gained from the universal use of this technique. Yet this was what the committee recommended [31, para. 523.15].

The committee was concerned that perinatal mortality was much higher in the lower than in the upper social classes. Despite the great increase in births in hospital and in the use of advanced equipment since the 1950s, the gap had widened. Likewise, preferential allocation of medical resources to the less favoured regions had failed to reduce their relative excess mortality rates. Yet the committee apparently accepted the professional view that 'intervention by a professional service is able to a significant extent to reverse and counteract the influence of the adverse social and economic environment' [31, para. 314] and it obligingly recommended more of the same treatment. Despite the beliefs of obstetricians: 'we believe that an expansion of consultant obstetric posts would help to reduce the mortality rates' [31, para. 152] and 'I would give top priority to improving facilities for intrapartum care' [31, para. 66], there is no evidence whatsoever that a given input of obstetric resources in any area brings about a related reduction in perinatal mortality. If the largest hospitals were indeed the best equipped and staffed, their mortality record did not show any benefit from the extra investment. There was, therefore, no evidence that the expansion of obstetric and allied staffs for intrapartum care which the committee recommended [31, paras 523.29, 523.35] would save more babies' lives, particularly where the need was greatest, although it would, of course, strengthen the professions concerned.

Like the Cranbrook and Peel Committees, the Short Committee recommended that midwives should be helped to regain their former status [31, para. 249], while the implication of other recommendations was to relieve them of responsibility and undermine their confidence, for all deliveries were ultimately to be in hospitals where an obstetrician would dictate labour ward practice, [31, para. 523.13] and in the interim all deliveries should have twenty-four hour cover by a doctor with obstetric experience [31, para. 523.30] and by a paediatrician if the need for resuscitation was anticipated [31, para. 523.18]. Midwives were expected to persuade women that hospital was safest, but this required emphasizing, indeed exaggerating, the potential dangers of birth – 'putting them in fear that everything is going to go wrong' [31, para. 56] – and consequently undermining their own and the mother's confidence.

The committee's purpose was to gather information material to reducing perinatal mortality. Since, like its predecessors, it was satisfied to accept unsupported assertions and did not insist on seeing justifying evidence, its recommendations relating to place of birth endorsed and intensified a policy which, by all the evidence, had not been instrumental in reducing perinatal mortality in the past and would not be so in the future. Unlike its predecessors, the members of this committee were laymen and might have been expected to make impartial judgements. Their very partial expert medical advisers ensured that their recommendations conformed with the interests of the dominant professions, and not with those of mothers and babies.

It is significant that when in 1980 an article was published pointing out that actual results belied the assertions made [28], the expert advisers found themselves unable to answer the challenges and produce supporting evidence. They left it to Mrs Short to bluster her way through an irrelevant defence [34, 35]. But exposure of the unsound basis of the recommendations was overlooked and did not detract from the reliance placed on the report by those who made and implemented policy.

Nor was it allowed to influence the committee's deliberations when, three years later and misguided as to causal relationships by the same expert advisers, it investigated how far its recommendations had been implemented and what effects had been produced.

THE 1984 FOLLOW-UP REPORT TO THE SHORT REPORT

The committee noted with satisfaction the further fall in perinatal deaths [36, para. 6]. It was led to

> believe that one factor had been the considerable interest generated at all levels by the 1980 Report, which stimulated revision of policies and practices, and monitoring systems. . . . Perhaps the most significant factor has been the medical specialisation and the deployment of new techniques which have ensured higher survival rates for low birthweight babies than was generally thought possible a decade ago.

(Its expert advisers should have told it, however, that the relative contribution made by the low weight subgroup to the overall perinatal mortality rate did not fall.) Satisfaction was marred, however, because mortality in Britain had not fallen as fast as in some other countries and because, within Britain, disparities between the social classes and between the regions had again widened, not narrowed as the obstetricians' 1980 optimistic boast [31, para. 314], already quoted, had promised.

The committee was pleased that the concentration. of deliveries in obstetric hospitals had progressed, but was disappointed that fewer isolated GP units had been closed than it had hoped, for it still accepted obstetricians' assertions that 'Small hospitals with inadequate facilities are dangerous places to have a baby where there is no paediatrician to resuscitate' [36, para. 36], despite the very good safety record these actually achieved.

Because their management techniques make childbirth more painful for the mother, obstetricians are always anxious to compensate by offering pain relief for which specialist anaesthetists are often required. Since the need for them may be irregular but urgent when it arises, their services can most conveniently be provided in the larger general hospitals, which constitutes a further reason for concentrating deliveries there. To obstetricians this is an emergency safeguard of transcending importance and one which the Faculty of Anaesthetists would willingly supply. Hence they added their weight to the crusade against delivery in smaller hospitals and, of course, at home, not only in submissions to the investigating committees of 1980 and 1984, but in a widely circulated document in 1987, *Anaesthetic Services for Obstetrics – A Place for the Future* [37]. These specialists in high technology overlook the fact that very few mothers who deliver with low technology midwifery care ever need pain relief beyond the sort midwives have been safely administering for decades. With undrugged babies, the need for specialist resuscitation is likewise rare.

Had it not endorsed widespread obstetric management, the committee would not have had to urge extension of anaesthetic and paediatric cover; in particular, it would have had less need to deplore the continued shortage of facilities for neonatal intensive care [36, para. 50]. There had been a small increase in obstetric and paediatric medical staff, but the committee acceded to the hardly disinterested plea from the RCOG and the BPA (British Paediatric Association) for more resources and recommended a great expansion of consultants in both fields [36, para. 60].

In 1984, the committee found 'There is still room for the more carefully defined and better use of the skills of both midwives and GPs in maternity care which the Committee recommended in 1980' [36, para. 39]. The competence and responsibility of general practitioners were hardly reinforced by the 1970 Peel recommendation [23, para. 249], repeated in 1980 [31, para. 523.63], that all pregnant women should be seen at least twice by a consultant obstetrician, given that there is absolutely no evidence that this improves outcome for such women, although it increases the power of obstetricians. Opportunities for midwives had been slightly increased through the few low-risk birth rooms which had been set up in consultant units, but 'there had been little progress with the introduction of "domino" schemes as recommended by the Committee in 1980, in which community midwives come into hospitals to deliver mothers to whom they have given antenatal care' [36, para. 37]. Since 1984, progress in these directions has been no less sluggish. Only limited provision had been made for more midwifery training courses for entrants without nursing qualifications [36, para. 65].

The committee's proposals for co-ordinating bodies, District Maternity Services Committees and Regional Perinatal Working Parties, had by 1984 met with a poor response and had achieved little [36, paras 73–5]. Only 63% of the 192 health districts had set up a Maternity Services Liaison Committee. Where they had not done so, the reasons were either that existing committees, of which there were already too many, fulfilled the proposed function or that the obstetricians would not co-operate. Where they had done so, the committees were mostly dominated by obstetricians or other leading officials from the establishment, the lay representation being small and ineffective [38].

At government level, the Maternity Services Advisory Committee (MSAC) was set up as proposed in 1981 and in its early reports had 'fulfilled many of the [Social Services] Committee's expectations [36, para. 72]. This was probably not surprising, since the MSAC obviously accepted the same advice, with the same disregard of impartial analyses of actual results, as the Social Services Committee had done, for in its study of intrapartum care the obstetricians' unfaltering creed was duly repeated: 'The practice of delivering nearly all babies in hospital has contributed to the dramatic reduction in stillbirths and neonatal deaths and to the avoidance of many child handicaps' [39, p. v].

Conscious of the prevailing ignorance, the Social Services Committee pleaded in 1980 for more research to determine 'how antenatal care can most effectively reduce perinatal mortality and morbidity' [31, para. 523.9]. In 1984, it was still seeking 'systems designed to measure the effectiveness of current and future methods of early diagnosis' [36, para. 14]. It had apparently not been made aware of the impartial and authoritative evaluations of many of the components of routine antenatal care published in 1982 [40]. It was thus prevented from recommending appropriate reforms in practices.

Reforms, which the committee did recommend in 1980 and which most districts had taken some steps towards implementing by 1984, concerned 'humanising obstetric care' [36, para. 40] – providing a more comfortable and homely environment in antenatal clinics and labour suites, with more flexible visiting, and allowing the mother to have a lay companion throughout labour, to adopt alternative postures for birth and to keep her baby by her side. The humanizing process may, however, have been less in response to the committee's recommendations than to pressure from consumers' organizations (pages 185–9, 234–8).

THE WINTERTON COMMITTEE: ITS 1991 REPORT

The Department of Health and Social Security had been separated into its constituent Departments, each having its own all-party House of

Commons Select Committee. In 1991 the Health Committee, with Nicholas Winterton as Chairman, embarked on a further comprehensive inquiry into the Maternity Services, which was to take a year to complete. It did so at the instigation of the well-informed member Audrey Wise, who drew attention to current reasons for dissatisfaction.

Five themes were embraced: preconception care, antenatal care, delivery/birth, postnatal care and neonatal care. The committee's invitation to submit relevant material produced an enormous response covering all aspects of the field. Around 450 memoranda, many long, detailed and well referenced, were received from organizations representing both the professional providers and the lay receivers of care, from bodies concerned with medical and social research and with the evaluation of services, as well as from individual providers and receivers of care and individual researchers. The committee broadened its understanding of the problems by visiting a sample of maternity hospitals and clinics, not only in the United Kingdom, but also in Sweden and Holland.

Besides digesting the written material submitted, the committee as usual called many of those represented to the House of Commons to give oral evidence and answer questions raised by committee members. The scholarly quality of the submissions describing the experience of mothers, their consistency and sincerity, convinced the committee that maternal satisfaction is not a trivial consideration, distinct from and much subordinate to safety, but indeed has lasting implications for physical, as well as psychological and social, welfare. For the first time in any such inquiry, paramount importance was given to organizing the maternity service so as to give precedence to the human needs of the service receivers over the professional interests of the service providers, wherever these do not happen to coincide.

The committee began with the important step of widening the field of its specialist advisers. It retained only the paediatrician, Professor Osmund Reynolds, and made five fresh appointments, including two obstetricians, Dr Naren Patel and Professor Philip Steer, and also two midwives with research and administrative experience, Caroline Flint and Rosemary Jenkins, and one General Practitioner much involved with maternity care, Dr Luke Zander.

Unlike its predecessors, the committee did not start with the negative assumption that childbirth is a dangerous physiological procedure depending for safe outcome on medical management. Instead, influenced in the direction pointed to by recent research, it began with the positive premise that 'healthy mothers and babies are the product of a generation of healthy parents' [41, para. 4]. It elicited evidence from sources with relevant expertise about the social, environmental, behavioural and pathological factors known to be associated with health and pregnancy outcome. It was quickly convinced that poor health and unsatisfactory pregnancy outcomes were far more strongly associated with low socio-economic status than with the medically directed maternity services. In particular, it heard that the research findings of the Institute of Brain Chemistry and Human Nutrition showed the greater chance of having a baby of low birthweight (the seed of much future disadvantage and the perpetuation of deprivation) was in mothers whose nutritional intake, both during pregnancy and before conception, was relatively deficient, a deficiency associated with poverty [42, p. 301] (page 121). The elimination of poverty, certainly the elimination of relative poverty, has, however, defied achievement in most countries throughout most ages.

In its 1991 Report, *Maternity Services: Preconception* [41], the committee recognized the practical difficulties of improving the standard of life of the socially deprived; the most effective strategies would seem to be the same as those relevant to improving the health of the whole population [43] and to lie in well-targetted health education and the liberal provision of information and advice to persuade people of the benefits of a healthy diet, of avoiding tobacco, other drugs and excessive alcohol, of family planning and responsible sexual behaviour. The committee was not impressed that medically organized preconception clinics could play a significant role (page 132).

THE 1992 REPORT OF THE WINTERTON COMMITTEE

Turning to the other four themes of its inquiry, the committee sought to reconcile the conflicting evidence and opinions submitted by the users of the maternity service and its providers.

From the consistency and sincerity of the submissions representing women's views the committee discerned their strong desire 'for the provision of continuity of care and carer throughout pregnancy and childbirth and that the majority of them regard midwives as the group best placed and equipped to provide this' [44, para. 49]. Most women want a wider choice of place of delivery than the existing concentration on obstetric hospitals permits. Unlike its predecessor, the committee was more convinced by the impartial statistical analysis of the results of maternity care [45, pp. 587–93] (Chapter 8) than by the unsubstantiated, but constantly repeated, assertions of obstetricians. It concluded 'that the policy of encouraging all women to give birth in hospitals cannot be justified on grounds of safety . . . it is no longer acceptable that the pattern of maternity care provision should be driven by presumptions about the applicability of a medical model of care based on unproven assertions' [44, para. 33]. The policy of withdrawing the options of delivery at home or in small maternity units was misguided and regrettable [44, paras 74–86].

Women also want more say in the type of care they receive at all stages, care which should always let them feel in control of their own bodies [44, paras 50–55]. They want more reliable information about the advantages and disadvantages of specific procedures and freedom to give or refuse informed consent and thus feel active partners in the process. From their written submissions it appeared that the medical providers of care had in recent years come some way towards acceding to the aspirations of women and to granting that maternal satisfaction is important for successful outcomes, but their oral evidence revealed some reservations:

> The witnesses from the RCOG did not cite continuity of care or, until they had been encouraged to commit themselves several times, even mothers' satisfaction when asked to give their criteria for good maternity care. Although they lent their support to the principle of providing 'the maximum choice to the mother' the RCOG added the rider 'consistent with the best possible level of care'. . . . in practice the RCOG do not, in the face of conflicting evidence, acknowledge the possibility of any disadvantages to a hospital birth. [44, para. 181]

In their written memorandum the Royal College of General Practitioners (RCGP) also acknowledged women's aspirations, in particular for continuity of care, but in oral evidence claimed that GPs, few of whom attend actual deliveries, are best placed to provide this. The committee discerned in the RCGP's attitude 'a continuing adherence to a somewhat medicalised and paternalistic pattern of service delivery' [44, para. 184].

The provisions for birth which the Department of Health is responsible for organizing manifestly do not facilitate the realization of its stated aim of making 'the event a satisfying and happy one for her [the mother], her partner and her family'. Although the Royal College of Midwives (RCM) enthusiastically accepts women's aspirations, these apparently are not to supersede the right of midwives to make 'full use of their professional skills' [44, para. 180].

Weighing up the evidence it had received, the committee found that the service providers were insufficiently alive to women's criteria for successful care and that compliance with these criteria had been hindered through being 'far too heavily influenced by territorial disputes between the professionals concerned for the control of the women they are supposed to be helping' [44, para. 191].

The committee found no evidence to support the present regimens for antenatal care and recommended that, for the majority of women whose pregnancies are normal, it should be community based, under the direct control of midwives who are the specialists in normal childbirth, with more emphasis on social support than medical treatment (page 119). For the minority of cases where complications are detected, midwives should have direct access to obstetricians, the specialists in abnormality, who should treat more of these patients, effectively and at less expense, in day clinics rather than as hospital in-patients. The RCGP understandably expressed its disquiet at relinquishing its role as middlemen [44, paras 194–219].

In their evidence concerning intranatal care, obstetricians, as ever expecting emergencies, were adamant that all women should be delivered in large obstetric hospitals 'where immediate and skilled help is available'; they remained unmoved by actual results which show that these facilities do not ensure better overall outcomes. The RCM, rejecting the 'potential disaster' model of birth, placed less emphasis on the need for emergency facilities and wrote that 'a home confinement service should be an integral part of the maternity service'. The place of birth is intimately associated with the kind of intranatal management practised there: hospitals reflect obstetricians' belief that interventions are necessary to ensure a safe outcome even at the sacrifice of women's satisfaction; home and GP units reflect midwives' belief that most births will have a safer outcome without interventions. In this conflict the committee identified '. . . the potential for a damaging demarcation dispute between the professional groups' . . . and an 'urgent necessity for the NHS and the Royal Colleges to address and resolve this dispute' [44, para. 232].

The committee accepted that there is no evidence that several of the commonest interventions do succeed in improving outcomes for mother or baby, yet women are subjected to them without proper explanations. It concluded that

. . . until such a time as there is more detailed and accurate research about such interventions as epidurals, episiotomies, caesarean sections, electronic fetal monitoring, instrumental delivery and induction of labour, women need to be given a choice on the basis of existing information rather than having to undergo such interventions as routine. [44, para. 96]

Nearly all interventions involve the administration to the mother of medication of some sort, which may pass through to the baby with some degree of harm. The BPA expressed the view that 'All of the babies born in consultant obstetric units require paediatric medical care during the newborn period'. Therefore, all such units should have paediatric medical staff and facilities present for immediate resuscitation at birth and then to screen the baby for defects before discharge. The committee thought that in most cases these tasks could be safely undertaken by appropriately trained midwives as part of their routine. To the extent that illness in babies is the consequence of intranatal interventions, paediatric supervision for neonates should rarely be needed in places of birth where interventions are not practised, but where the need does arise, the committee recommended that community midwives should have direct and speedy access to specialist advice, though keeping the GP informed of such referrals [44, paras 227, 239, 243].

In contrast to their eagerness to control care of the mother before and during delivery, obstetricians have shown far less concern for her postnatal care, although she may have problems in recovering from physical and psychological damage resulting from delivery and in adjusting to the new demands on her, including the establishment of breastfeeding.

Although doctors know that breastfeeding brings the immediate advantage to the baby of increasing its resistance to gastro-intestinal and respiratory infections [46, 47] and so its chance of survival, and the later advantage to the mother of reducing her risk of breast cancer [48], they are content to leave assistance with breastfeeding to midwives whose training covers this aspect of care. Some midwives carry out their responsibility enthusiastically and conscientiously, others less so, conniving in practices which are actually obstructive and giving little encouragement to unconfident mothers to overcome their reluctance. Breastfeeding is successfully initiated and maintained in a relaxed environment, which is not easy to create in hospital and is not furthered by the disruption of impending discharge. Its advantages last as long as breastfeeding is continued. Although mothers are more likely to carry on breastfeeding for longer if they get off to a good start, which may depend on the quality of their postnatal maternity care, how long they will continue to do so will depend more on attitudes in society, over which maternity care has only distant influence. The committee was impressed by experience in Sweden where about 90% of mothers, far more than in Britain, were known to be still breastfeeding after six weeks and recommended that midwife managers should set challenging targets against which to measure the success of British midwives in supporting mothers in this health-promoting practice.

The lying-in stay in hospital has been reduced for 35% of mothers to two days or less, further care being transferred to community midwives. Early discharge brings attractive economies for the service and greater pleasure for many mothers, but is less welcome for those unable to make satisfactory domestic arrangements. The committee recommended greater flexibility in hospital discharge policies to accommodate the varying needs and better co-ordination of the professions whose function is to provide remedial services which should be evaluated [44, paras 244–57].

It is widely accepted that, if they are to survive, the very small and immature babies, as well as the very sick, need the high technology of intensive care. This service, expensive in equipment and staffing, is provided in most obstetric hospitals in units separate from the postnatal wards where normal babies are nursed beside their mothers. Neonatologists, however, have come to realize that the emotional disadvantages of separating babies from their mothers manifest themselves in physical disorders and that this applies equally to sick babies. The committee therefore approved the development of transitional care nurseries, where successful treatment can be carried out nearer their mothers, for those who are judged to need more than 'normal' but less than 'special' or 'intensive' care. If sufficient midwives were available to give this intermediate care, fewer babies would need to be segregated for special treatment, releasing cots to meet the rising demand for intensive care, and the committee recommended measures to ensure this sufficiency [44, paras 258–62].

The rising demand for intensive care comes largely from the greater numbers of babies, born live after short gestations often following intranatal interventions or as multiple births. Only a very small proportion of all babies have the most serious complications. Facilities for treating these are most economically concentrated in a few units in regional or sub-regional centres, which inevitably are not near the homes of many patients, who have to be transferred there before or after delivery. The advantages of close contact between mother and baby are no less great for the babies concerned than for other babies, but doctors believe the life-saving benefits of this care far outweigh its emotional and social costs and other disadvantages.

The neonatal paediatricians who made submissions to the Winterton Committee were firmly of the opinion that the impressive decrease in mortality rates for babies of low birthweight and ever shorter gestation was due to the impressive technological developments in neonatal intensive care, which had happened in several countries over the same period. Research studies have indicated better survival rates for infants of very low birthweight born in or transferred to the larger, most specialized Neonatal Intensive Care Units (NICUs) than in the smaller NICUs or Special Care Baby Units (page 205–6), a benefit later confirmed when outcomes are considered in relation to the pathological state of the infants treated [49]. The committee was persuaded by the neonatologists' confidence and recommended that projected organizational changes to the NHS should not be allowed to impair the provisions for specialist neonatal care, which must have adequate staffing and pathology services. It did, however, recommend also that the survivors of intensive care should be followed up through childhood and the results 'made widely available, so that the outcome of intensive care is clearly known' [44, paras 264–304]. Reasons to suspect that the neonatologists' inferences – that intensive care is the undoubted and overriding cause of the improved survival of low-weight and immature babies – may not be a correct or complete interpretation of the evidence will be considered in Chapter 8 (page 362–5).

The Winterton Committee had to point out that the policy of appointing more obstetricians, recommended by the Short Committee and duly implemented, had still failed to narrow the gap between the perinatal mortality rates of the highest and lowest social classes or of the most and least favoured geographical areas, despite obstetricians' repeated claims that it could do so (pages 210, 221). The committee put more reliance on 'other forms of social advance and support for mothers' and on providing them with continuous care from a single health professional rather than the shared care currently offered [44, paras 307, 309].

The committee could not find evidence of lack of safety or greater cost in unattached GP maternity units, and recommended that the policy of closing them for such alleged reasons, despite their popularity with mothers, should be abandoned [44, para. 312], again a complete reversal of the Short Committee's advice (page 207). It approved the midwifery-managed maternity units recently set up in obstetric hospitals and recommended the further development of this compromise service [44, para. 324]. It is, however, obvious from the high rate of transfers into the consultant units that the proximity of these enables obstetricians to continue exerting a powerful influence on the attitudes and behaviour of staff regarding the need for interventions in the midwifery units, as happens also in integrated GP maternity units [50].

Although the committee proclaimed the need for 'a cultural shift within the obstetric specialty . . . away from demanding that women go to obstetricians and a willingness among obstetricians to go to women' and the need for obstetricians to be open to a 'non-medical model' of care [44, para. 319], it did not go so far as to recommend reducing the provision of consultant units. It merely recommended, as the Short Committee had earlier done (page 213), the further spread of 'humanizing' modifications to the labour ward environment and wider consent for women to choose their own most comfortable positions in labour [44, paras 319, 325–8].

The implementation of these changes would imply reassessment of the roles of the care providers. The status of midwives should be raised: they should work as salaried professionals, expected to carry out their job from start to finish, not interrupted by the dictates of the clock. Any conflict in the needs of mothers and midwives should be reconciled by the adoption of team midwifery (pages 76, 106). Midwives should be given the right to have their own caseloads, to take full responsibility for the women under their care, to establish and manage their own maternity units within and outside hospitals and to admit women directly to NHS hospitals [44, paras 339–45].

The system for paying general practitioners has contributed to the fragmentation of maternity care by encouraging them to undertake antenatal and postnatal but not intranatal care (pages 8, 200). The committee recommended that the system should be redesigned, so as to focus on the needs of the mother and baby and to stop discouraging the doctors who would otherwise be willing and competent to supervise deliveries. Duplication of care with midwives should be avoided. The committee deplored the biased advice frequently given to women, which concealed the option of delivering anywhere other than in an obstetric hospital, and urged that safeguards be introduced to prevent victimization of women who tried to insist on giving birth at home. At the time of the Report GPs were not empowered to purchase maternity care on behalf of their patients. The committee felt that such action would probably prevent the reorientation of the maternity services which it was recommending and asked that no precipitate decision should be made to give GPs this power [44, paras 346–50].

The committee received conflicting opinions about the need for and supply of consultant obstetricians. Much of the 'substandard' care to which many of the unsatisfactory outcomes of maternity care are attributed is blamed on there being too few consultants whose other duties leave them too little time adequately to train and supervise their juniors. As in previous inquiries and with the same unjustified optimism (pages 201, 204, 210), a senior consultant claimed that

> The single factor that could make the largest contribution to lowering perinatal morbidity and mortality and increasing the quality of care for each mother and baby in the District General Hospital is a dramatic increase in appropriately trained 'manpower'. [44, para. 353]

This claim is refuted by much of the evidence reviewed by the committee. The Report illustrated its unreliability by publishing statistics for three sample areas which show that in 1990 the place with the lowest ratio of consultants to deliveries had also the lowest rates for caesarean sections, for inductions of labour and for perinatal mortality [44, para. 354].

To overcome the apparent shortage of consultant obstetricians on the wards would need, according to the RCOG, some 300 extra appointments involving a very high cost, expenditure which would be justified only if it could be shown, by impartial evaluation, to result in a commensurate 'health gain'. In any case, the current shortage of recruits to the specialty (page 70) would make it difficult to fill these extra posts.

The shortage of obstetricians would be eased if they were relieved of their duties as gynaecologists and to this end the committee made the bold proposal that separate posts be created for each sub-specialty [44, para. 368], so challenging one of the objectives of the founders of the RCOG (page 58). Such a divorce might make it easier for obstetricians to accept a 'non-medical' model of care as recommended. Another route for easing the shortage might lie in the adoption of new working practices, which might be less discouraging for junior staff, and particularly women, from staying in the profession. The committee recommended that such possibilities be investigated [44, para. 373].

The committee was more persuaded that the availability of medical and nursing staff was indeed inadequate to meet the present needs of babies in the special and intensive care units and recommended that the proposals of the professional bodies concerned for greatly increased numbers of appointments be adopted. Much of the demand for this kind of care, however, follows the interventions of obstetric intranatal management and might well be reduced if, as recommended here, more women were cared for by midwives during pregnancy, labour and birth.

In considering the steps necessary to make the future maternity service more responsive to women's needs, the committee sensed that a corner had already been turned: obstetricians, midwives and general practitioners now seemed more ready to admit that they had in the past paid too little attention to women's reactions to the care given. To reach objectives of making services more effective in improving health would require the redeployment of human and financial resources, changes in the training of young doctors to 'concentrate on the normal and those aspects of abnormality capable of being dealt with at general practitioner level', and restructuring the training course for specialist obstetricians to expedite their attainment of the status of independent practitioners. While their present basic training should be adequate to prepare midwives for the role being recommended, this would have to be reinforced by appropriate in-service training, in particular for the resuscitation of the newborn, a function which neonatologists showed reservations about ceding to midwives [44, paras 394–415]. Midwives understand best what will be required of their education, so the midwifery profession should retain control over all aspects of its training courses. These should not, as current legislation threatens, be subsumed into nursing education, whose needs are based on a different philosophy (pages 74–5) [44, paras 416–17].

The committee emphasized the need for evaluation of both existing practices and new ones, particularly those concerning midwives' care, which should be introduced first on a small scale so as to ensure that they merited later universal adoption. But for evaluation competent researchers and reliable statistics are needed. The committee highly applauded the research work of the National Perinatal Epidemiology Unit since its institution in 1978, culminating in the publication in 1989 of its evaluation of the practices in maternity care [51], and recommended that appropriate funding be continued. The committee noted with frustration that in the maternity service a commendable history of good official record keeping broke down after 1985 and urged that this lapse be remedied as soon as possible [44, paras 418–36].

The establishment of local Maternity Services Liaison Committees was recommended by the Short Committee in 1980, but by 1990 these were still proving an ineffectual mechanism for enabling the users of care to influence the provisions made (page 213) [42, pp. 277–81]. Nevertheless the Winterton Committee thought that, strengthened by more lay members and with a lay chairperson, they could become an integral part of the planning process, with the specific objectives of monitoring service delivery, eliciting and passing on users' reactions, promoting clinical audit and quality assurance and ensuring adequate facilities for transitional care for the not too sick babies and for the resuscitation of mothers and babies [44, paras 318, 445, 471].

In its publications [39], the Maternity Services Advisory Committee, the central co-ordinating body set up in 1981 as proposed by the Short Committee, largely echoed the establishment's opinions for which the Winterton Committee could find no justification. For the future, the more productive duty for it was proposed of preparing a protocol, identifying specific health care targets for the maternity service and monitoring the providers' specific plans for meeting these, which should involve '. . . a radical reconsideration of the deployment of human and financial resources' [44, paras 394–5].

Clearly, the Winterton Committee's proposals implied radical restructuring of the maternity service. The immediate response of the Department of Health was to set up an Expert Maternity Group to consider further the practical implications of the changes involved, its ten members including administrators as well as representatives of provider and user bodies. Its recommendations were to determine future policy.

REPORT OF THE EXPERT MATERNITY GROUP, 1993: *CHANGING CHILDBIRTH*

Following the recommendations of the Winterton Report, the Expert Group began its nine months' work, accepting the newly proposed principle that

the woman must be the focus of maternity care. She should be able to feel that she is in control of what is happening to her and able to make decisions about her care, based on her needs, having discussed matters fully with the professionals involved. [52, p. 8]

Before it reported, the Expert Group was aware of the material, representing many points of view, presented for discussion at a consensus conference organized for the Department of Health by a policy research group, the King's Fund Centre. It was much influenced by the statement about the deliberations of this conference drawn up by an independent panel of twelve members [52, pp. 97–106]. The panel confirmed that women want a maternity service that offers safety, continuity of care and carer, is kind, inspires confidence, responds to individual needs, and enables them to feel in control. It should make possible informed choice of options and the consensus was that, even when professionals believe that the mother's choice may increase the risk of harm to herself or her baby, they do not have the right arbitrarily to impose their views. Ceding this right marks an abrupt reversal of medical maternity policy and practice in Britain – a right which still seems to be firmly upheld in the USA (page 245).

In its report the Expert Group accepted that, while safety must remain the cornerstone of maternity care, no one feels more strongly about safety than the baby's mother who, entrusted with carrying her own case notes, should be kept fully informed about all matters relating to their care, including whether the benefits of proposed interventions are proven or merely assumed: she should choose the professional who would be responsible for leading and providing continuity of care and carer throughout. The person chosen would often be a midwife and the choice would be facilitated through team midwifery, schemes for which should be further developed and refined until a satisfactory network is provided in all areas (page 76). Although it is not widely known or hitherto acted upon, no law prevents midwives from admitting women in labour to hospital maternity beds. The Group recommends that this freedom should be exploited. 'Within 5 years, 75% of women should be cared for in labour by a midwife they have come to know in pregnancy.' [52, 2.3, 2.4]

Where the woman's lead professional is an obstetrician, he/she would have more time to build a continuing relationship, once relieved of the responsibility for most women with a normal pregnancy. The Market and Opinion Research Institute (MORI) survey commissioned specially by the Expert Group found that the GP is currently seen by women as giving the most continuous care before and after delivery. Where the GP is chosen as the lead professional, he/she should be encouraged to maintain the skills necessary for intrapartum care as well, though difficulties in honouring other practice duties would have to be resolved (page 8).

The Expert Group deplored duplication of antenatal examinations given by doctors and midwives, 'welcomed the move towards more antenatal care in the community', but did not pronounce on the Winterton Committee's proposal that shared care between hospital and GPs should be abandoned. Like the Short and Winterton Committees, it was unconvinced of the effectiveness of formal routine antenatal check-ups and called for an assessment of the service in successfully identifying fetuses at risk (pages 134, 207). It obviously felt that the published reviews already undertaken [53, 54] had not gone far enough in reforming policy or practice. It expressed more faith in the benefits to be gained from informal parent education sessions. It agreed that guidance and support through the range of tests and investigations for the detection of fetal abnormality are desirable. Unlike the Winterton Committee, however, it doubted that day units for such tests have in all cases effectively reduced antenatal inpatient admissions and recommended that their role be reassessed before further investment is made in this service (pages 118, 217) [52, 2.5].

It was apparent to the Expert Group that most women were given little choice about the place of birth, yet the MORI survey showed that, of the 98% who gave birth in an obstetric hospital, 72% would have appreciated a choice; despite prevailing propaganda, 22% of these would have considered a home birth and 44% a midwife-led domino delivery, respectively equal to 16% and 32%, and together nearly half, of all birthing women [52, 2.6]. This illustrates that the professionals first to give advice, usually GPs, had not studied the recent analyses of results, in this history and other publications, but clung uncritically to their indoctrinated, but insupportable, beliefs that out-of-hospital births are dangerous. They were in fact continuing to purvey unsound, biased advice, not the 'clear, unbiased advice' required in the Group's stated objective. The Expert Group enjoined service providers to 'review their current organisation to ensure that real choice about place of birth is available', which is not the most forceful way of reforming GPs' ill-informed attitudes and 'ensuring that women receive information about the full range of options for place of birth available in their locality'.

To meet obstetricians' constant fear that out-of-hospital deliveries will frequently but unpredictably need emergency treatment (which, as many quoted reports show, is not always immediately available in hospital either), the Group recommended the presence of two attendants, the prompt co-operation of obstetricians and GPs if asked for help, and the inclusion of an appropriately trained member in the front-line ambulance crew to help the midwife during transfer to hospital of a mother or baby in trouble [52, 2.7].

For the births planned for hospital delivery, the Group favoured including in her case notes the woman's own birth plan, so that her

desires, about interventions and anaesthesia for example, may as far as possible be accommodated [52, 2.8]. The Group reiterated the desirability of separating mothers as little as possible from their babies and of delaying their discharge until the mother feels fit to cope at home [52, 2.9].

If once home either mother or baby seems unwell, the midwife should consult the GP or have direct access to a paediatrician if specialist care seems necessary. The Group hoped that a continuing relationship with a known midwife would make breastfeeding easier to establish and maintain and would in due course facilitate a smooth transfer of care to the Health Visitor. All the professionals concerned should be alert to the possibility of women developing postnatal depression, which under the present regimen afflicts 10–15% of women and needs specialist treatment [52, 2.9]. This high proportion may, possibly, be related to intranatal interventions and, if so, would be reduced by the decrease in interventions which should follow the proposed increase in midwife-led deliveries.

GPs, who had been largely ousted from intranatal care, were recognized by the Expert Group as performing a pivotal role before and after birth, though they were now to be required to give properly informed, impartial advice, but they were not given effective guidance as to how to ensure that this would be done. Their position would be strengthened by the more appropriate training recently proposed [55] and by a better targetted system of payment which the Department of Health was recommended to devise [52, 2.10].

Those midwives who have already been organized in teams were reported as finding their new responsibilities and practices more satisfying. As explained by the Department of Health's solicitors, midwives' legal responsibilities should be borne directly by midwives and not fall unfairly on obstetrician or GP colleagues. The Expert Group was favourably impressed that midwives were being prepared for the duties they were to fulfil by the advances now embodied in modern midwifery education:

> Midwifery education emphasises a balance of clinical skills and knowledge, the need for intellectual development, knowledge of the human sciences and the need to use scientific evidence in practice. Importantly, a high premium is placed on interpersonal and communication skills. [52, 2.11] (page 77)

Obstetricians, who had worked so hard to secure domination of all maternity care for themselves, faced the prospect of most of their empire being handed over to midwives and some of it to GPs. No further mention was made of the need for all pregnant women to be seen at least twice by a consultant obstetrician (page 212), but obste-

tricians were to go on attending any woman who expressed a preference for their care and, in addition, retain the management of women
with a high risk, complicated pregnancy and delivery [52, 2.12]. The
Expert Group, however, did not presume to specify what conditions
constituted 'high risk', conditions for which obstetricians had in recent
years developed increasingly inclusive criteria though without reference
to actual results (pages 104, 110–11).

Like the Winterton Committee, the Expert Group foresaw the need
for the relevant professional bodies to redesign the role of senior house
officers, stressing their need for training more strongly than their service
commitments. Some of these would have to be undertaken by senior
obstetricians, some by midwives, and both professions would have to
be involved in teaching the young recruits, whose training should equip
them, whether working eventually as GPs or consultant obstetricians, to
provide a full range of maternity services.

Again like the Winterton Committee, the Expert Group placed great
hopes on the re-constitution in every Health Authority of strengthened
Maternity Services Liaison Committees (MSLCs) with significant lay
input [52, 3.2]. MSLCs would be better able to carry out their duties if
they, like women, had access to satisfactory systems of information and
communication, letting them know how the services were actually
being used and how they might be. The Department of Health was
urged to develop such systems [52, 3.3–3.7]. The future role proposed
by the Winterton Committee for the Maternity Services Advisory Committee was not specifically mentioned.

The Expert Group, expecting positive moves towards woman-centred
and community-based care within five years without the existing
wasteful duplication of resources, shifted ultimate responsibility for the
conduct of maternity care from the professional providers to the purchasers acting on behalf of the users when it stated:

> Purchasers have a key role in ensuring that providers implement
> practices of proven benefit and abandon those which have been
> demonstrated as ineffective. When the benefit or effect of a practice
> is unclear, it should be systematically evaluated. Existing patterns
> of practice and organization of services should not be exempt from
> evaluation. . . . New patterns of service should be designed to
> allow evaluation of both their effectiveness and their acceptability
> to women using the service [52, 4].

The Expert Group conceded that implementing its principles would
require many changes to the planning and monitoring of services, to the
roles of the providing professions, their education and training and,
most fundamentally, to their attitudes, now having to recognize the
central role of the mother. It set out ten practical indicators by which

progress should be measured towards its targets which should be reached within five years. However difficult the transition might seem to be, the Expert Group cherished the hope that by then 'the principle embodied in this report will have become so widely accepted and its practices so commonplace that *Changing Childbirth* will have done its work and can take its place on the shelf of history' [52, 5]. There are, however, reasons to doubt that as it stands it is explicit and decisive enough to achieve its aims.

DISABLING FLAWS IN *CHANGING CHILDBIRTH*

Women have reason to be extremely grateful for the far-reaching proposals for reform of the maternity service embodied in these recent reports. The recommendations of the Winterton Committee, if implemented, would revolutionize maternity care, first in Britain and perhaps later in the rest of the world. In turn, the vetting committee set up by the Department of Health, the Expert Group, supported most of and did not specifically reject any of the Winterton recommendations and so close the door to very desirable reforms. It did not, however, deal with a few of the most radical proposed changes. Most importantly, it left the issue of safety unresolved and this leads to inherent contradictions.

On the question of the safest place for birth, the Expert Group referred to the arguments for and against hospital delivery which had continued for decades and concluded weakly and illogically that the 'inability to reach agreement after this length of time suggests that there is no clear answer' [52, 2.6.3]. This, of course, is to assume, wrongly, that the argument has turned around impartial interpretation of the evidence of actual results and to ignore that one side has always had superior political power and a very strong vested interest to support.

The statistics analysed here in Chapters 7 and 8 show clearly that, for any defined risk group, the disadvantages in hospital of obstetric interventions and the unfamiliarity of the setting outweigh any advantages afforded by the proximity of facilities for coping with unforeseen emergencies and severe complications. Reforming the maternity service to give mothers more choice can certainly be justified on grounds of democratic freedom to indulge their own preferences, but the Expert Group has denied women its explicit support in the more decisive issue, that non-hospital births are safer. Having itself dismissed the validity of conclusions drawn from statistical evaluations of past results, can the Group reasonably expect the purchasers and providers of care to honour the validity of conclusions to be drawn from the future evaluations of practices which it prescribes?

In pregnancy and childbirth, women would like the advice given to them to be consistent. This implies wide agreement among the professionals giving the advice. This history of maternity care shows that, at least for several centuries, the opposing philosophies of what promotes safety in childbirth have prevented wide agreement between advisers from different professions, except when one profession has succeeded in dominating the others. But the philosophy the dominant profession has propagated has always lacked the support of factual evidence that it is effective. Certain procedures and treatments have now been evaluated by reputable scientific methods and the resulting conclusions should command general acceptance and compliance. The vast volume of consistent evidence from many sources supports the validity of the hypothesis that in most cases childbirth is safest with the least interference, but until this conclusion is universally accepted, the advice given by members of different professions is bound to be inconsistent. Advice may be consistent but uniformly wrong. There is obvious danger in pressing birth attendants to put consistency before what in the light of evidence is accuracy. The Expert Group gave no direct indication, though many indirect indications, that it accepted the non-interventionist philosophy, but the strategy it proposed for propagating its wider acceptance lacks conviction that it will prove effective, most doubtfully within the brief target time-scale set.

In sharp contrast to the 1970 Peel Report which pointed to a future of less choice of where, and less control of how, mothers could give birth, the recommendations contained in the Reports of the House of Commons Winterton Committee in 1992 and the Department of Health's Expert Group in 1993 point to a future of increased choice and control for mothers. To some women, choice can be a welcome privilege, to others a less welcome burden. To help them choose well and wisely, women are to be furnished with as much impartial information as will enable them to judge which of the basic philosophies of childbirth the maternity services should support. Many of the less assertive women would not make this choice for themselves, but would choose only the adviser whose status they most respected and follow his/her advice. Some would choose the adviser who shouted loudest or whose ill-informed message spread the greatest fear. Therefore, the important first step is to rid the advisers of their long-standing bias, and whether the action proposed to implement the stated objective, 'Clinical practice should be based on sound evidence and be subject to regular clinical audit', will be enough to achieve this remains to be seen. The 'sound evidence' available to it should have empowered the Expert Group to declare against the obstetric management of childbirth with its proven disadvantages or at the very least to let it judge that the balance of probabilities lay strongly against obstetric management in hospital.

Pregnancy and childbirth offer women both an experience which they all share and a wide variety of individual experiences. To meet their many needs and desires, common and individual, maternity services should offer a range of options, which should be flexible in operation. The Expert Group, like the Winterton Committee, stressed the need for flexibility and so left many details to be decided locally. Local policies, however, often reflect only the views of the most powerful service providers, in effect those who habitually support obstetric management and are less open to re-education by the measures proposed by the Expert Group.

The Winterton Committee identified territorial disputes between obstetricians, general practitioners and midwives and urged the Colleges concerned to resolve their differences [44, para. 232]. The Expert Group gave no practical advice about how mutual respect and clinical co-operation should come to prevail, without sacrifice to mother or baby. Perhaps it accepted that this reconciliation had already been achieved in the joint statement in 1992 (to which it did not refer) by the Presidents of the Royal Colleges representing obstetricians, midwives and general practitioners since it repeats some of the views expressed there:

> Clear and unbiased information about the options for antenatal care and the place of delivery should be provided wherever a woman makes first contact with the health service. The woman's own views and preferences should be a very significant factor in formulating any programmes of care. It has to be recognised that these may not always coincide with the opinions of her professional adviser.

Doubt that this verbal agreement would be readily matched by practical action was quickly cast by obstetricians' contentious reception of the *Changing Childbirth* Report.

Neither did the Expert Group disclose its reaction to the Winterton Committee's recommendation (which meantime is being ignored) that no more small rural maternity units should be closed unless the case for doing so, on grounds of safety or cost, is overwhelming [44, para. 312]. Nor did it elaborate on the Winterton proposal for separate careers for obstetricians and gynaecologists [44, para. 368].

All but one of the professions providing maternity care accepted the Report of the Expert Group. The RCOG, however, was apparently unhappy that so much trust should be placed in midwives who are not trained to diagnose general morbidity in mothers. Discounting the mountain of information amassed by the Winterton Committee and the Consensus Conference, a Birmingham obstetrician complained to the press that the report of the Expert Group had suggested major alterations in current practice without objective review of available evidence.

The RCOG therefore asked that action to give effect to its recommendations and those of the Winterton Committee be delayed until November 1993, so that issues could be further considered. No authoritative statement of policy promptly followed this reconsideration, but the Department of Health wanted all concerned to go on debating the proposed changes. It wanted health authorities over the next nine months to develop strategies for implementing the changes, which could be reflected in purchaser/provider contracts for 1995/96 [56]. Some recommendations had already been implemented in some places by the end of 1993, but it is still uncertain whether the RCOG, probably with the support of obstetricians world wide, will be able to use its considerable political powers to frustrate the intentions of these epoch-making reports and prevent the general implementation of the changes they recommend. No convincing strategy was proposed for removing the intellectual confusion and professional bias in which medical minds have become steeped after decades of unremitting brain washing.

PAYING FOR MATERNITY CARE

In Britain before 1900 most users had to pay for their own intranatal care. The richer ones could afford to buy the services of doctors with the possibilities of instrumental delivery and anaesthesia. The less rich were deprived of this luxury, a deprivation which was in truth a benefit, although not widely appreciated as such. The very poor could be helped by charities which organized domiciliary midwifery schemes and supported lying-in hospitals. For the destitute there were the Poor Law Infirmaries.

After 1900, provision for the poor became less meagre and less harsh. The community accepted its responsibility to pay, through the local authorities, for free antenatal care in municipal clinics, for more midwives and more maternity beds in municipal hospitals. But the unwelcome stigma of poverty attached to these free provisions which deterred many women from using them. Maternity benefit payments from compulsory health insurance made it easier for the recipients to buy their own intranatal care, even at some financial hardship.

The National Health Service swept aside these social deterrents by making maternity care free to all. Medically organized care was accepted as being so advantageous to welfare that financial cost was no longer the limiting criterion. Doctors were given a generous budget to organize the service as they thought best and obstetricians thought extension of hospital facilities best. Cost accounting was very confused; track was soon lost of what the separate elements of the service cost and out of which budget they were financed.

Without question, the simpler the treatment, the fewer the interventions, the less it costs, but it was easy to argue, although not to prove, that the simple treatments were less safe. For those who have to pay, care in any institution is far more expensive than care at home. But for the individual client who saves her normal maintenance costs, as well as the cost of incidental equipment and materials, a free stay in hospital for delivery is net financial gain. It now paid poorer women to enjoy on equal terms the promised greater safety that had formerly been the privilege and prerogative of the rich. This inducement helped to break down their traditional opposition to hospitalization.

Published accounts are such that it is extremely difficult accurately to apportion costs between the different arms of the maternity service. One unpublished calculation, making the best use possible of available national data, estimated that if the proportion of deliveries in hospitals, GP units and at home had stayed for the next twenty-five years as they were in 1958 – 49%, 12% and 36% respectively – and if 1983 costs had applied throughout, the bill paid by the public sector for maternity care would have been £1.7 billion less than it actually was, equal to an average annual saving of some £68 million [57]. Over the same period there would have been an average annual saving of 12 000 babies' lives. On this showing, official policy has cost the community dear. The actual magnitude of the overspend depends on the actual, but unreckoned, costs at each place of delivery, but that it was large is undoubted.

Local studies in England in 1979 [58] and in Scotland in 1981 [59] involved much guesswork in quantification, but agreed in finding average costs for deliveries highest in obstetric hospitals, lower in GP units and lowest for those at home. Yet health authorities contrive to justify closing small maternity hospitals by adducing the higher cost of treatment there. This result can only be achieved by spurious accounting methods.

In addition to the higher current costs incurred in institutional care, there are the considerable costs on capital account of providing and maintaining the accommodation, as well as the necessary technical equipment. The average cost per patient treated is less, the greater the number of patients over whom the capital costs can be spread. Capital costs are likely to be much higher for accommodation in a large, generously equipped specialist hospital than in a small, sparsely equipped maternity unit. But if the small unit is sufficiently underused, the average cost per patient treated may well work out at a figure higher than in the specialist hospital serving the same population. If Health Authorities favour large obstetric units, booking policy can be engineered to ensure that calculated costs in the small hospitals appear excessive, so furnishing a persuasive reason for closing them. It can be argued that, since a specialist unit, with indivisible high-cost technological equipment, has in any case to be maintained to deal with complicated cases and its overhead costs cannot be reduced, then the only way in which an overspent Health Authority can cut its costs is to close the small peripheral hospitals. Centralizing deliveries in the large obstetric unit reduces the average cost per case there, but especially in rural districts it transfers extra transport costs to the mothers concerned and their families.

More expensive facilities can only be cost-effective if their use achieves better results than are possible by alternative means. The obstetric hospitals claim the lion's share of maternity expenditure because the treatments they provide cost more. A study in 1991, combining data on the costs of procedures and hospital stay, found the total cost to be over three times as high after caesarean as after vaginal deliveries, with spontaneous vaginal deliveries carrying much the lowest cost [60]. Obstetricians have never been able to show that high rates of caesarean section or instrumental delivery are associated with low rates of mortality or morbidity, rather the reverse. On the other hand, since it costs three times as much to treat babies if they have respiratory distress syndrome, the expensive therapies of administering surfactant to such babies, and corticosteroids to their mothers may both save lives and reduce the cost of neonatal intensive care [62] for the babies concerned [61]. More survivors, however, are likely to need prolonged neonatal care for other conditions associated with prematurity [62] and go on to have more than average needs for paediatric care [63] (page 124).

Cost accounting in the maternity service remains as confused as ever. It has to be conceded that, since maternity care is in most cases only one of the many medical services provided in hospitals, isolating its separate cost presents complex problems. Nevertheless, the Winterton Committee was astonished that so little effort had apparently been made to solve the problems and establish the costs, far less the cost-effectiveness, of the maternity service in total or of its component procedures. It summarized its scathing judgement and its unfavourable impression of the chaotic state of the hospital information systems thus:

> No significant progress has been made towards costing the maternity services in a way which would enable those responsible for delivering them to make informed decisions about whether they met their targets (which are themselves ill-defined and often inappropriate) in a cost-effective manner. We are convinced by this inquiry that much of what is done in the name of maternity services is a waste of money, while many important needs remain unacknowledged and unmet. [44, para. 419]

In other countries the cost of maternity care to the user is covered by contributory or State-funded insurance schemes. In the Netherlands, the Sick Funds will reimburse a woman for non-teaching hospital care only if she has an agreed high risk condition. In other countries, like the USA and Australia, insurance schemes aid and abet obstetricians: they will cover the high costs of a caesarean section, even an unnecessary one, but not, in Australia, the much lower costs of a home confinement.

THE INVOLVEMENT OF VOLUNTARY AGENCIES

Alongside the growing acceptance in the early 20th century of public responsibility for maternal and child welfare, voluntary associations with the same concern were founded, typically by compassionate members of the more privileged classes in the interests of the less privileged. Some women from the working class, however, were similarly motivated and campaigned through the Women's Co-operative Guild for local authorities to initiate schemes to help mothers, for example, to secure that the financial Maternity Benefit under the National Health Insurance Act was paid directly to them as from 1913 [64].

The National League for Health, Maternity and Child Welfare was formed in 1905 and in 1915 opened its first maternity centre, an antenatal clinic in London, for the purpose of 'supervising the antenatal as well as the postnatal care of infants and the education of the mothers' [65, p. 8]. The voluntary associations were concerned to improve the nutrition and social conditions of childbearing women and their children, but they were anxious also to secure access for them to the presumed benefits of medical care which otherwise they could not afford.

The origin and growth of the National Childbirth Trust

Financial barriers to medical care were removed in Britain after the inception of the NHS in 1948. Obstetricians were poised to put into operation the schemes of technical management which, they believed, were the key to reducing mortality, accompanied by the propaganda designed to convince everyone that they were right. But many women found the means a high price to pay for the promised end and some dared to doubt the validity of the new philosophy. Their natural instincts were in accord, rather, with gentler, non-interventive methods taught by Grantly Dick-Read (page 96). To promote his teaching, one young mother, Prunella Briance, whose baby had just died after conventional obstetric care, was moved to found in 1956 the Natural Childbirth Association of Great Britain, which later became a charitable trust and changed its name first to the National Childbirth Association and then in 1961 to the National Childbirth Trust (NCT). It aimed to teach pregnant women skills in relaxation and breathing, which should reduce tension and anxiety, and in the relief to be gained from massage and different postures in labour. It aimed to build up their confidence through emotional support. Such preparation was carried out in small antenatal classes, for which a modest fee was charged and which were led by women who supplemented their personal experience of child-birth by successfully completing the training course for teachers devel-oped by the Trust. It aimed also to persuade medical authorities to facilitate home births or at least to provide a homely environment for institutional births, including allowing the presence of husbands or other lay companions [66, pp. 2–3]. It understood the benefits to be gained from breastfeeding, before these were quantified by recent research [46–48], and sought to encourage and sustain the practice by developing a training course for breastfeeding counsellors. It under-stood, better than the official maternity service, that birth itself is only a major event in a continuous process which could be made more rewarding for mothers and their families by support which its network could give throughout early parenthood.

The NCT's early successes in influencing medical authorities were inconspicuous. These pressed on undaunted with implementing inter-ventive obstetric policies and spreading appropriate obstetric propa-ganda. The Trust's antenatal preparation (page 107), which had soon been widened to incorporate other approaches to natural childbirth, like the psychoprophylaxis of Lamaze and Sheila Kitzinger, had to be widened further to prepare women for the procedures most of them were actually going to experience. With obstetricians on its panel of advisers, the NCT's objective was no longer to dispute the rightness of their principles of managing childbirth, so long as the management was carried out humanely; it sought co-operation and complementing rather than confrontation between providers and users. In the words of one second generation member 'They [the antenatal classes] gave me the confidence to go with my body to give birth, and the information I needed to understand the doctor and know when intervention was jus-tified' [67, p. 2].

Not all its members were so satisfied with the medical care they were given and the NCT had to revert to a less conciliatory stance. The infor-mation volunteered continuously by its members emphasized again that what the maternity services were providing was often not what the mothers felt to be in their or their baby's best interest. It then sought more actively to influence 'policies and the provision of services . . . by encouraging individual users . . . to speak up for what they want, by the appointment of NCT representatives to health committees, by the publication of information and original research, . . . by teaching or training NHS personnel, by raising public awareness and influencing opinion on a range of maternity issues' and by encouraging NCT members to contribute to birth and parenthood education in schools. In 1991 it submitted to the Winterton Committee its own carefully balanced analysis of its first hand evidence of users' experience of maternity care and its proposals for improvement, a submission which the committee obviously found compelling [42, pp. 231–77].

The origin and growth of the Association for Improvements in the Maternity Service

Prunella Briance was not the only enterprising woman to be so disturbed by the intranatal care she received in hospital as to organize a protest movement against it. In 1958, wondering whether her unhappy prenatal and intranatal stay in hospital was unique, Sally Willington tried repeatedly for a year before she found a newspaper willing to print her letter, asking if other women had shared her experience, for in the 1950s childbirth was not a subject to be discussed in the public press. Once the taboo was broken, letters flooded in from all parts of the country, confirming the complaints of loneliness; of lack of sympathy, privacy, consideration and rest; of having to deliver in a supine position; of being separated from the new baby; of the complete disregard of mental care or the personality of the mother. These letters gave rise to a voluntary organization, originally called the Society for the Prevention of Cruelty to Pregnant Women but from 1960 the Association for Improvements in the Maternity Services (AIMS), to fight for the redress of grievances [68].

Professionals brushed aside complaints as coming from women who had been drugged and could not remember events clearly. But the Ministry of Health was moved to publish a report in 1961 entitled *Human Relations in Obstetrics* [69], enjoining hospital authorities to remedy the causes of complaint publicized by AIMS. How far reforms were implemented depended on individual hospitals or consultants. The evidence gathered by the House of Commons Social Services Committee showed that many had still not been implemented by 1980, or indeed by 1984.

At first, the improvements AIMS wished to achieve were more technical developments more competently applied. But as interventions became more widely used, their disadvantages became apparent. As the induction rate multiplied in the early 1970s, AIMS joined with the Patients Association and other consumer groups to secure wide publicity for the issue that obstetric practice was putting convenience before safety. For whatever reason, the induction rate levelled off in the mid-

1970s before beginning a substantial decline (page 156). By the 1980s, AIMS had come to accept that it was dangerous not only to perform interventions incompetently but to perform them routinely and changed its objectives accordingly. Almost too late it realized that normal childbirth was most likely to be possible in the family home under the care of a midwife.

To spread its message, the members of AIMS organized local groups and maintained contacts with likeminded movements in other countries. Helping women to get the kind of care they want and to make effective complaints about unsatisfactory care meant that its volunteer officers had to keep knowledgeable and up to date about obstetric and midwifery practices, so that the information AIMS in turn dispensed in leaflets and in its quarterly journal was reliable. It was thus well prepared to give the Winterton Committee its detailed account of women's grievances and its proposals for remedies, which tallied closely with those from other consumer groups [70, pp. 465–510].

The Maternity Alliance

Stimulated by the Short Report of 1980 [31], the Maternity Alliance, a voluntary alliance of 70 national member organizations covering a wide range of maternity interests, was formed to campaign for the rights of mothers, fathers and babies and to secure improvements in the services, and also in the social and financial support given from before the child's conception through until its first birthday. It spreads information on matters of concern by organizing conferences and by producing occasional reports on specific issues, as well as a regular bimonthly (quarterly from 1994) bulletin, *Maternity Action*. The enquiries it most frequently receives relate to financial support and employment rights at work and its detailed submissions, written and oral, to the Winterton Committee drew special attention to these needs [42, pp. 80–108]. It is particularly concerned with the needs of the most socially disadvantaged women, including those with disabilities and from racial minorities, and believes that a maternity service, organized to meet their needs, would also meet the needs of most other women. Such a service would be dominated by midwives giving social support, rather than by obstetricians giving medical treatment.

Consumer groups with specific purposes

Pressure by AIMS and the NCT had been powerless to prevent the near total hospitalization of birth, but birth at home had not been outlawed, though professional propaganda gave the impression in many quarters that it had. It fell to a consumer group in Durham to found the Society to Support Home Confinements, which performed the immensely important service of establishing the precise steps a woman must take to obtain the home birth which she wanted and for which the NHS was legally bound to supply attendants.

Certain women, convinced by their experience of the inadequacies of orthodox obstetrics, have been motivated to organize groups which offer women alternative approaches and treatments in pregnancy and delivery. One of these is the Active Birth Movement, founded by Janet Balaskas, pioneering a fresh concept of antenatal preparation for natural childbirth (page 187). Another is the Pre-eclamptic Toxaemia Society (PETS), set up by Dawn James, a young mother disillusioned by birth attendants' ignorance about this condition, their unhelpfulness to women affected and the apparent inefficacy of the medical treatments currently prescribed. From the personal experiences of its members and from the medical literature, PETS aims to evaluate these treatments and has found that far better results are obtained from following an ample, high protein diet in pregnancy, as laid down by the American obstetrician, Tom Brewer (page 114). Another voluntary organization, Action on Pre-eclampsia, was founded in 1992 by parents who had lost babies through this illness, with the objectives of spreading general awareness and encouraging research, of building bridges between the profession and the public.

Affected users have identified other areas of need which have been overlooked or inadequately covered by conventional maternity services and have organized voluntary groups to supply the missing care to the victims. They have done this both directly, through arranging empathetic support, information and advice from fellow sufferers, and indirectly through persuading the professional providers of maternity care, clinical and administrative, to amend their practices, which have shown too little sensitivity to the emotional consequences of the unsuccessful outcomes of childbirth. The pain suffered by parents whose babies die before or after birth has in too many cases been aggravated by the uncaring treatment they have received and this neglect has prompted the foundation in recent years of helping associations like the Stillbirth and Neonatal Death Society (SANDS), the Miscarriage Association, Support After Termination For Abnormality (SATFA) and British Victims of Abortion (BVA). The additional problems associated with multiple births are focused by the Twins and Multiple Births Association (TAMBA); the Association of Breastfeeding Mothers (ABM) and the La Leche League of Great Britain (a branch of the American foundation) campaign in various ways to make the practice of breastfeeding more widely accepted in society. Foresight –

the Association for the Promotion of Preconceptual Care – aims to forestall problems by establishing links between environmental and dietary factors and unsuccessful outcomes. The Brook Advisory Centres provide a resource for preconception, antenatal and postnatal care for women, particularly very young women, who are deterred from using the NHS provisions but whose need for advice, particularly on family planning, is great. Financial support given by government sources to such charitable, non-governmental organizations is likely to prove a rewarding investment.

Community Health Councils

Towards counteracting the danger that the NHS would be managed to suit the dominant service providers, the doctors, statutory bodies were established to represent the users' interests. In the 1970s lay Community Health Councils (CHCs) were set up in every health district. In practice their power in any department has been limited. Although individual councillors have been sympathetic to the complaints of users and alive to the shortcomings of the maternity service, the CHCs have not halted, far less reversed, official policies for concentrating births in large hospitals, closing smaller units and making home births difficult to arrange.

CONSUMER GROUPS ABROAD

As in Britain, childbirth has been taken over by obstetricians and home birth has become rare in all developed countries except Holland. As in Britain, consumer movements have grown up to protest against the medicalization of an essentially physiological function and the hospitalization of what should be a healthy family event and to campaign for the restoration of the home as at least an optional place of birth and the midwife as a usual birth attendant. Such is the power of professional propaganda in instilling fear that only a small minority of mothers and midwives have enough confidence to risk leaving the professed protection of doctors' care. Nevertheless, the first International Homebirth Conference, organized jointly by AIMS and held in London in 1987, was able to draw representatives of consumer groups in twenty-eight countries, from Japan to Brazil, from Canada to New Zealand, from most countries in Western Europe and one country in Eastern Europe. A second International Homebirth Conference was held in Sydney, Australia, in 1992 and a third is planned to take place in Italy.

It is characteristic of women's organizations that they tend to be small and local and find it difficult to fight with a united voice. In the

USA there are many groups with similar objectives: for example, the American Foundation for Maternal and Child Health, New York; the Association for Childbirth at Home, International, California; the International Childbirth Education Association, Minnesota. The InterNational Association of Parents & Professionals for Safe Alternatives in Childbirth (NAPSAC, Missouri) aims to promote education about the principles of natural childbirth, the implementation of family-centred care at home, in maternity centres and in hospital and to act as a forum facilitating communication and co-operation among parents, medical professionals and childbirth educators. It produces its own and publicizes other relevant literature [71].

In the face of the caesarean epidemic in the 1980s, women anxious to avoid this operation, either as an initial or repeat procedure, formed protest groups and their mission was supported and given practical help by the International Cesarean Awareness Network, based in Syracuse, New York. It is the universal experience of protest organizations of consumers that they are hampered by shortage of funds in carrying out their work; most of their members have limited means and they do not hold out the prospect of profits to commercial sponsors.

The need for information to counter medical propaganda is met also by journals, such as *The Birth Gazette* (Tennessee), *Mothering* (New Mexico) and *Cesarean Prevention Clarion*, as well as by the internationally respected *Birth*. Despite all this activity towards achieving a system of maternity care which is biologically sound, with psychological and sociological advantages, and costs less in terms of lives, health and money, it has done little to dent the entrenched monopoly of obstetricians and their associated professional beneficiaries.

The consumer protest groups in other countries are modestly organized and financed. Homebirth Australia sought for several years to co-ordinate the efforts of different local groups and collect relevant statistics on a voluntary basis from the attending midwives. It produced a regular newsletter and in 1990 and 1992, in collaboration with the AIHW National Perinatal Statistics Unit, statistical analyses of the data for the years 1985–7 and 1988–90. Unlike results from every other source, the later Australian ones did not show lower mortality for birth at home than in hospital. Numbers were small and may have been incomplete, but neither this deficiency nor any other factor could be found to provide a convincing explanation for the surprising results. A new organization, Homebirth International Australia, was set up in 1993 to join

... with others around the world for the purposes of information, support and solidarity in the belief that every woman has a right to birth where and with whom she chooses and that her choices do not financially disadvantage her or her standard of care or put her or her birth attendant outside the law. [72]

ENFORCING PROFESSIONAL DISCIPLINE

Legislation in Britain has made the services of birth attendants legal monopolies. Restraints on abuse by doctors of their privilege lie in the hands of employing authorities, with powers of dismissal in cases of incompetence, and the General Medical Council (GMC), with powers of deregistration in cases of professional misconduct. Both employing authorities and the GMC are dominated by doctors. As regards the maternity service their standards are set by obstetric specialists, the pursuit of whose invasive practices is accepted as medically right, albeit without the explicit consent of the mother, and even in face of her explicit disagreement. Consequently, many cases of incompetence or misconduct, as judged by the victims and lay observers, escape the official retribution and are condoned by the professional watchdogs as long as they do not challenge established opinion and the status of the obstetric profession.

Attitudes are quite different if the conduct or expressed beliefs of a doctor do challenge current accepted practices. A consultant obstetrician whose views disputed the correctness of modern obstetric practice was suspended from her hospital appointment in 1985 on charges of professional incompetence and was not re-instated for fifteen months until after a quasi-legal public enquiry had completely exonerated her. The specific charges concerned matters on which orthodox obstetric opinion was not unanimous and so they could not finally be upheld, but a less courageous and tenacious person, who insisted on her right to have the enquiry in public and provoke widespread interest and sympathy, would not have carried on the protracted struggle to final vindication against what amounted to an attack on an alternative philosophy and its proponents [73]. Another obstetrician, who in 1979 expressed her support of natural childbirth, was gradually relieved of her hospital duties until, despite her continued protests, she was declared redundant in 1984 and finally dismissed in 1989, although paid full salary until then. She had to wait to be publicly exonerated of professional incompetence by her employing Health Authority until 1990, after an industrial tribunal found that she had been wrongfully dismissed [74].

In Australia persecution was even more ruthless. In the State of Victoria the obstetric establishment contrived a case against one of the two general practitioners, who continued to carry out home deliveries, mostly to the complete satisfaction of his clients, with an associated perinatal mortality rate well below average. His medical judges found

his clinical care in two cases negligent and caused him to be dereg-
istered. His legal appeal to the Supreme Court of Victoria in 1984 was
heard by a judge who obtained his clinical information from the same
source from which the initial accusation had originated and did not ask
for substantiating evidence for the assertions made. He accepted as
decisive that 'The Royal Australasian College of Obstetricians and
Gynaecologists has officially announced its strong disapproval of home
births under Australian conditions, and has officially adopted a policy
of discouraging them' [75]. Impartiality was impossible. The doctor's
deregistration was upheld. More recently, hostile action was taken by
the same establishment to restrict the practice of the remaining general
practitioner willing to attend home births.

The midwifery profession in Britain benefited from legal protection
under the *Midwives Act* which from 1910 forbade women who were not
certified midwives to attend women in childbirth 'habitually and for
gain' except under the direction of a medical practitioner. This in due
course got rid of competition from unqualified handywomen. The
restriction was later extended to any unqualified attendant, except in an
emergency. By the 1980s the practice of domiciliary midwifery had itself
been all but stamped out. Women had great difficulty in finding a competent and co-operative midwife for a home confinement. But when in
1982 two unqualified fathers sought to get round this obstacle by
supervising the delivery of their own healthy babies without professional assistance, they were successfully prosecuted for breaking this
law [76]. Public sympathy, however, was with the fathers and this tactic
for asserting professional monopoly was not repeated.

Although the maternity service would not willingly provide the care
requested, it was necessary to prevent a precedent which might encourage the re-emergence of the unqualified birth attendant. Ostensibly this
was to protect the safety of mother and child. Effectively it was to
protect the jobs of obstetricians, for protecting the jobs of domiciliary
midwives was by then hardly a live issue. In approving the prosecu-
tion, the Royal College of Midwives, whose Vice-President at the time
was the District Nursing Officer involved in one of the cases, gave a
further tacit illustration of the acceptance by the profession's leaders of
their subservient role [77].

Since midwives were first registered, rules have been laid down and
frequently updated to govern their conduct. Supervisors, after 1936
usually experienced midwives, have been appointed by local health
authorities to ensure that standards are maintained. Rules are notoriously capable of more than one interpretation and an individual supervisor's interpretation will depend on which school of thought she
favours.

In any case all eventualities cannot be foreseen. Strict adherence to the rules can conflict with the midwife's other duty, to judge what is in the mother's (or baby's) best interest in a given contingency. A midwife whose action, though sensible and beneficial, does not conform with her supervisor's interpretation of the rules risks incurring official disapproval, with immediate and often lengthy suspension without pay, midwives being more ruthlessly treated in this regard than suspended doctors. Deregistration can follow if the adjudicating panel shares the supervisor's view. The threat acts as a powerful deterrent to midwives who would like to implement their radical principles and avoid performing interventions they disapprove of.

The power of the supervisor extends, and in the 1980s was used obstructively, over those few midwives who, frustrated by the constraints of the State system, set up as private practitioners, offering continuity of care and home delivery. Disciplinary proceedings were instituted on flimsy pretexts, even when the mother and child were both safe and well. In one case they were pursued to ultimate deregistration ordered by the adjudicators after a hearing which amounted to a travesty of justice [78]. The authorities disavowed any intention of witch-hunting, but to the disinterested observer their actions looked like another use of legal procedures to protect the interests of the dominant birth attendants, the obstetricians and their supporters. In this case the deregistration was later annulled on appeal to the High Court.

Reacting to the patent unfairness of existing procedures, the Association of Radical Midwives continues to agitate for reform of the way the Professional Conduct Rules 1987 are operated and to propose changes to redress the unfairness [79].

Repression of midwives has been more severe and of much longer standing in other countries where obstetricians have dominated maternity care. Midwives' independent practice has been beset with restrictive regulations and they have been maligned with false accusations and harried with prosecutions for alleged incompetence and criminal responsibility on pretexts which, if applied to the practice of doctors, specialist or non-specialist, would have found most of them guilty.

In America the legalization of midwives who have not also completed a training in nursing is a matter for each State and a matter for constant campaigning. Legislation is introduced, modified and rescinded in States on a continuing basis, so that the overall situation keeps changing: by 1989 in nine States 'direct-entry' midwives (not certified nurses) were prohibited, in eight States they were clearly legal and in the rest they were covered by a wide variety of legal statutes [80]. In 1988 only 3.4% of American babies were delivered by midwives, but this is four times as many as in 1975. In Canada midwives were legally barred from practising until, after a tremendous fight, their practice was legalized in one Province in 1989 and in two others by 1994. With the removal of this legal barrier, ambitious programmes for educating direct-entry midwives were initiated.

In 1987 a hospital paediatrician was instrumental in having a charge of manslaughter brought against a midwife after a home birth in Queensland, Australia, but no negligence could be found and all charges were dismissed [81]. The process of attrition continues, the same paediatrician instituting in 1991 a similar process, in similar circumstances, this time against a highly qualified, British-trained midwife and her lay colleague, with a similar outcome [82].

LITIGATION

Dissatisfaction with the results of professional self-discipline and with official complaints procedures which yielded neither explanations nor apologies has led individual victims of medical misfortune to sue doctors directly. The custom started and spread in the United States before becoming adopted in Britain in the 1980s to such a degree as to necessitate huge increases in subscriptions required for medical defence insurance. Of all specialists, obstetricians have been most often the object of litigation. In self-defence they attribute this to the over success of their propaganda which has raised to an unrealistic level parents' expectations that the outcome will be satisfactory in every respect, that fetal distress can be accurately diagnosed, that interventions can overcome all problems, that these are necessary and always beneficial. Review of the medical notes of disputed cases, however, found most blame to lie in the misuse of forceps and misinterpretation of fetal heart trace records by junior staff who in turn blamed inadequate training and supervision by senior staff for the complicated deliveries they had to do [83].

Some litigants complain that the interventions undertaken were in fact unnecessary and harmful. Others complain that not enough intervention was undertaken or that it was of the wrong kind or too late and these are the complaints that Courts seem most prone to uphold. They accept, without evidence, obstetricians' claims that birth by caesarean section reduces the risk of intranatal hypoxia (lack of oxygen) and so of death or brain damage to the infant. Fear of litigation is given as one of the chief reasons for the rising incidence of this operation (page 167). High caesarean section rates do not correlate with low perinatal mortality rates and they are likely to raise rates of maternal mortality and morbidity (Chapters 4, 7, and 8).

Likewise Courts are impressed by the visible record of the reactions of the fetal heart and perhaps have not yet been told that the fetal distress inferred from the trace from an electronic monitor, a fertile indication for emergency caesarean sections, is all too often not borne out by the condition of the newborn infant (pages 124, 178). Nevertheless, since Courts are likely to judge the absence of this trace as evidence of negligence, fear of litigation is given as justifying the continued use of this kind of monitoring. It is apparently one thing to introduce a new piece of technology, but quite another to take it out of service, even when it has been shown to bring no benefit. And once legal precedents have been created, reversal of damaging practices is made even more difficult.

The Winterton Committee recommended that the problem of litigation could be reduced by improved education of the care-givers and a more effective complaints system [44, para. 448]. Probably the problem would be more greatly reduced if the maternity service and the education of the care-givers were reformed in accordance with the committee's other recommendations and based on the alternative philosophy of childbirth. Midwives are seldom sued for negligence, though they all have insurance cover. Moreover, since it is by no means certain that all cases of brain damage originate at the time of delivery, charges against the professionals present then may well be wrongly directed. The incentive for parents to obtain funds to cover the very high cost of the lifetime's care for their brain-damaged children by suing the obstetricians would probably be reduced if provisions existed to meet this need in some less harassing way.

In America the dangers of engaging the support of lawyers began in the 1980s to have more sinister ramifications. A body of legal thought developed that a viable fetus has rights distinct from the mother and it is the duty of the obstetrician to overrule the parents in the protection of these rights, to the length of obtaining Court orders to force women to be detained in hospital and undergo obstetric procedures, in particular caesarean section, against their will.

Support for this extension of obstetric jurisdiction is not lacking. A survey of attitudes within the American medical profession towards the legal enforcement of fetal rights found that nearly half of the 57 senior university and teaching hospital obstetricians consulted thought that 'mothers who endangered the life of the fetus by refusing medical advice should be detained to ensure compliance'. A quarter advocated State surveillance of women who stay outside the hospital system in the third trimester and 22% said home births should be illegal [84]. On the other hand the American Medical Association is opposed to granting legal sanction for obstetric intervention against the patient's will and in 1994 the Ethical Committee of the RCOG proposed a similar motion for agreement in Britain.

Concern for the fetus and its rights is rapidly dissipated when the fetus becomes a child and mother and child cease to be material for obstetric practice. The longer term possibility, with its profound social implications, is not addressed that forcibly depriving the mother of responsibility in pregnancy and delivery will irreversibly damage her innate responsibility to care for and nurture her child.

CONCLUSION

In the course of the 20th century, the public has had to become concerned with several aspects of maternity care. Policies have been determined and implemented through government departments and parliamentary committees, and the strongest voice influencing these has been that of the professional provider of care who has gained increasing domination, the obstetrician. By far the weakest voice was always that of the users of maternity care, even although for over thirty years they have organized voluntary groups to advance their interests, until at last in 1992 and in 1993 the British users' voice was listened to with the attention it deserved, first by a parliamentary committee and then by a Department of Health committee. Both committees recommended revolutionary changes, implementation of which obstetricians have acted, and may continue to act, to delay. In most recent decades Courts of Law have been appealed to in cases of dispute, but these too have depended on the dominant professionals for advice which could be unsound and biased, so that legal impartiality has also been surrendered.

REFERENCES

1. Interdepartmental Committee on the Physical Deterioration of the Population (1904) *Report*, HMSO, London.
2. Local Government Board (1910) *Report for 1909–10* (supplement on infant and child mortality), HMSO, London.
3. Local Government Board (1913) *Report for 1912*, HMSO, London.
4. Local Government Board (1914) *Report for 1913*, HMSO, London.
5. Local Government Board (1915) *Report for 1914–15* (supplement), HMSO, London.
6. Local Government Board (1917) *Report for 1915–16*, HMSO, London.
7. Local Government Board (1918) *Report for 1917–18*, HMSO, London.
8. Medical Officer of the Local Government Board (1915) *Memorandum on Health Visiting and on Maternity and Child Welfare Centres*, HMSO, London.
9. Campbell, J.M., Ministry of Health (1923) *Notes on the Arrangements for Teaching Obstetrics and Gynaecology in the Medical Schools*, Reports on Public Health and Medical Subjects No. 15, HMSO, London.
10. Campbell, J.M., Ministry of Health (1923) *The Training of Midwives*, Reports on Public Health and Medical Subjects No. 21, HMSO, London.

11. Campbell, J.M., Ministry of Health (1927) *The Protection of Motherhood*, Reports on Public Health and Medical Subjects No. 48, HMSO, London.
12. Campbell, J.M., Ministry of Health (1929) *Infant Mortality*, Reports on Public Health and Medical Subjects No. 55, HMSO, London.
13. Campbell, J.M., Cameron, I.D. and Jones, D.M., Ministry of Health (1932) *High Maternal Mortality in Certain Areas*, Reports on Public Health and Medical Subjects No. 68, HMSO, London.
14. Campbell, J.M., Ministry of Health (1924) *Maternal Mortality*, Reports on Public Health and Medical Subjects No. 25, HMSO, London.
15. Shaw, W.F. (1954) *Twenty-five Years. The Story of the Royal College of Obstetricians and Gynaecologists 1929–1954*, Churchill, London.
16. Ministry of Health (1930) *Interim Report of the Departmental Committee on Maternal Mortality and Morbidity* (Chairman Sir George Newman), HMSO, London.
17. Ministry of Health (1932) *Final Report of the Departmental Committee on Maternal Mortality and Morbidity* (Chairman Sir George Newman), HMSO, London.
18. Towler, J. and Bramall, J. (1986) *Midwives in History and Society*, Croom Helm, London.
19. *Maternity in Great Britain* (Survey undertaken by a Joint Committee of the Royal College of Obstetricians and Gynecologists and the Population Investigation Committee) (1946) Oxford University Press, Oxford.
20. Gillie, A.K. (1956) in *Proceedings of a Conference on General Practitioner Obstetrics*, College of General Practitioners, London, pp. 2–3.
21. Ministry of Health (1956) *Report of the Committee of Enquiry into the Cost of the National Health Service* (Chairman C. Guillebaud), HMSO, London.
22. Ministry of Health (1959) *Report of the Maternity Services Committee* (Chairman The Earl of Cranbrook), HMSO, London.
23. Ministry of Health (1970) *Domiciliary Midwifery and Maternity Bed Needs: the Report of the Standing Maternity and Midwifery Advisory Committee* (Sub-committee Chairman J. Peel), HMSO, London.
24. Department of Health and Social Security (1971) *Report of the Expert Group on Special Care for Babies*, Reports on Public Health and Medical Subjects No. 127 (Chairman W. Sheldon), HMSO, London.
25. Department of Health and Social Security (1974) *Report of the Working Party on the Prevention of Early Neonatal Mortality and Morbidity* (Chairman T. Oppé), HMSO, London.
26. Department of Health and Social Security (1976) *Fit for the Future: The Report of the Committee on Child Health Services* (Chairman D. Court), HMSO, London.
27. Richards, M.P.M. (1978) A place of safety? An examination of the risks of hospital delivery, in *The Place of Birth* (eds S. Kitzinger and J. Davis), Oxford University Press, Oxford.
28. Tew, M. (1980) Facts not assertions of belief. *Health Soc. Serv. J.*, 12 September, 1194–7.
29. Sinclair, J., Torrance, G., Boyle, M. *et al.* (1981) Evaluation of neonatal-intensive-care programs. *N. Engl. J. Med.*, **305**, 489–93.

30. Royal College of Physicians of London (1988) *Medical Care of the Newborn in England and Wales*, Royal College of Physicians of London, London.

31. House of Commons Social Services Committee (1980) *Perinatal and Neonatal Mortality; Second Report from the Social Service Committee, 1979–80* (Chairwoman, R. Short), HMSO, London.

32. Banta, D. and Thacker, S. (1979) Electronic fetal monitoring: is it of benefit? *Birth Family J.*, **6**, 4.

33. Prentice, A. and Lind, T. (1987) Fetal heart rate monitoring during labour – too frequent intervention, too little benefit? *Lancet*, **ii**, 1375–7.

34. Short, R. (1980) No evidence from Marjorie Tew. *Health Soc. Serv. J.*, 28 November (letter), 1521.

35. Tew, M. (1980) Misuse of statistics. *Health Soc. Serv. J.*, 12 December (letter), 1596.

36. House of Commons Social Services Committee (1984) *Perinatal and Neonatal Mortality Report: Follow-up; Third Report from the Social Services Committee, 1983–84* (Chairwoman, R. Short), HMSO, London.

37. Association of Anaesthetists (1987) *Anaesthetic Services for Obstetrics – A Place for the Future*, London.

38. Garcia, J. (1987) The role and structure of the Maternity Services Liaison Committees. *Health Trends*, **1** (19), 17–19.

39. Maternity Services Advisory Committee (1984) *Maternity Care in Action. Part II Care During Childbirth (Intrapartum Care); A Guide to Good Practice and a Plan for Action*, HMSO, London.

40. Enkin M. and Chalmers, I. (eds) (1982) *Effectiveness and Satisfaction in Antenatal Care*, William Heinemann, London.

41. House of Commons Health Committee (Chairman N. Winterton) (1991) *Maternity Services: Preconception*, vol. 1, HMSO, London, pp. i–xxxiv, paras 1–143.

42. House of Commons Health Committee (Chairman N. Winterton) (1991) *Maternity Services: Preconception, vol. II, Minutes of Evidence*, HMSO, London, pp. 1–291.

43. Department of Health (1992) *The Health of the Nation*, HMSO, London.

44. House of Commons Health Committee (Chairman N. Winterton) (1992) *Maternity Services*, vol. 1, HMSO, London, pp. i–xciii, paras 1–453.

45. House of Commons Health Committee (Chairman N. Winterton) (1992) *Maternity Services, vol. II, Minutes of Evidence*, HMSO, London, pp. 338–650.

46. Lucas, A. and Cole, T. (1990) Breast milk and neonatal necrotising enterocolitis. *Lancet*, **336**, 1519–23.

47. Howie, P., Forsyth, J. *et al.* (1990) Protective effect of breast feeding against infection. *Br. Med. J.*, **300**, 11–16.

48. United Kingdom Case Control Study Group (1993) Breast feeding and risk of breast cancer in young women. *Br. Med. J.*, **307**, 17–20.

49. The International Neonatal Network (1993) The CRIB (clinical risk index for babies) score: a tool for assessing initial neonatal risk and comparing performance of neonatal intensive care units. *Lancet*, **342**, 193–8.

50. Tew, M. (1984) Understanding intranatal care through mortality statistics, in

Pregnancy Care for the 1980s (eds L. Zander and G. Chamberlain), Royal Society of Medicine and Macmillan Press, London, pp. 115–25.

51. Chalmers, I., Enkin, M. and Keirse, M. (1989) *Effective Care in Pregnancy and Childbirth*, Oxford University Press, Oxford.

52. Department of Health (1993) *Changing Childbirth. Report of the Expert Maternity Group* (Chairman Lady Julia Cumberlege), HMSO, London.

53. Hall, M. (1989) Critique of antenatal care, in *Obstetrics* (eds A. Turnbull and G. Chamberlain), Churchill Livingstone, Edinburgh, pp. 225–33.

54. Chamberlain, G. (ed.) (1990) *Modern Antenatal Care of the Fetus*, Blackwell, Oxford.

55. The Royal College of General Practitioners and the Royal College of Obstetricians and Gynaecologists (1993) *General Practitioner Vocational Training in Obstetrics and Gynaecology*, RCGP/RCOG, London.

56. Page, L. (1993) Changing childbirth. *MIDIRS Midwifery Res.*, **3**, 385–7.

57. Horvath, M. (1985) Place of Birth and Perinatal Mortality, unpublished research, Worlingworth, Woodbridge, Suffolk.

58. Stilwell, J. (1979) Relative costs of home and hospital confinements. *Br. Med. J.*, **2**, 257–9.

59. Gray, A. and Steele, R. (1981) The economics of specialist and general practitioner maternity units. *J. R. Coll. Gen. Pract.*, **31**, 586–92.

60. Clark, L., Mugford, M. and Paterson, C. (1991) How does the mode of delivery affect the cost of maternity care? *Br. J. Obstet. Gynaecol.*, **98**, 519–23.

61. Mugford, M., Piercy, J. and Chalmers, I. (1991) Cost implications of different approaches to the prevention of respiratory distress syndrome. *Arch. Dis. Child.*, **66**, 757–64.

62. Sittlington, N., Tubman, R. and Halliday, H. (1991) Surfactant replacement therapy for severe respiratory distress syndrome: implication for nursing care. *Midwifery*, **7**, 20–4.

63. Skeoch, F., Rosenberg, K. *et al.*, (1987) Very low birthweight survivors: illness and readmission to hospital in the first 15 months of life. *Br. Med. J.*, **2**, 579–80.

64. Oakley, A. (1984) *The Captured Womb*, Blackwell, Oxford.

65. National League for Health, Maternity and Child Welfare (1915) *Annual Report*.

66. National Childbirth Trust (1986) *Facing the Future: Annual Report for 1986*, London.

67. Brownlie, A. (1986) *NCT Annual Report for 1986*.

68. Willington, S. (1985) Origins of A.I.M.S. *Assoc. Improvements Maternity Serv. Q. J.*, Conference Bulletin.

69. Ministry of Health (1961) *Human Relations in Obstetrics*, Central Health Services Council, HMSO, London.

70. House of Commons Health Committee (1992) *Maternity Services, vol. III, Minutes of Evidence*, HMSO, London, pp. 338–650.

71. Stewart, D. (1981) *The Five Standards for Safe Childbearing*, Napsac Reproductions, Marble Hill, Missouri.

72. Elaine Odgers Norling (1993) Personal communication. Homebirth International Australia, Sydney.

73. Savage, W. (1986) *A Savage Enquiry*, Virago Press, London.
74. Dyer, C. (1990) Miss Pauline Bousquet clears her name. *Br. Med. J.*, **300**, 1674.
75. Supreme Court of Victoria, Melbourne, Before the Honourable Mr Justice Fullagar, Between John Stevenson and the Medical Board of Victoria, Judgment, 27th June 1984 (Causes Jurisdiction No M25 of 1984).
76. Robinson, J. (1982) Guilty: the crime of giving birth. *Assoc. Improvement Maternity Serv. Q. J.*, Autumn.
77. 'The Court Press' (1982) *Assoc. Improvements Maternity Serv. Q. J.*, Autumn.
78. Lady Pickard (1988) The Case of Jilly Rosser: hearing before the Professional Conduct Committee of the United Kingdom Central Council for Nursing, Midwifery and Health Visiting. *Assoc. Radical Midwives Mag.*, **39**.
79. Flint, C. (1989) Professional conduct machinery – some necessary changes. *Assoc. Radical Midwives Mag.*, 40.
80. Becker, E., Long, M. *et al.* (1990) *Midwifery and the Law*, A *Mothering* special edition, Mothering Publications, Albuquerque.
81. Jakel-Kuchel, J. (1987) Homebirth in the courts. *Homebirth Aust., Newslett.*, 15.
82. Idle, M. (1991) Personal communication. Cairns, Queensland, Australia.
83. Ennis, M. and Vincent, C. (1990) Obstetric accidents: a review of 64 cases. *Br. Med. J.*, **300**, 1365–7.
84. Kolder, V., Gallagher, J. and Parsons, M. (1987) Court-ordered obstetrical interventions. *N. Engl. J. Med.*, **316**, 1192–6.

Evaluating the results of maternity care: statistical instruments

6

In the 20th century in all countries, medical and social resources have increasingly been devoted to providing a maternity service which is intended to make the birth safer for mother and child. But there has never been a concomitant allocation of statistical resources to measure to what extent the service provided, as a whole or in its constituent parts, has achieved its intended objective. Such evaluation as is available has had to be done by indirect methods. It is fragmentary but the pieces can be fitted together to indicate a consistent and convincing picture.

REQUIREMENTS FOR EVALUATION

Before any evaluation is possible measurements have to be recorded describing the desired outcome on the one hand and the factors which may have contributed to it on the other. Lack of the necessary money and skills are cogent practical reasons which limit the quantity of relevant data which have been collected (pages 27–31). This in turn limits the scope for evaluation.

The desired outcome of maternity is primarily the survival of mother and child and simple records of death rates in Britain have for a long time been reasonably complete and reliable (pages 5–6). Death is certain and unambiguous. The second desired outcome of maternity is healthy survival. Morbidity (illness and handicap) are much less straightforward to identify and measure. Hence records of morbidity rates are much less complete and reliable.

Less complete and reliable also are records which measure the factors already identified as influencing outcome, and there may be other factors not yet so identified. These factors may be divided into two distinct, though not always independent groups. One group is made up of biological and social factors which go towards describing the physical condition of the mother and infant at the time of the pregnancy and birth. Many of these, such as maternal age and fetal gestation, can be categorized and quantified and from those known before the onset of labour the risk status of the impending birth can be predicted.

The other group is made up of factors which go towards describing the nature of the antenatal, intranatal and postnatal care received by the mother and the neonatal care received by the baby. Many of these can readily be described by quantity, but quantity is not a reliable proxy for the more critical parameter, quality. For example, the number of antenatal attendances does not describe the quality, far less the effectiveness, of the care received and should not be presumed to do so.

THE BASIC ARITHMETIC OF MORTALITY RATES, ACTUAL AND STANDARDIZED

The absolute numbers of the factors described only begin to have meaning when they can be related to each other. They become instruments for making comparisons when they can be converted into rates, ratios which show the actual number of objects or events in a subgroup of the category of interest as a proportion of the total number of objects or events in that category. Values for both numerators and denominators are needed to calculate ratios. Correct interpretation of the statistical results of maternity care depends on understanding first how a mortality rate is made up, an insight apparently not enjoyed by obstetric propagandists.

A mortality rate per 1000 births is simply the number of deaths divided by the number of births in the same place and period, with the fraction multiplied by 1000. But it is also an average of the specific mortality rates in the component subgroups, weighted by the proportion that each subgroup makes up of the total. This can most easily be demonstrated by an example, as in Table 6.1(a), using data from the 1958 Perinatal Mortality Survey, for which 88% of the births were classified by grade of maternal toxaemia and place of actual delivery. (The unclassified births are omitted from the calculation.) For simplicity of exposition, the grades of risk are compressed into three subgroups at low, moderate and high risk and the data for general practitioner units (GPUs) and home are combined because they are so similar.

Table 6.1 Perinatal mortality rates (PNMR) per 1000 births: to show how they depend on the proportion of births and the specific PNMR in subgroups of risk on account of maternal toxaemia

Risk group	Total births (15 009 = 100%)			Hospital births (7625 = 50.8%)			GPU/Home births (7384 = 49.2%)		
	Proportion of total P	Specific PNMR R	Product P × R	Proportion of total P	Specific PNMR R	Product P × R	Proportion of total P	Specific PNMR R	Product P × R
(a)									
		Actual			Actual				
Low	0.87	26.9	23.4	0.82	38.4	31.5	0.92	16.3	15.0
Moderate	0.06	42.6	2.6	0.07	51.9	3.6	0.04	26.2	1.0
High	0.07	88.8	6.2	0.11	107.1	11.8	0.04	35.7	1.4
All	1.0	32.3	32.2	1.0	46.5	46.9*	1.00	17.4	17.4
(b)									
		Actual			Hypothetical or standardized				
Low	0.87	26.9	23.4	0.87	38.4	33.4	0.87	16.3	14.2
Moderate	0.06	42.6	2.6	0.06	51.9	3.1	0.06	26.2	1.6
High	0.07	88.8	6.2	0.07	107.1	7.5	0.07	35.7	2.5
All	1.00	32.3	32.2	1.00	44.0	44.0	1.00	18.3	18.3

Source: reference [9] Table 30 (births with no or insufficient information excluded).
*Small error due to rounding.

The overall mortality rate per 1000 births was 32.3, the weighted average of the rate in hospital, 46.5, where 50.8% of the births took place, and in GPU/home, 17.4, with 49.2% of the births ($0.508 \times 46.5 + 0.492 \times 17.4 = 32.3$). The proportions of births at moderate and high risk were higher in hospital, but so also were the mortality rates there at each grade of risk. Indeed, the mortality rate for the low-risk group in hospital (38.4) was marginally higher than for the high-risk group in GPU/home (35.7).

The validity of the claim that disparities in mortality rates at different birth places are accounted for by disparities in the predicted risk composition of the births at each place can only be verified if data describing the relevant risk compositions are available. When such data, together with the specific mortality rates in each subgroup of risk, are known, the actual mortality rates can be standardized by the direct method, that is, recalculated to show what they would have been if each place had had the same proportion of births at each level of risk. When this is done, as in Table 6.1(b), it shows that the hospitals' total mortality rate would have been slightly reduced, from 46.5 to 44.0, and the GPU/home rate would have been slightly raised, from 17.4 to 18.3, but the discrepancy between them would have been reduced only by 11.7%, from 29.1 to 25.7. With higher rates in all the specific risk groups, the persisting discrepancy is arithmetically inevitable. Less than one-eighth of it could have been due to the greater proportion in hospital of births at higher risk on account of toxaemia.

If in each subgroup of risk the number of births, but not the number of deaths, is known for each place separately, although the specific mortality rates are known for all places combined, the other more complicated indirect method of standardization has to be used. The method is illustrated in Table 6.2, using data from the 1970 British Births survey which omitted to publish figures of deaths which would have allowed embarrassing comparisons of risk-specific mortality rates between places of birth to be immediately made (page 331).

A weighted average will be higher the greater the proportion it includes at high risk, and conversely. If, over time, proportions in subgroups change, the weighted average must, in the absence of counteracting influences, change in the appropriate direction. The perinatal mortality rate associated with home births is the weighted average of two distinct subgroups: one made up of women who have normal midwifery care and the other made up of women who, although biologically or socially at high risk, reject care of any kind or whose precipitate delivery forestalls arranged care. Typically, perinatal mortality rates are very low for the former group, but very high for the latter group, largely the teenage and unmarried mothers having unwanted

Table 6.2 To illustrate an indirect method of standardizing perinatal mortality rates (PNMR) per 1000 births in different places of delivery: indirect standardization is necessary when the actual number of deaths in each subgroup of risk at each place of birth is not known, although the number of associated births and the overall PNMR for each subgroup are known. Using the known data, the number of deaths expected in each subgroup is calculated on the assumption that the births at each place shared the same average mortality experience. The ratio between the actual total of deaths at each place, also known, and the sum of the expected deaths shows the percentage relationship of the PNMR in each place to the overall average

Risk group maternal parity	Overall PNMR (known)	Hospital		GPU/Home	
		Births (known)	Expected deaths (calculated)	Births (known)	Expected deaths (calculated)
A	B	C	B × C/ 1000	D	B × D/ 1000
0	21.3	4249	90.5	1154	24.5
1	18.0	3018	54.3	1776	32.0
2	21.7	1663	36.1	969	21.0
3	19.1	922	17.6	499	9.5
4 +	34.1	1304	44.5	262	8.9
All births	21.4		243.0		95.9
Actual deaths (known)			310		23
Standardized PNMR overall PNMR × actual deaths/expected deaths			21.4 × 310/243.0 = 27.3		21.4 × 23/95.9 = 5.1
(Actual PNMRs (known)			27.8		4.9)

Source: reference [15], Table 5.9.

and concealed pregnancies [1, 2]. As long as many births took place at home, the former group predominated and the weighted average mortality rate reflected mainly their experience and was low. But as the policy of hospitalization was implemented, the proportion having planned deliveries at home was progressively reduced, leaving the uncared-for deliveries to make up an increasing proportion of the diminishing total. The weighted average rate increasingly reflected their experience and rose. Even leading obstetricians rushed to welcome the new trend as eventually vindicating their accusations of the lack of safety in domiciliary midwifery [3, 4], but in their eagerness they allowed themselves to be misled by what was simply an arithmetic artefact.

Techniques of standardization are useful when average mortality rates between two places or two periods have to be compared, but interpretation of outcomes is simpler and conclusions more reliable if the data permit specific rates at each different level of risk to be calculated and then compared.

RISK ASSESSMENT

Since the chance of a safe outcome varies with the predicted risk status of the birth, the effectiveness of any service can be fairly measured only if account its taken of the predicted risk status of the births which have actually received it. If the effectiveness of alternative services or alternative treatments is to be compared, the groups of births receiving them should have comparable risk status. Once the necessary information about any single risk factor has been collected, births, with the associated deaths, can be categorized in subgroups and it is simple to calculate specific death rates for each subgroup of risk. When births in any subgroup have received different treatments, differences between the specific death rates offer a measurement of differences between the effectiveness of the treatments.

One risk factor by itself, however, is an inadequate indicator of a birth's overall risk status, which is determined by the combined effect of many, often interdependent, factors, some of which influence the degree of risk in the same direction while others influence it in the opposite direction. For example, risk increases with maternal age and also with parity. A woman who has already borne several children is likely to be in an older age group. Hence much of the risk associated with age is accounted for by high parity and vice versa. Risk is higher where socio-economic class is lower. Mothers of low social class tend to have larger families. Hence much of the risk associated with high parity is accounted for by low social class and vice versa. On the other hand, mothers of low social class tend to be younger, so that risk from one factor tends to counteract risk from the other.

A group of mothers receiving a particular treatment is likely to be made up of women at different degrees of risk on account of the various factors. If the outcome for these mothers is to be compared with that for another group having an alternative treatment, the combined predicted risk status from all known factors must be similar for the two groups. Several methods for achieving this comparability have been developed.

METHODS OF EVALUATION

The method which at present commands the most respect when the effectiveness of different treatments is to be compared is the randomized controlled trial. If, in a prospective study which includes sufficient numbers, subjects are allocated at random to receive one or other treatment, it is likely that similar distributions of each single risk factor among the treatment groups will be achieved. Each group will be found to contain similar proportions of subjects in each subgroup of maternal age, parity, social class, infant birthweight and other relevant risk factors. Thus any difference in outcome between the groups can be attributed to the unequal effectiveness of the treatments and not to an excess proportion at high predicted risk on account of any biological or social factor in one of the groups.

If it had no drawbacks, if its conditions could always be fulfilled, the randomized controlled trial would be the ideal method of eliminating risk bias in the composition of groups on which the effectiveness of alternative treatments is to be tested. Unfortunately, there are drawbacks. Bias proves hard to eliminate.

In practice, a trial is proposed when an interested researcher has reason to suspect that one treatment is more beneficial than its alternative, or when a disinterested researcher wishes to settle an issue on which the care providers have conflicting opinions. Thus an element of bias may underlie the trial at its inception.

If the treatment to be tested is a drug, then it is possible to avoid bias by blinding the participants, both clinicians and subjects, to whether the active drug or a placebo, an inactive alternative, is being given and taken. If the treatment to be tested is a procedure, then the stratagem of blinding to avoid bias is obviously impossible, unless the outcome to be measured is distant in time from the procedure, which leaves no identifying physical marks and remains unknown to the outcome evaluator.

Prospective trials bring problems at every stage. In the first place, it may be difficult to command the necessary resources of finance and skill in planning and administration and a badly planned or conducted trial is likely to produce useless results. The informed consent of participating subjects should be obtained, but this involves making them aware of uncertainties about the correct treatment. Those who are left believing that one of the alternatives is really better will be unwilling to be randomized to the other. Those who agree to enter the trial with open minds may feel like guinea pigs and in some way behave differently from people not conscious of being watched. Their reaction may prejudice the validity of generalizations proposed from the trial's results. If, during the course of the trial, the belief spreads that one procedure is superior, subjects randomized to the suspected inferior procedure may cease to comply with it.

Participating clinicians, who really believe that one procedure is better at least for certain patients, may not allow all candidates to be randomized. If their own initial experience in the trial leads them to favour one procedure, they may feel obliged to depart from stipulated protocols before the trial has collected sufficient material to support a valid conclusion. Likewise, ethics committees, which have to be consulted about research proposals, may intervene to bring the trial to an end, if too many adverse outcomes appear to be occurring to one side.

To the degree to which bias creeps in to the implementation of a randomized controlled trial, its initial purpose of eliminating bias in confounding risk factors is defeated and the validity of its results must be doubted. For in order to retain the virtue of randomization, the results must be measured in the groups as randomized to the treatments being studied. But the findings have practical value only if all, or nearly all, the subjects allocated to a treatment actually have that treatment; otherwise the comparison of outcomes ceases to have meaning. If after all subjects allocated to treatment A have actually had treatment A and all subjects allocated to treatment B have actually had treatment B, and the result is better for treatment A than treatment B by a margin too great to be due to chance, then it is properly accepted that A is the superior treatment. But if some subjects allocated to treatment A do not have it, or worse still have treatment B, while some subjects allocated to treatment B do not have it, or worse still have treatment A, then the better result for the group randomized to treatment A says little or nothing about the relative effectiveness of the treatments actually received.

It might have been possible to mount a randomized controlled trial to show whether birth was safer in a specialist obstetric hospital than in a non-specialist hospital or at home if this had been done around 1950, before obstetricians' propaganda had persuaded nearly everyone that it was so. Later it would have been quite impossible to ensure the impartial conduct, and hence the impartial results, of a trial once the majority of participants, both the users and providers of the service, had become heavily biased about the expected outcome, as was to happen.

It might just be possible in a geographically defined area where the necessary options were available, to conduct a randomized controlled trial to compare safety in different places of birth if certain conditions could be fulfilled. First, subjects would have to be limited to women whom obstetricians predicted to be at low risk and, in their view, less certain to require specialist care, so that the participating obstetricians would be less likely to depart from the prescribed protocol. Second, sufficient numbers of such women would have to be found who were truly indifferent as to where they laboured and were willing to be randomized to any place. Third, sufficient numbers of birth attendants would have to be willing to carry out their service without bias in the allocated place. It is, however, far from obvious who would undertake the responsibility for initiating such a trial and ensuring that its protocols were strictly observed.

To mount a prospective randomized controlled trial of the safest place of birth would be at any time an ambitious and onerous undertaking. More feasible would have been the conduct of such trials to test the effectiveness of the specific procedures, the elements of specialist obstetric care, before they became adopted as standard practice on the unsupported assumption that they were effective and suitable for general use. Although feasible and necessary on both clinical and ethical grounds, such trials were very rarely carried out. The results of trials carried out belatedly to establish and quantify the benefit from treatments already in general use have rarely supported the original claims for them, as is shown by the examples quoted in this book and elsewhere [5]. But even if advance trials had been done, they would still have been open to misinterpretation.

A trial comparing one obstetric procedure with another may lead to conclusions about the relative benefits of one of them, but the conclusions may apply only within the setting in which the trial took place. A lonely example of such a randomized trial found a marginal and short-term benefit for continuous electronic monitoring over intermittent auscultation of the fetal heart among a large number of deliveries in a hospital committed to active obstetric management and adherence to set time limits for progress in labour [6]. It cannot be assumed that the result would have been the same if the comparison had been between continuous electronic fetal monitoring in a specialist hospital and intermittent auscultation in the more relaxed and permissive setting of the non-specialist hospital or family home. The same uncertainty overhangs the trial in an obstetric hospital which demonstrated the apparent benefit of the administration of syntometrine in preventing postpartum haemorrhage [7].

PROSPECTIVE AND RETROSPECTIVE STUDIES

Because of its reputed capability of eliminating selection bias, the prospective enquiry is frequently claimed to be a more accurate research method than retrospective analysis of existing results. The result of a prospective enquiry may not, however, be representative of normal experience. It is a well recognized social phenomenon that, when people are conscious that their behaviour is being observed, they perform to a higher standard than usual – the so-called Hawthorn effect. It is another well recognized phenomenon that a study carried out to evaluate a procedure in whose invention the researcher is personally involved yields better results than can be achieved by other practitioners who do not have the same high interest in demonstrating its success. Participants may not be equally motivated and unequal motivation may distort results. It may not be possible to replicate the findings of a prospective study under normal conditions when specific motivation is absent, so they would not necessarily provide the most reliable guide for future policy.

This source of distortion is avoided by statistics, like routinely collected official data, which describe the normal experience of large, unselected populations. On the other hand, retrospective analysis of existing results, of what actually happened, is bedevilled by the difficulty of identifying comparable risk groups from the data available. One technique frequently adopted is to match a study group exposed to one kind of treatment with a control group whose members have, as far as possible, the same risk characteristics, believed to be relevant, as members of the study group but who were exposed to a different treatment. The outcome for each of the matched groups is then compared and differences are attributed to the unequal effectiveness of the treatments. The possibility remains that the risk factors controlled for do not include factors material to outcome but not yet identified as such. Here an unequal result may reflect, not unequal effectiveness of treatments, but an unequal distribution of the unidentified factor.

The matched control method has frequently been used to study outcomes in different places of birth and outcomes following specific treatments in the same place of birth. Relevant examples are quoted elsewhere in this book. The method, of course, can only be used by researchers who have access to detailed information in case records, which are confidential, and to computing facilities for sorting out and analysing the extracted data. For researchers not so privileged, official publications of routinely collected data relating to maternal and perinatal outcome offer most scope for informative retrospective analysis, although insufficient use has been made of the opportunities presented.

In some of these documents relating to England and Wales, the actual place of birth is cross-classified with up to two risk factors simultaneously: maternal age and parity or maternal age and birth legitimacy [8, 9]. The report of the 1958 perinatal survey published separate cross-classifications of mortality by place of birth, both actual and intended, with maternal parity, social class and toxaemia, with fetal gestation and with infant birthweight [10]. Reports of the Confidential Enquiries into Maternal Deaths covering the years 1964 to 1975 cross-classified mortality rates by intended place of birth with maternal age and with parity [11–14].

From such data, specific mortality rates at different levels of predicted risk can be calculated for each place of delivery. With remarkable consistency, these always turn out to be higher for births in obstetric hospitals (Chapters 7 and 8). The standard response of obstetricians to this finding is that the available risk factors by themselves do not adequately measure the cumulative risk from all risk factors, implying that if there were such a measure it would show that the excess predicted risk of births in hospital would more than account for their apparent excess mortality.

The concept of cumulative scores as tools for both prospectively directing practice and retrospectively evaluating the success of treatment appealed to doctors and researchers in several departments of medicine and surgery in the 1970s. But the concept proved to be more attractive in theory than in practice. Determining the factors rightly to be included and weighting their usual relative importance where known presents many problems; an overall score may obscure and distract attention from an individual component factor of greater significance in a particular circumstance. In the field of maternity care several prospective scores were used experimentally in restricted contexts, but none proved satisfactory enough to be suitable for general adoption. The British Births 1970 survey [15] offered the only large data base for which an attempt was made to use retrospective scores for evaluation.

RISK SCORES – INSTRUMENTS FOR THE RETROSPECTIVE ANALYSIS OF DATA

Towards providing such instruments, the analysts of that survey constructed two composite risk scores (pages 332–8). Some of the problems encountered will become obvious in the following description of their application. The first of these, the antenatal prediction score, is summarized in Table 6.3. It combined the risks associated with the maternal biological and social characteristics of age, parity, social class (as measured by husband's occupation or by marital status) and aspects of obstetric and medical history – risks present at the start of pregnancy. Where a previous pregnancy had been by caesarean section, or where the mother already had hypertension (high blood pressure) or diabetes, the current pregnancy was deemed to require specialist obstetric care and deserve a score of four points on each count which applied. Risk on account of the other factors was graded on three levels, low, moderate and high, measured by point values of 0, 1 and 2 respectively. The point values were based on the specific mortality rates in the subgroups of the factors found in the perinatal survey of 1958, when the overall average rate was 35 per 1000 births.

Table 6.3 Antenatal prediction score: weights given to different risk factors

Maternal risk factor	Level of risk		
	Low	Moderate	High
Age	0	1	2
Parity	0	1	2
Social class	0	1	2
Obstetric history			
Previous stillbirth			4
Neonatal death			4
Abortion			4
Caesarean section			4
Co-existing disease			
Hypertension			4
Diabetes			4

Source: reference [15], pp. 39–42.

For example, the perinatal mortality rate associated with maternal ages 20–29 was lowest at 30 and was given the risk score of 0; the rate associated with maternal ages under 20 and 30–34 was 37 and was given the risk score of 1; the rate at maternal ages over 35 was 52 and was given the score of 2. The parity and social class factors were similarly divided into three grades of risk. Scores of 2 were given when the mother had already borne more than three children or belonged to the lowest social class or was unsupported, subgroups which in 1958 had perinatal mortality rates of 52 and 42 respectively. Scores of 4 were given when the mother was already hypertensive, or had had a caesarean section, or a stillbirth or neonatal death, conditions which in 1958 carried perinatal mortality rates of 47, 66 and 77 respectively. Clearly, the score values were approximate and could not be proportional since the lowest value was set at 0.

The second of the composite risk scores constructed, the labour prediction score, summarized in Table 6.4, enables the process of analysis to be taken much further, for it adds to the risks known early in pregnancy the risks from the most serious complications which may develop during pregnancy and from conditions identified during labour as having an important influence on its outcome. Thus the labour prediction score computed for each birth purports to give a fairly complete measurement of its cumulative predicted risk status shortly before delivery.

Again the risk from most of the factors listed was graded in up to

Table 6.4 Labour prediction score, singleton pregnancies: weights given to risk factors

Risk factor	Level of risk		
	Low	Moderate	High
Antenatal prediction score	0	1	2
Previous caesarean section			4
Hypertension/toxaemia	0	1	2
Antepartum haemorrhage	0		2
Duration of pregnancy	0	1	2
Duration of first stage of labour	0	1	2
Fetal distress (heart rate)	0	1	2
(meconium)		1	
(both signs present)			2
Breech presentation			4

Source: reference [15], pp. 151–4.

three levels quantified with scores of 0, 1 or 2. The risks reflected in the antenatal prediction score were summarized in three grades corresponding to perinatal mortality rates of 15, 26 and 43 respectively in 1970, when the survey average had fallen to 21. Pregnancies lasting between 37 and 42 weeks scored 0, those lasting over 42 weeks scored 1, while those lasting less than 37 weeks scored 2; the associated mortality rates for these three groups were, however, 10, 18 and 171 respectively.

Births following antepartum haemorrhage from any cause scored 2 and births without history of bleeding scored 0; the specific perinatal mortality rates (in 1970) were 60 and 17. Where diastolic blood pressure remained normal or rose moderately, the score was 0 or 1; where it rose greatly or the mother's urine contained protein, the score was 2. The perinatal mortality rates in these three subgroups (in 1970) were, however, respectively 19, 18 and 34.

The duration of the first stage of labour was divided into three subgroups of risk: up to 12 hours, 12–24 hours and over 24 hours, scoring 0, 1 or 2. This grading was obviously based on the obstetricians' misconception, which suited their system of management (pages 158–60), that risk increases the longer the first stage of labour lasts. The relevant mortality rates in the 1970 survey were not published, but in 1958 they were 32, 28 and 38 respectively, the risk being lowest between 12 and 24 hours [10, p. 157]. Risk increases with fetal distress, of which the signs are taken to be a heart rate slower or faster than normal, scoring 1 or 2, and the presence of meconium (faeces passed by the fetus) in the amniotic fluid, by itself scoring 1; the presence of any two signs of distress scored an extra 2 points. Neither survey quantified mortality by these signs of fetal distress. Breech presentation, which is associated with many fetal problems and high mortality and is said to need intrapartum care by an obstetrician, was given a score of 4 points.

Although risk from a previous caesarean section had been included with a score of 4 in the antenatal prediction score, an extra 4 points was added on this account to the labour prediction score. The risk was grossly exaggerated, for the mortality rate in 1970 for births following a previous section, at 22, was only slightly higher than the survey average of 21, a smaller excess than had been found in 1958.

Shortcomings of scores

As in the antenatal prediction score, the values for individual risks in the labour prediction score were approximate and they did not always represent the known gradient of risk in the specific factors. As between factors, a score of 2 could represent mortality rates ranging (in 1970) from 34 (hypertension) to 171 (short gestation), while a score of 4 was given to the lesser risk of previous caesarean section (22). The risks which in obstetricians' opinion were highest and which were most likely to secure specialist care tended to be overvalued in the scoring system. As a result, the predicted risk status of the births in specialist hospitals would tend to be overstated. Nevertheless, despite all the imperfections in their composition, the two prediction scores in conjunction with the detailed survey data supply instruments of analysis far more useful and reliable than any other data available before or since in enabling account to be taken of differences in predicted risk status when comparisons are made retrospectively of the outcome of birth in different places of delivery.

Comparing like with like

The prediction scores were used to give each birth in the 1970 survey points appropriate to its degree of risk in respect of each of the factors listed, its total score giving a measure of its total risk as predicted either in early pregnancy or in labour. Births with the same total scores were deemed to be at the same total risk. Therefore groups of births with the same score could properly be compared. The births, with the associated deaths, could then be cross-classified by risk score and place of delivery, so that specific mortality rates at each level of risk at the same stage of pregnancy or labour at each place of delivery could be compared. Hence, any inequality between the mortality rates for births with the same score, particularly the more complete and more immediate labour prediction score, should be a fair measure of the unequal effectiveness of the intranatal care given at each place.

At last it was possible to compare like with like, as obstetricians have always insisted that it should be. Or at least it would have been possible if the data had been published frankly in the survey report. In fact, frankness was lacking.

The distribution of births by antenatal prediction score at each place of birth was published, but without the associated deaths. Nevertheless, using other information in the report, a close estimate can be made of mortality rates in the broad groups of low, moderate and high antenatal risk (Table 8.5). For the labour prediction score, neither the distribution of births nor associated deaths was published by place of birth. These data were eventually released privately in response to a persistent campaign carried out by the present author, five years after the publication of the survey report in 1978 and thirteen years after the data were collected in 1970. Only then, in 1983, was it possible for enquirers not privy to the survey material to compare like with like, but by then maternity policy had become too deeply entrenched to be influenced by the facts revealed (Table 8.6 and pages 330–8).

Validating scores as instruments for retrospective analysis

Both prediction scores were validated in that they correlated very strongly with specific perinatal mortality rates and respiratory depression ratios (the percentage of babies born alive but taking more than three minutes to establish regular respiration). The higher the scores, the higher were these rates [15]. The labour prediction score also correlated strongly with infant birthweight: the percentage of births weighing less than 2500 grams increased as the score rose [15]. Critics, seeking to cast doubt on the general applicability of the belatedly revealed results when labour prediction scores were used to analyse the 1970 survey data and quantify comparable mortality rates at each place of birth [16, 17], have pointed out that the score has not been validated in relation to any other data set [18]. But this does not mean that it would not have been, if anyone had had access to a suitable data set and had bothered to undertake the exercise. In any case, the pro-specialist bias built in to the score would have tended to paint an over favourable picture of the results of hospital care by exaggerating the predicted risk status of the births there. Other criticisms of the completeness of the labour prediction score will be discussed and refuted when the results of this analysis are considered in Chapter 8.

STATISTICAL SIGNIFICANCE

The larger the number of subjects in groups for which an outcome, in particular one following different medical treatments, is to be compared, the more likely are the findings to be representative of general experience following these treatments. But since collecting data is always expensive, the number of subjects included in surveys or trials is always restricted. Since the 1930s, statistical theoreticians have developed techniques which make it possible to estimate from samples of different sizes how probable it is that a difference in outcomes observed between the limited groups being compared reflects the same difference as would exist between the sections of the total population of which the study groups are samples. The probability is, by definition, not a certainty and therefore must be less than 100%. It is conventional to accept a probability of 95% or more as 'statistically significant'. This means that when the appropriate calculation has established that the observed superior outcome in one sample group over the other would have occurred in at least 95 samples out of 100 from the total population, then that difference can be accepted as reflecting the general experience, in particular that one of the medical treatments concerned gives truly better results than the other. (Occasionally each of two medical treatments tested has only a trifling effect on overall outcome, so the 'statistically significant' superiority of one may have negligible medical significance.)

If the outcome following one of the treatments is apparently the better, for example the mortality rate is lower, but the appropriate statistical calculation cannot establish that the difference observed between the study samples would have occurred in as many as 95% of other samples from the same population, then the apparently better outcome is not statistically significant and cannot be used to support the hypothesis that the treatment in question is superior. The treatment in question may indeed be superior, but the study samples have been too small for this superiority to be identified. If statisticians have a good estimate of how much the mortality rate is likely to be lowered by a new treatment, they can calculate how many subjects should take part in each arm of a trial in order for a result at the desired degree of significance to be established.

A statistically significant difference is denoted by the symbol $p < 0.05$', or '$p < 0.01$', or '$p < 0.001$', or '$p < 0.0001$', representing a 95%, or 99%, or 99.9%, or 99.99% probability (p) that it is real. To carry out tests of statistical significance requires certain conditions to be fulfilled and certain data to be available. Often these requirements cannot be met. This lack reduces, but does not destroy, the value of statistical evidence which does exist.

CORRELATION

When an association is observed between two conditions there is always a temptation to assume that one condition is the cause of the other. The temptation is very strong if the apparent correlation is much desired and it has proved irresistible to successive generations of obstetricians who have all too eagerly attributed improvements in outcome to their own treatment. The Central Midwives Board, giving their views to the Cranbrook Committee in 1956, betrayed the same flawed reasoning when they said: 'The Board are confident that the history of the midwifery service over the last 50 years, which shows a steady reduction in the maternal and perinatal mortality rates, and a vast improvement in the service provided for the expectant and nursing mother, reflects great credit on the midwife . . . [19]

The association may be observed between different places, for example mortality may be high in some districts and low in others, while the level of hospitalization may likewise vary between the districts and people are prone to infer a causal relationship if this would accord with their cherished beliefs. Wrong inferences about causal relationships are even more frequently made, and for the same reason, when the observed association is between changing values over time. For example, the mortality rate in a given area may fall over a period during which the rate of some other variable, like hospitalization, rises and people are prone to assume that the former trend has been caused by the latter. However, correlations between time series in which there is a trend in each of the related variables (and this is the case in most time series) are more likely than not to be spurious [20]: the secular decline in mortality rates could as readily be shown to correlate with the secular increase in motorway mileage or the secular decrease in cinema attendances. If one variable is dependent on another, any change in the independent variable will be associated with an appropriate change, in direction and quantity, in the dependent variable and the relevant data have to be analysed to see whether or not this condition is met. The first step is to calculate the proportional changes in each variable year by year.

There are different methods of calculating the degree of correlation between the variables. A product moment correlation coefficient can be calculated from the pairs of values of the variables relating to each place or to the values of the proportional changes over time, but the calculation can be laborious unless an appropriate computer program is available. A simpler and better known method, which reaches an almost identical result, is Spearman's rank correlation [21]. For cross-sectional analysis by area, this requires the values for each variable in each place to be ranked in order of size and for analysis over time the values of the proportional annual changes in each variable to be similarly ranked. (Table 8.8 illustrates an example of ranked data in two time series.) A simple statistical procedure is applied to the two sets of ranked values to calculate a correlation coefficient which at one extreme will be positive (+) and high if the two rank orders correspond closely and at the other extreme will be negative (–) and high if one rank order is approximately the inverse of the other. Between the extremes, the correlation coefficient may be less strongly positive or less strongly negative. In all cases, the next step is to establish, by means of a test of statistical significance, whether and at what level of confidence the resulting correlation coefficient is unlikely to be due to chance and, hence, whether it indicates the possibility of a causal relationship between the variables.

It will certainly not do so if, although significant in magnitude, it is opposite in sign to what the particular hypothesis being tested requires: for example, if the larger values in the independent variable are required to correlate with the larger values in the dependent variable but in fact correlate with the smaller values (and vice versa). If the sign is in the desired direction but the magnitude is statistically insignificant, the hypothesis of a dependent relationship between the variables has not been supported by the data used, but the possibility of some small dependency nevertheless existing has not necessarily been ruled out, although it is low if the value of the coefficient is low.

But even if the correlation coefficient has the correct sign for the hypothesis and is significant in magnitude, this in itself is no proof of causality. It only admits advance to the next of the further steps in analysis which must be passed before a true causal relationship can be identified, for the apparent relationship may not be directly causal, but may operate through another intermediate variable to which the given variables are each related. This is the explanation of the wrongly imputed causal relationship between frequent attendances for antenatal care and low perinatal mortality (page 110). It is very often the explanation of apparent correlations in time series.

The correlations which obstetricians and others claim between increasing medical care, or specific obstetric interventions, and decreasing mortality are quickly shown to be spurious. They all fall at the first hurdle, so that the further analysis is never necessary.

REFERENCES

1. Tew, M. (1981) Effects of scientific obstetrics on perinatal mortality. *Health Soc. Ser. J.*, **91**, 444–6.
2. Campbell, R., Macdonald Davies, I. and Macfarlane, A. (1984) Home births

in England and Wales; perinatal mortality according to intended place of delivery. *Br. Med. J.*, **289**, 721–4.

3. Russell, J.K. (1981) Should home births be ruled out? *The Times*, 21 January.

4. Chamberlain, G. (1981) Danger at home for new babies. Comment reported in *The Observer*, 15 June.

5. Chalmers, I., Enkin, M. and Keirse, M.J.N.C. eds (1989) *Effective Care in Pregnancy and Childbirth* (2 vols), Oxford University Press, Oxford.

6. Macdonald, D., Grant, A., Sheridan-Pereira, M. *et al.* (1985) The Dublin randomised controlled trial of intrapartum fetal heart rate monitoring. *Am. J. Obstet. Gynecol.*, **152**, 524–39.

7. Prendiville, W., Harding, J., Elbourne, E. *et al.* (1988) The Bristol third stage trial; active versus physiological management of the third stage of labour. *Br. Med. J.*, **297**, 1295–1300.

8. Registrar General, *Statistical Review of England and Wales Part I, Annual for the Years 1965 to 1973*, HMSO, London.

9. Office of Population Censuses and Surveys, *Birth Statistics, Annual for the Years 1974–92*, HMSO, London.

10. Butler, N.R. and Bonham, D.G. (1963) *Perinatal Mortality*, Churchill Livingstone, Edinburgh.

11. Ministry of Health/Department of Health and Social Security (1969) *Report on Confidential Enquiries into Maternal Deaths in England and Wales*, Reports on Public Health and Medical Subjects No. 119, 1964–66, HMSO, London.

12. Ministry of Health/Department of Health and Social Security (1972) *Report on Confidential Enquiries into Maternal Deaths in England and Wales*, Reports on Health and Social Subjects No. 1, 1967–69, HMSO, London.

13. Ministry of Health/Department of Health and Social Security (1975) *Report on Confidential Enquiries into Maternal Deaths in England and Wales*, Reports on Health and Social Subjects No. 11, 1970–72, HMSO, London.

14. Ministry of Health/Department of Health and Social Security (1979) *Report on Confidential Enquiries into Maternal Deaths in England and Wales*, Reports on Health and Social Subjects No. 14, 1973–75, HMSO, London.

15. Chamberlain, G., Philipp, E., Howlett, B. *et al.* (1978) *British Births 1970 Vol. 2, Obstetric Care*, Heinemann, London, Chaps 2 and 5.

16. Tew, M. (1985) Place of birth and perinatal mortality. *J. R. Coll. Gen. Pract.*, **35**, 390–4.

17. Tew, M. (1986) Do obstetric intranatal interventions make birth safer? *Br. J. Obstet. Gynaecol.*, **93**, 659–74.

18. Campbell, R. and Macfarlane, A. (1987) *Where To Be born? The Debate and the Evidence*, National Perinatal Epidemiology Unit, Oxford.

19. Central Midwives Board (1957) *Report*, Evidence to the Maternity Services Committee.

20. Granger, C. and Newbold, P. (1974) Spurious correlations in econometrics. *J. Econometr.*, **3**, 111–20.

21. Siegel, S. (1956) *Nonparametric Statistics for the Behavioural Sciences*, McGraw-Hill, New York, Chap. 9.

7 | Mortality of the mother

EVIDENCE FROM LONG AGO

If we go as far back as the Bible we find many catalogues of successive generations which chronicle the Israelites' successful implementation of the divine command 'Be fruitful and multiply' [1]. Births are frequently mentioned, but although there are several references to the obstetric problems of involuntary infertility, late motherhood, twin births and fetal malpresentations, there is only one reference to difficult labour ending in a maternal death [2].

... and Rachel travailed and she had hard labour. And it came to pass as her soul was in departing (for she died) . . .

However, the child of this hard labour, Benjamin, survived.

The record of Genesis almost certain implies an unduly favourable ratio of reproductive success to failure, but although subsequent references to the tribulations of childbirth have abounded, reflecting the many pregnancies that ended in loss, the number of live births continued to be more than sufficient to compensate for deaths at all stages from infancy to old age, so that the world's population has increased enormously. Increases in live births have soon made good temporary excesses of deaths arising from famines, plagues and wars.

Leaping from Biblical times to 17th century England, we find that in 1662 John Graunt estimated from the London Bills of Mortality that 'not above three [women] in two hundred died in childbed' and less than one in two hundred from 'the hardness of their labour' [3, p. 12]. These categories may correspond to the later classifications respectively of maternal death from all causes, direct and indirect, up to a month after the birth, and of the direct or 'true' causes only. In so far as these London rates may be regarded as equivalent to 15 and 5 per 1000 total births, or rather over that per 1000 live births, and as comparable with the official figures for the whole of England in the 19th century of around 5 per 1000 live births for all causes and just over half that for 'true' causes, they would indicate that child birth had become safer in these two hundred years, with the greater part of the improvement in the indirect or 'associated' causes [4].

If there was such a reduction in mortality it would be almost entirely due to the improvement in the quality of the mother and at best only marginally to an improvement in the quality of maternity care, which field the man-midwife was beginning to penetrate and influence (Chapter 2). Even if birth had been made safer in the hands of better educated attendants, male or female, the proportion of all births enjoying this attention was small. On the other hand, despite the obvious urban poverty, there had been a considerable rise in the average standard of living, which should have been reflected in some improvement in the average standard of maternal health (Chapter 1).

In the unquantified judgements of many observers, there was reason to doubt that birth was made safer by the interventions, whether of the rising obstetricians and accoucheurs or of the more impatient midwives. Graunt and some of his 17th century contemporaries, including the distinguished midwife, Jane Sharp, claimed that poor country women, poorly housed, had fewest problems in childbirth. The reason for this in the words of the eminent physician, William Harvey [3, p. 12], was that

> poor women often escaped the officious attentions which many midwives thought it their duty to give, and in consequence Nature was allowed unimpeded to take her course.

THE IMPORTANCE OF NUTRITION

The claim of safer birth for country women is supported from different times and places. In Kendal, a small country town in north-west England, a midwife kept detailed records of the 412 deliveries she attended between 1669 and 1674 without mentioning a single maternal death [5, pp. 88–90]. In the USA, the informative diary of a rural midwife, who practised in Maine between 1778 and 1812, recorded only four maternal deaths and few potentially fatal complications in the 996 women she delivered [6, p. 20]. An illiterate, untrained, but very competent midwife, who was described as officiating at every birth in the village of Juniper Hill in the English Midlands between 1880 and 1890, found that in this healthy community complications of birth were rare and no mother's life was lost in that decade [5, pp. 171–4].

The country women, although poor, were probably relatively well fed. It was to the good health of the country girls who flooded in to the expanding seaport of Liverpool that the Ladies' Charity there attributed the low mortality of the mothers for whom it provided a midwife, and if necessary a doctor, as well as food and other necessities. Its records for six of the years between 1799 and 1815 show only eight maternal deaths in 6100 labours [5, p. 150]. Perhaps it was the continuing influx of healthy country women which accounted for Liverpool's continuously favourable experience. The record of the Liverpool Lying-In Hospital and Dispensary for the Diseases of Women and Children for the years 1842–5 showed one maternal death in 341 labours. In the 1850s, the maternal mortality rate in the city's workhouse was 3.2 per 1000 live births and in the city itself it was 3.5 in 1873 and 2.9 in 1880, much lower than the national averages [5, p. 138].

The country environment seems to have been relatively successful at breeding a race of healthy, well-formed women who did not expect to need and did not receive significant intervention in childbirth. Townswomen seem to have been less robust of body and attitude and they had readier access to birth attendants who could try to ease their difficulties with what they thought were appropriate interventions.

THE EFFECT OF SURGICAL INTERVENTION

Men who favoured the surgical approach sought to speed the birth process with the assistance of instruments. Their female rivals deplored the results of their techniques, as indeed did their more restrained male colleagues. The midwife Sarah Stone (page 43) in the early 18th century alleged that 'more mothers and children had died at the hands of raw recruits just out of their apprenticeship to the barber-surgeon than through the worst ignorance and stupidity of midwives' [3, p. 31]. Later in the century the midwife, Margaret Stephen, declared 'that the practices of men attendants has caused far more deaths than they had prevented' [5, p. 124]. The celebrated man-midwife, William Hunter, condemned the use of forceps, because 'where they may save one, they murder twenty' [3, p. 31]. Frank Nicholls, physician to King George II, criticized male practitioners for frightening women into engaging them while 'by their own misuse of instruments they were themselves often guilty of the death of both mother and child' [3, p. 32]. Another midwife, Elizabeth Nihell [3, pp. 32–3], expressed the view shared by other opponents of the male practitioner that

> he used instruments unnecessarily to hasten the birth and save his own time, as well as to impress the family with his dexterity and justify charging a higher fee. Consequently more infants were lost than formerly, and if the mother did not die of the injuries she

might sustain or of resulting childbed fever, she was frequently left with fearful and lasting disabilities. Worse still, the male practitioner, adding insult to injury, was so adept at concealing his errors with a cloud of hard words and scientific jargon that the injured patient herself was convinced that she could not thank him enough for the mischief he had done.

Dr Charles White, a well known man-midwife of the period, 'pointed out that although the poor were often half-starved and diseased, their maternal death rate might still be less than that of patients delivered in lying-in hospitals or of the more affluent class attended by men' [3, p. 35]. Apparently these commentators considered that the dangers of obstetric interventions greatly outweighed the dangers of malnutrition.

Similar evidence relating to the mid-19th century, and backed with statistics, was produced by the Royal Maternity Charity of London to defend itself against medical criticism of its use of midwives rather than doctors in its work. It was able to show that 'although it served poor working class women, often living in unhealthy conditions, its maternal death rate was lower than the Registrar General's figure for the country at large' [3, p. 58]. In its eastern district, 4.5 per 1000 of the women attended between 1828 and 1850 died within a month of the birth, 3.3 per 1000 from puerperal (direct or 'true') causes. In its western, less impoverished district between 1852 and 1864 the figure was 2.2 for all causes. These rates compare very favourably with the national maternal mortality rate per 1000 registered live births (a smaller denominator than women attended and so giving a larger ratio), which was 5.4 between 1847 and 1854 and 4.75 between 1855 and 1864 [3, pp. 211–12]. The charity's mortality rate, like that of similar charities in Liverpool and elsewhere, was also lower than that achieved by male accoucheurs among their better-off patients who probably wanted and received more instrumental interventions.

Certainly birth at home, whether attended by midwives or doctors paid for by the patient or the charity, was much safer than birth in hospital, where the risk of puerperal infection, which carried a high case-fatality rate, was far greater. Since most births were at home and probably had an average mortality rate of less than 4, the small proportion of births in hospital must have had a very high rate to give a national overall average of around 5. A Scottish obstetrician, James Duncan, seeking to defend the superiority of hospitals, argued in 1870 that the official statistics must be wrong [3, p. 94]: the national average rate could not possibly be less than 8, and the charities' records must be defective for they made it seem that

educated accoucheurs lost five times as many patients and this would lead to the absurd conclusion that poor women, delivered in filthy slum dwellings by 'imperfectly educated' midwives or medical students, were at less risk than well-to-do patients attended in salubrious conditions by experienced accoucheurs.

Florence Nightingale pointed out that Duncan's figures supported the long-standing belief that maternal mortality was highest among the better off, despite their higher standard of living [3, p. 94].

OFFICIAL EVIDENCE

Adverse criticisms of the quality and effectiveness of accoucheurs' care continued to be made by informed commentators, for example in the Registrar General's annual report of 1876 and in evidence to the House of Commons Select Committee on Midwifery Registration 1891–3 [5, p. 167]. According to Dr W.C. Grigg, physician to Queen Charlotte's Lying-in Hospital, 'more cases of "injury and physical disaster" resulted from the imprudent use of forceps and turning [version] by medical men than from the negligence and ignorance of midwives' [3, p. 131]. According to Dr W.S. Playfair, consultant to the General Lying-in Hospital, 'not one medical man in a hundred in private practice used antiseptics in any regular and systematic manner' [3, p. 131], despite the compelling evidence by then accumulated that they were the principal vectors of the devastatingly infectious puerperal sepsis.

The Select Committee's terms of reference did not include the deregistering of incompetent medical practitioners of midwifery. They did, however, accept doctors' claims that the untrained midwife was the cause of much unnecessary maternal and infant mortality and morbidity. They had no means of allowing for the fact that the least competent midwives or handywomen worked among the poorest, least healthy mothers, whose troubles stemmed as much if not more from their physical condition as from the care they received. There were no data to compare the outcome for such women delivering in their homes with that for their counterparts delivering in hospital under medical supervision. The Select Committee's duty was to consider the registration of midwives and this they recommended in their report of 1893 [5, p. 167].

Some of the ignorant untrained midwives must nevertheless have been capable and successful at their job, like the midwife of Juniper Hill already referred to (page 271). Others must have been less praiseworthy and furnished the model for Sarah Gamp, the fictitious handywoman depicted so convincingly by Charles Dickens that she came to represent, in the public's imagination, the typical domiciliary midwife. Dickens presented a treasured gift to medical men which they used to good effect and without scruple in their propaganda war against their professional rivals, long after the *Midwives Act* of 1902 ensured that only trained, experienced midwives could legally practise.

MATERNAL MORTALITY BETWEEN 1900 AND 1935

Efforts to raise the competence of midwives were only one of many developments after 1900 which were intended to improve the maternity service and so, directly or indirectly, to reduce the mortality of mothers and infants (Chapters 2–5). Evaluating them, establishing which of them were successful and which not, identifying which were responsible for the changing patterns in mortality proved to be tasks too baffling for contemporary observers. Interpretations were inevitably biased by the preconceptions and professional interests of the judges. Mistaken identification of cause and effect relationships led to the unjustifiable policies that were to be followed with increasing obsessional zeal after 1950.

As far as maternal mortality was concerned, the measures put in train between 1900 and 1935 seemed, to the perplexity of all concerned, to have been completely unsuccessful.

The failure of the maternal mortality rate to yield one decimal point to the sustained attack which has been directed against it, but its tendency rather to react in the opposite direction, has endowed it with an air of mystery and malignity. The 1933 figure of 5.8 per 1000 [total births] is 7 per cent higher than the figure for the preceding year and 15 per cent higher than that of 20 years previously. [7]

The apparent rise in mortality may or may not have been real. The numerator of the rate may have been augmented through more comprehensive compliance with the legal requirement of death registration and the greater willingness of doctors to certify deaths to a direct or 'true' maternal cause or to mention maternity as an indirect or 'associated' cause [8]. On the other hand, the denominator of the rate was also augmented after 1929, when the law required stillbirths to be registered and maternal mortality was henceforward calculated in relation to total births, instead of only live births as previously. A larger denominator results in a lower calculated rate. In 1929 the rate from all causes, direct and indirect, was 5.82 per 1000 live births but 5.59 per 1000 total births; from direct causes only the corresponding rates were 4.33 and 4.16. [4]

The rate may have been inflated because the figure for deaths included those following abortion, of which those due to criminally induced abortion were hardly the fault of the maternity service. It could not be discerned from the statistics whether procured abortion with fatal consequences was becoming commoner, but it was suspected that more women were trying to limit the size of their families by this dangerous method. The trend towards smaller families had, apart from the post-war upsurge in births in the early 1920s, been continuous from the 1860s to the 1930s and methods of contraception were often not known. 'In 1861–69 the average family contained 6.16 children; by 1900–9 the number had fallen to 3.30; and in 1934–7 it was 2.04, the lowest on record.' [9]

On the other hand, as families became smaller, a greater proportion of births would be first births, which carry a higher risk to the mother than second and third births. More than compensating for this, however, would be the reduction in fourth and later births, which carry a much higher maternal risk, so that on balance smaller families should have led to falling maternal mortality.

Whether or not the rates by 1935 were fairly comparable with those of earlier years, they certainly did not suggest any improvement over the rate of 5.6 from all causes between 1901 and 1905, which was as high as in the 19th century. The rate had fallen to 5.0 between 1906 and 1910, and stayed around that level until 1925, except in 1918 when the rate from indirect causes was raised by the influenza epidemic in that year. From 1926 it rose again to reach 5.8 in 1933 and was still 5.7 in 1934. The trend in mortality from direct causes only followed the same pattern, reaching a peak rate of 4.4 per 1000 births in 1934 [10].

MATERNAL MORTALITY IN OTHER COUNTRIES

Rising rates of maternal mortality were experienced over the same period in other countries where medical involvement in midwifery was increasing, despite efforts to combat the trend. In Scotland the rate continued to rise between 1900 and 1930 and in 1935, at about 6 per 1000 live births, was still higher than it had ever been between 1850 and 1920 [11]. In Australia the rate was 5.06 in 1910 but 6.0 in 1936 [12].

In the United States, the rate rose steeply after 1915 and fluctuated between 7 and 9 for a few years around 1920 before settling for a decade around 7, so that by 1935 it was still higher than it had been in 1915. Throughout this period it was much lower among the white population, whose standard of living was relatively high and whose birth attendants were more likely to be doctors, than among the non-whites, whose standard of living was relatively low and whose attendants were more likely to be midwives or untrained helpers. The standard of living was rising for both populations between 1915 and 1935, but it was only among the non-whites that the maternal mortality rate fell [6].

A similar pattern of mortality was experienced in several other countries: New Zealand, Belgium, Netherlands, Denmark and Sweden all recorded rates as high or higher in the early 1930s as they had been thirty years before [13].

There have always to be reservations about making international comparisons of maternal mortality rates because of possible differences in the way they are calculated. The available figures suggest, however, that the United States and Australia, with their higher standard of living on the one hand and their greater medical involvement in maternity care on the other, had higher maternal mortality over these years than had England. Within the British Isles, England with its higher standard of living had lower maternal mortality than Scotland and Ireland. In turn the English rates were higher than in Sweden and the Netherlands where stricter attention to asepsis procedures was more successful in keeping down deaths from puerperal infections and added to the advantages of good standards of living [13].

SEEKING THE CAUSES OF MATERNAL MORTALITY

In England, official enquiries were undertaken to identify the cause of the disturbing facts. In the first of these [14], reported in 1924 by Dr Janet Campbell, Medical Officer at the Ministry of Health (pages 196-7), the circumstances leading to death were investigated in a sample of cases and blame was laid on the incompetence of the professional birth attendants, on the unwise behaviour and poor health of the mother and on her unsatisfactory social environment in that order of importance. A substantial proportion of deaths was judged to have been avoidable if the attendant and/or mother had acted more wisely. If they had followed the best established practice, it was argued, the death rate could have been immediately reduced, but making them familiar with the best established practice was obviously not something that could be immediately achieved.

Further reports by the Ministry of Health confirmed these findings. In one, published in 1932, it was stated that

> We are, however, convinced that the primary essential for the reduction of a high maternal mortality is sound midwifery, before, during and after childbirth . . . at least half the deaths which have come under review could have been prevented had due forethought been exercised by the expectant mother and her attendant, a reasonable degree of skill had been brought to bear on the management of the case and adequate facilities for treatment been provided and utilised. [15, p. 134]

The study of maternal mortality in New York City, 1930–2, by the New York Academy of Medicine, judged two-thirds of the deaths to have been preventable and reached the same verdict as to cause:

The incapacity of the attendants, either in judgement or skill, contributed significantly to the large number of avoidable deaths. Their failure to provide proper prenatal care has already been pointed out. The prognosis of delivery was frequently incorrect. Labor was often improperly conducted. The physicians were apparently ignorant of indications and contra-indications for interference. Operative procedures were undertaken when there was no indication or plain contra-indication. Labour was terminated by rapid traumatising delivery when non-interference was called for. Operative procedures were performed on potentially infected patients. Attendants were tardy in obtaining proper consultations. There was failure to treat severe complication with all the means which should have been available. Difficult obstetrical operations were performed by physicians whose training and experience could not be considered adequate. [16, p. 215]

A second American report, in 1933, of a survey covering eleven states by the White House Conference on Child Health and Protection [17] likewise blamed mothers for not availing themselves of prenatal medical care and doctors of underdiagnosing or overdiagnosing complications and following the diagnosis with unnecessary interventions. They were more ready to intervene, despite their inadequate surgical skills, because of the false confidence antiseptics and anaesthetics now gave them, because both they and the mother wanted the labour to be shorter and because they could charge higher fees for interventions – the kind of judgement familiar to the 18th century critics in England, as just described, and relevant to experience in several countries in the late 20th century, as will be described.

Between 1910 and 1921 in one Boston maternity hospital the rate of operative deliveries increased from 29% to 45% and the trend continued upwards. The conference estimated that three-quarters of the caesarian sections were unnecessary and without them the maternal mortality rate would have been 10% lower [6, p. 162].

One leading obstetrician, Eardley Holland, found a similar picture in Britain since 1915.

A striking change in the last fifteen to twenty years is the remarkable widening in Britain of the indications for intervention during labour and the great increase in the number of operative deliveries (induction of labour, forceps and caesarean section). This has occurred in spite of efforts to frustrate it on the part of leading teachers and textbooks. [7]

Another eminent obstetrician observed that deaths from these operations, often undertaken in response to wrong antenatal diagnosis, merely replaced the deaths from obstructed labour which they were intended to forestall. The net effect of antenatal care had in many cases been simply to transfer mortality 'from one column to another' [18]. National records were not kept of the frequency with which caesarean section was resorted to, but deaths with mention of this operation increased steadily from 88 in 1922 to 182 in 1937 and 190 in 1944 [10, 19].

In both Britain and the USA, obstetricians, who obeyed the Papal encyclical *Casti Connubi* of 1930, had to attempt to save the infant's life, if necessary at the expense of the mother's, although there was no evidence that this was more likely to be done by operative deliveries.

IMPROVING THE EDUCATION OF DOCTORS

Some leading obstetric teachers in both Britain and the USA still cautioned against over-enthusiastic intervention undertaken on insufficient indications without regard to the risks involved. They interpreted the failure of medical care to bring down mortality as demonstrating that practitioners needed to be taught greater technical competence to carry out the interventions more safely and also, and even more importantly, they needed to learn to judge when the interventions were appropriate. '. . . the way in which it [maternal mortality] can be remedied is, to a certain section of the medical profession at all events, perfectly clear. . . . The necessary personnel has not been trained.' [7].

The efforts made by medical schools to improve the midwifery education of aspiring doctors in the limited time available in the curriculum were able to concentrate more on the former of these needs, which more nearly coincided with the skills required for gynaecological and other surgery, than on the latter, which could only be acquired after considerable practical experience of normal as well as abnormal childbirth. Thus undergraduate educational constraints caused the acquisition of technical skills to be stressed at the expense of the learning of judgement. Judgement to be learned during post-graduate appointments in hospital, an environment not conducive to giving experience in normal births. This emphasis on technical skills accorded with the preferences of other obstetric teachers who were still convinced that birth was mainly a pathological process and were captivated by the promise of applying the advances of science to assert man's mastery over nature's limitations in human biology.

FINDING FAULTS IN THE MOTHER

Professionals, searching for an explanation of the persistently high maternal mortality, discerned that some of the damaging factors lay in the mother. Sometimes her behaviour was blamed for an 'avoidable' cause of death. Usually her fault lay in not attending clinics for any or enough antenatal care or in not following the advice she was given there. While this may have been a valid criticism in specific instances, evidence had not been collected to confirm that in general the advice, diagnoses and treatments resulting from antenatal care did lead to fewer deaths (Chapter 3).

Sometimes the danger arose from the mother's poor physique and state of health. Only some morbid conditions were susceptible to immediate remedy by medically directed advice and care. All too often the women having babies in the first decades of the 20th century had deformed pelves resulting from their childhood experience of malnutrition which caused rickets. They were destined to have difficult labours. Medical care could not reverse the deformity for that generation of women, but their chance of a safe outcome might be improved by appropriate and competent obstetric intervention.

As always, ill health and deformity more often affected women from the lower social classes who were less well fed and less well housed, especially if they had been so all their lives. But average standards of living had continued to rise since 1870. Women of childbearing age shared the general improvement in health and this should have made them fitter to reproduce. Moreover, their tendency to have smaller families should have saved them from the most dangerous pregnancies. The natural factors, therefore, predisposed to reduced mortality, but for some reason mortality in childbirth did not fall.

At the same time, pregnant women were receiving more attention from the medical profession than other subgroups in the adult population and more than they had received in the past. Apparently it was failing to produce the desired result. Critical obstetricians conceded that interventions carried out unnecessarily or incompetently were harmful and recommended improved education in midwifery. Beneficial results from this would, however, take some time before they would be reflected in reduced mortality. No one dared to suggest that an immediate improvement might be achieved by challenging clinical freedom and imposing rigid criteria which would limit when and by whom the potentially harmful interventions could be undertaken. No one suggested that less medical care should be provided; the recommended treatment was more of the same but to be delivered in future with greater competence.

FINDING FAULT IN THE GENERAL PRACTITIONER

Obstetricians were most disposed to blame bad results on their non-specialist colleagues, the general practitioners, who had the least training. Formerly doctors had blamed the incompetence of midwives, who did not, indeed could not, attempt surgical interventions, although whenever there were data on which to make comparisons, the midwives came out with better results (page 273). After the *Midwives Act* of 1902, increasing numbers of them had the formal training approved by doctors and the circumstances in which they were obliged to call for medical aid were more precisely defined. However, those whose judgement and self-confidence had been undermined by the training process were becoming more inclined to call a doctor on slighter signs of possible complication. They were thus inviting interventions and unwittingly exposing more women to their dangers. An analysis of the records of midwives attached to the Queen's Institute of District Nursing between 1905 and 1925 showed that 'the rise in the proportion of cases to which midwives called the doctor was not accompanied by the expected decrease in the maternal death-rate. On the contrary the death-rate actually rose in step with it' [3, p. 190].

By 1936, half of the 16 000 registered and practising midwives worked on a salaried or subsidized basis for maternity charities, nursing associations, hospital outpatient departments or local authorities. 'Many of their patients were overburdened and living in insanitary conditions and, in country areas, far from medical aid, yet . . . many of such organisations averaged a maternal death rate of only half, or less than half, the national rate.' [20] Presumably these midwives did not call in a doctor so often. It was hard to go on blaming midwives for the high mortality. Doctors should have recognized that the beam was in their own eye.

Their colleagues in Canada viewed experience there with the same purblindness [21]. In Saskatchewan, in 1919, the Medical Officer of Health reported that the 50% of the province's women who gave birth without either doctor or nurse attending had a much lower maternal mortality than the other half. In Manitoba, the Minister reported in an article that in the period 1921–7 maternal mortality in the province was three times as high for hospital as for non-hospital births and that mortality among the non-hospital cases was highest in the more prosperous districts with most doctors and lowest in a sparsely populated district without a resident doctor or public health nurse. In Ontario, in 1928, an investigation found that mortality was higher in the Red Cross hospitals than in medically unserviced areas, where indeed the rate was less than 80% of the rate in Ontario as a whole. Reactions to this evidence were perverse in the extreme. In Saskatchewan, the information was kept from the public; in Manitoba, the Minister of Health went on to draw the extraordinary conclusion that the absence of medical service in the unorganized districts no doubt contributed largely to the high maternal mortality rate; the Director of the Ontario

Red Cross was satisfied that 'if every case of maternity in Canada were conducted in hospital, our general maternal mortality rate would be much lower than it now is'.

AN UNEXPECTED ADVANTAGE OF BEING POOR

The women in the specific investigations referred to were apparently representative. Women in the lowest social class were likely to be the least physically fit and at highest risk of mortality, while at the same time they were least likely to have any medical attention before, during or after delivery. Yet an analysis of maternal mortality by social class carried out by the Registrar General [22] for the years 1930–2 showed that, paradoxically, it was these women who had the lowest maternal mortality for all the direct causes except abortion and postpartum hae-morrhage (Table 7.1). Their increased risk of dying from puerperal sepsis as a result of their poorer and less hygienic living conditions was apparently more than offset by their reduced risk as a result of their fewer contacts with doctors. The experience of previous centuries, just recounted, was repeated.

The poorer women died less often from severe toxaemia and eclamp-sia than did women in higher social classes, although their uptake of antenatal care gave fewer opportunities for the warning signs to be detected and remedial treatment given. They were least likely to enjoy the ten- or twelve-day lying-in period recommended by doctors and so were least likely to die of phlebitis ('white' leg, *phlegmasia alba dolens*). In contrast, women in the highest social classes (I and II) were appar-ently deprived of all their natural advantages of better health and a better environment by what was thought to be the best of medical care.

Table 7.1 Maternal mortality at the social extremes: rates per 1000 births

Cause of death	Social class		
	I and II	V	All
Puerperal sepsis	1.45	1.16	1.29
Toxaemia (all)	0.81	0.68	0.99
Abortion (all)	0.51	0.57	0.55
Postpartum haemorrhage	0.50	0.60	0.49
Other accidents of childbirth	0.47	0.40	0.44
Phlegmasia alba dolens (phlebitis: 'white leg')	0.40	0.26	0.31
All direct causes	4.44	3.89	4.13

Source: reference [22], Table 11.

SPECIFIC CAUSES OF MATERNAL DEATH

As the 20th century progressed, puerperal sepsis continued to be the greatest single cause of maternal death, as it had been throughout the 19th. This happened despite the incontrovertible evidence that it was a contagious disease and its incidence could be greatly reduced by rigorous attention to hygiene. Rigorous attention to hygiene could, however, be irksome for birth attendants and complete decontamination after contact with a case could even require their abstention from work for a period. Conscientious efforts to provide a germ-free environment in hospital, to cleanse a woman from germs she might be harbouring anywhere in her body, made the decontamination process, which included pubic shaving and administration of enemas, distressing to mothers also. The control of infection was in reality complicated. The painstaking work of 20th century microbiologists in several countries had distinguished several different varieties of causative agent, besides the haemolytic streptococcus, which could reach the victim by different routes [23]. For such reasons the rules of hygiene must, in many places, have been misdirected or disregarded, for sepsis following childbirth and abortion continued to make up nearly half of the direct causes of maternal mortality [24].

The opportunities were being increased by the lesions resulting from obstetric interventions, especially if incompetently performed, which were becoming more frequent in Britain following antenatal care and overdiagnosis [25]. The two American studies already quoted found that 'nearly half the women died after an operation done unnecessarily, improperly, or with insufficient care for asepsis' [6, p. 161]. Such interventions were one of the reasons why in both England and the United States, infection rates remained higher for deliveries in hospital than at home.

As in any battle, the outcome depends on the relative strengths of the attackers and the defenders. The incidence of puerperal sepsis is determined by two opposing factors: the virulence of the attacking causative agent and the resistance of the defending hosts. The strength of each factor may increase or decrease independently at different times, either one reinforcing or offsetting the other. Neither can be objectively measured, so it cannot be certainly known how much changes in incidence and case-fatality rates depend on one or the other. It is not well understood what causes streptococci to become more or less virulent, or indeed more or less susceptible to bactericidal assaults. It is better understood that resistance of the hosts depends directly on the state of their general health and there is independent evidence of improvements in this throughout the 20th century.

Though the virulence of the causative agents may have diminished, the better health of the women was almost certainly increasing their resistance to the disease. In England, in 1919, it killed 57% of the women who contracted it, but in 1929 only 49% [26, 27], while some hospitals reported much lower case-fatality rates in the 1930s [28]. In Scotland, the case-fatality rate for puerperal sepsis rose until 1928, after which it began an uninterrupted decline, although the rate of notification of the disease increased until 1934 [11]. If these falling case-fatality rates were representative of all British experience, then the incidence must have been increasingly greatly to account for the persistently high maternal mortality in relation to the number of births.

As for the other causes of maternal death, there was little or no progress towards alleviating them either. Some of those associated with haemorrhage were prevented by blood transfusion, administered in the larger obstetric hospitals and in outside confinements by 'flying squads', mobile units with skilled obstetric teams based at the larger hospitals. But any successes from the techniques then available must have been offset by additional failures, for the mortality rate hardly changed.

Antenatal care, as delivered, did not succeed in reducing the dangers of eclamptic toxaemia, the second greatest single cause of maternal death. Contemporary obstetrician observers did not attempt to explain why it was the mothers in social classes I and II, who had the most antenatal care, who suffered the highest mortality from this cause (Table 7.1).

THE MIRACULOUS DECLINE IN MATERNAL MORTALITY AFTER 1935

The depressing, frustrating scene was suddenly transformed. A slight fall in the death rate in 1935 was followed by a more definite fall in 1936 and the downward trend suddenly gathered pace and continued thereafter. By 1945, in England and Wales, maternal mortality was half what it had been ten years earlier. By 1950, it was half what it had been in 1945.

The astounding transformation was started, not through an advance in the scientific understanding of obstetrics, but through the opportune application to maternity care of a fundamental advance in pharmacology. When, in 1936, the drug Prontosil (page 92) was introduced experimentally on all cases infected with haemolytic streptococci at the Puerperal Fever Clinic of Queen Charlotte's Maternity Hospital, London

> The change in the overall clinical picture was dramatic . . . it was usual to see the temperature drop to normal within a day or two; threatening signs of peritonitis disappear; and positive blood cul-

tures become negative. One patient, who was very ill on admission and whose blood culture showed more than 3000 streptococci per c.c. on each of the first three days in hospital, had a negative blood culture and a normal temperature on the fourth day. Nothing like this had been seen in ten years' work on puerperal fever [23].

In the latter part of 1936, the drug became available for general use and at once the death rate from sepsis began its sharp descent. Prontosil was quickly superseded by the chemically simpler and even more effective derivative, sulphanilamide. The death rate due to sepsis in childbirth and abortion, which had risen from 1.30 in 1923 to 2.03 in 1931, fell to 1.35 in 1936, then to 0.58 in 1940, to 0.37 in 1945 and 0.13 in 1950. After 1939 it ceased to be the greatest single cause of maternal mortality. Its relative importance in childbirth deaths shrank from around 40% before 1936 to around 5% in 1950, but it continued to account for over 60% of the deaths following abortion. For although the death rate from sepsis in childbirth was reduced by 1950 to one-tenth of its level in 1936, the corresponding ratio in abortion was only one-fifth, which suggests that women having abortions were less likely to be treated with the new drug [24].

OTHER CAUSES OF DEATH

The sudden and steep reduction after 1936 in mortality from sepsis was followed at last after 1940 by a gentler reduction in mortality from toxaemia. The death rate, which had fluctuated between 0.73 and 0.86 in the 1930s, fell to 0.65 in 1940, to 0.46 in 1945, and to 0.26 in 1950 [24]. Despite this decline, toxaemia superseded sepsis as the most frequent cause of maternal death after 1939.

The favoured treatment to prevent toxaemia from developing into the highly dangerous eclampsia – sedation, rest and dietary control – had hardly changed since the 19th century, but thorough antenatal care could detect the warning signs – the rise in blood pressure and the presence of protein in the urine – and should have enabled preventive treatment to be given, if indeed treatment was effective. For reasons which puzzled obstetricians, antenatal care for thirty years had failed to reduce mortality. It is very unlikely that the changed trend from 1940, a time of social disruption and reduced medical staff in maternity care, was due to vigilance suddenly becoming more effective. More likely it was due to the markedly improved health which pregnant women shared with the rest of the community during the war years. This hypothesis is supported by the later finding in Aberdeen that the incidence of pre-eclampsia declined between 1975 and 1982 in phase with other indicators of improving health, independent of any changes in care.

The third most important cause of maternal death was haemorrhage, antepartum or postpartum. The rate remained close to 0.5 per 1000 births until 1941, but then fell to 0.3 by 1945 and to 0.1 by 1950. Research in the early 1930s had led to a better understanding of the significance of anaemia in pregnancy, realizing at last Ballantyne's vision (page 88), but it was well into the 1940s before tests to measure the haemoglobin content of the pregnant woman's blood began to be part of antenatal care and it was even later before they were routinely carried out. The development of better techniques of blood transfusion to meet military needs also helped to reduce the maternal death toll from haemorrhage. But once again, improved maternal health probably made a most important contribution, for the effect of better diet and antenatal iron supplements would be to reduce anaemia.

The death rate from the miscellaneous group of 'other' causes closely copied the downward trend from toxaemia. The group included some conditions like placenta praevia, where the power to treat sepsis removed much of the iatrogenic danger from the preventive operations, so that these no longer simply transferred the cause of mortality from 'one column to another' (page 279).

The death rate from the indirect causes associated with childbirth or abortion, which was around 1.2 per 1000 births between 1931 and 1937, fell to 0.7 by 1940, to 0.5 by 1945 and to 0.3 by 1950. Some of these causes, like pneumonia, were directly responsive to the antibiotic drugs, but again improved maternal health bestowed greater resistance to disease. For example, the incidence of tuberculosis was already falling rapidly before the availability of streptomycin.

CHANGES IN THE 1940s

The pace of decline in maternal mortality accelerated in Britain during the war years despite the disruptions to social life. Arrangements were improvised to evacuate pregnant women, especially working class women, from the vulnerable cities and to open emergency lying-in hospitals scattered in country districts in whatever accommodation could be requisitioned and adapted.

In the event, more maternity beds were provided than were used, the mothers preferring to remain near their families. Apparently they considered social and psychological support in childbirth of greater importance than safety from air-raids. But for the thousands of women who were evacuated, the experience was healthy. Despite the primitive equipment, the shortage of medical staff and the inclusion of some abnormal cases, death rates for mothers and their babies were very low [29].

In Scotland, although there also it was not possible to select only low-risk women for evacuation, the maternal mortality rate per 1000 births in the emergency hospitals was 0.53, compared with the Scottish average of 3.7. 'Labours were surprisingly short and easy, while hae-morrhages, both prenatal and postnatal, practically never occurred and conditions like uterine inertia were unknown.'[11] For English evacuees experience was exactly the same: '. . . confinements were easier, uterine inertia was practically unknown and less interference was required' [29]. It was suggested that the good outcomes may have resulted from the mothers having been admitted a few days before labour and having a period of rest in healthy surroundings with good food, to allow them and their fetuses to build up their strength, the same beneficial effect that Dr Haig Ferguson had noticed forty years before in the refuge for young unmarried pregnant women (page 89). The improved environ-ment more than compensated for the reduced attention of obstetric staff. Circumstances forced the beneficial change in maternity policy that no-one would otherwise have dared to recommend.

The sharp downturn in maternal mortality that occurred in England and Wales, illustrated in Figure 7.1, after 1936 occurred also in other

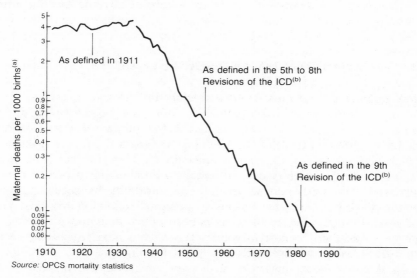

Source: OPCS mortality statistics

Figure 7.1   Maternal mortality; England and Wales 1911–84, United Kingdom 1985–90.
(a) 1985–90 per 1000 maternities. (b) ICD = International Classification of Diseases.
Note: the vertical axis is plotted on a logarithmic scale on which a straight line denotes a constant proportional rate of change – the steeper the gradient, the greater the propor-tional change. Source: OPCS mortality statistics.

countries. For example, in Scotland the rate fell from around 6 in the early 1930s to 4.7 in 1937–9, to 3.2 in 1943–5, and to 1.2 in 1949–51, a total decline of about 80% [11]. In the USA the rate by 1940 was about half of what it had been in the early 1930s and by 1950 about one-seventh [6, p. 162].

Everywhere the greatest single cause of decline was the virtual conquest of sepsis. In Scotland, the death rate in childbirth and abortion from this cause fell from 2.5 before 1936 to 0.14 in 1949–51, a drop of 94%. There were lesser but still large falls from other causes: from haemorrhages about 85%, from eclampsia about 76% and from phlebitis ('white leg') about 59% [11].

The reasons for these declines were everywhere the same. On the one hand, standards of living were continuing to rise and mothers' health to benefit, not only from the better diet and living conditions they currently enjoyed, but also from the nutrition they had enjoyed as fetuses and throughout childhood, which was better than had been available to the previous generation. In addition, some advances in medical science could now be incorporated in life-saving medical treatments which greatly reduced the adverse side-effects of obstetric interventions undertaken hopefully to make good inefficiencies in the natural process. Moreover, exposure of their shortcomings had spurred practitioners, specialists and generalists, to use greater care in carrying out the interventions.

MATERNAL MORTALITY AND SOCIAL CLASS

How quickly the reforms enabled doctors in England to reverse their negative record of 1930–2 (Table 7.1) could not be measured in the same way, because the war prevented the taking of the decennial census in 1941 and by 1951 the NHS had removed the financial barriers which had previously deterred women in the lowest social class from having medical maternity care, although to some extent cultural barriers remained. The 1951 analysis of maternal mortality by social class no longer offered proxy comparisons of outcome following maximal and minimal obstetric care. In fact, the pattern which emerged was unclear; the rate was then highest in social class V, but next highest in social class II, although lowest in classes I and II combined [30]. Apparently medical care, or its absence, no longer overrode the results to be expected from the good health of mothers in social class I and the poor health of mothers in social class V. Scottish data make it possible to compare maternity mortality by social class in the years 1939–40, before the NHS, and in 1944–50, partly before, partly during the NHS [11]. Local authority arrangements may have made it easier for poor Scotswomen than their English counterparts to have medical maternity attention. By 1939–40, Scottish doctors may have become more careful. For whatever reason, maternal mortality was then lowest in social classes I and II (2.73), higher in classes IV and V (4.21), but higher still in class III (4.59) and highest of all for unmarried mothers (6.18). By 1944–50, this rank order was nearly the same, but the range between the extremes was much reduced, for classes I and II showed the least relative decline (to reach 1.61) and unmarried mothers the most (to reach 1.92). This was only slightly higher than classes IV and V (1.89) and actually lower than class III (2.14). If abortion is excluded, the rate in 1944–50 was lower for the unmarried (1.20) than in classes I and II (1.54).

Some of the outstanding improvement for the unmarried may have been due to their receiving more intensive care from local authorities or to the Welfare State having greatly eased their financial and social handicaps. Even so, their standard of living would be much lower than for the married women in social classes I and II and they almost certainly received less obstetric care. Yet their mortality rates in 1944–50 were lower for most specific causes which obstetric care is intended to help: for eclampsia and toxaemia 0.33 as against 0.48 in classes I and II, for accidents of birth 0.21 as against 0.30, for puerperal embolism and thrombosis 0.08 as against 0.25, for antepartum haemorrhage 0.08 as against 0.13. The class I and II women must have been exposed to some harmful influence which outweighed their natural advantage over the unmarried women. Was it an excess of obstetric care? It is of interest also that even in 1939–40, when the unmarried women suffered more serious deprivation and their mortality rate was much the higher for most specific causes, it was nevertheless substantially lower for antepartum haemorrhage and accidents of birth [11].

MORTALITY OF CHILDBEARERS AND WOMEN OF CHILDBEARING AGE

In England and Wales, between 1935 and 1950, maternal mortality from sepsis fell by 89%, from all other direct causes by 71% and from indirect causes by 72%. Over the same period, mortality for all women aged 15 to 44 fell by around 51% [24, 31]. Without medical maternity care, a healthier cohort of women should have been able to reproduce with less risk than formerly and their improved health status should have accounted for the larger part of the decline in maternal mortality. Was the relatively greater decline in mortality for childbearers than for the childbearing age-group a measure of the positive contribution of maternity care?

Until 1935, maternity care seemed to have made a negative contribution to safe childbirth, for until then some factor had prevented the mortality of mothers falling in line with that of other subgroups of the population, in particular women of childbearing age. The factors to which the childbearers were uniquely exposed were maternity and maternity care; the more maternity care was delivered, the more the nearly constant rate of maternal mortality diverged from the falling death rate of the relevant age-group. Certainly, the principal killer was puerperal sepsis and maternity carers were the chief vectors of the infecting organisms. The damage inflicted by the surgical interventions of doctors was more serious than the naturally occurring lesions of parturition and increased the mother's susceptibility to infection. The advent of a curative drug enabled them to cover up and make good much of the damage they inflicted.

Obviously the magnitude of relative changes between specified years depends on the values at the starting year. Because the maternal mortality rate had not fallen between 1870 and 1935, while the age-group mortality had done so steadily, it would be more accurate to relate the 1950 values to an earlier year than 1935. Available statistics make it possible to compare the changes in death rates from direct maternal causes, puerperal sepsis and others, and the approximate changes in the death rate for women aged 15–44 between 1891–5 and 1950 [24, Table XIX, 27, Table VIII, 31, Table 4]. The contrasting experience before and after 1935 is shown in Table 7.2.

Thanks to the striking changes after 1935, over the sixty-year period the risk of dying as a result of pregnancy and childbirth (84%) had fallen rather more than the risk of dying from all causes (78%). This could have been the result of different and complementary factors. The medical components of antenatal and intranatal care may have combined to reduce the incidence and seriousness of complications of maternity more effectively than medical care reduced the incidence and seriousness of other causes of death. The social component of current and past antenatal care, through the dietary supplements it

Table 7.2 Percentage declines in mortality rates in England and Wales

Period	Direct maternal causes			Women aged 15–44
	All	Puerperal sepsis	Others	
1891–1935	25	29	21	55
1936–1950	79	89	71	51
1891–1950	84	92	77	78

Sources: references [24, 27, 31].

provided and through persuading mothers to take better care of themselves, may have made pregnant women the healthiest in their age-
group and better able to withstand threats to well-being. Although the
age-group as a whole benefited from the welfare provisions, from the
extra milk and vitamins available to them as children and to their
mothers twenty years before, the childbearing women benefited particularly from the prevention and cure of deficiency diseases which
impaired skeletal and pelvic development and led to future reproductive problems with increased risk of mortality in childbirth. Women in
this age-group had become fitter for living, but more particularly fitter
to reproduce.

Professor McKeown's analysis led him to conclude that before 1950
improved health and survival for the population as a whole was due,
not to medical treatment, but to increased resistance to disease (page 4).
Reduced susceptibility to disease should have meant that pregnant
women needed less intervention than hitherto. In fact, as the obstetrician, Eardley Holland, observed, they were subject to more [7]. Part
of the risk attached to interventions was removed or reduced by the
newly acquired control of sepsis and more effective administration of
blood transfusions; part of it could be reduced by more competent
operators, but it is extremely doubtful that improvements in the
training of doctors in midwifery and obstetrics, which had been so difficult to bring about (Chapter 2), could have appreciably raised the
standards of the average practitioner before 1950, especially in view of
the withdrawal of new graduates from maternity work between 1939
and 1945. Indeed, a speedy reduction in mortality was not expected
from the recommended improvements in education: 'The whole process
will take time and the country must be asked to wait patiently until the
standard of midwifery practice has been remarkably raised' [7].

Yet hardly had the educational reforms begun when maternal mortality started to fall and kept doing so by unprecedented amounts. As
they have done on other occasions, obstetricians succumbed to the
temptation to infer a cause and effect relationship in a situation where
they desperately wanted one to exist and to conclude that their good
intentions had been so promptly and generously rewarded. It is totally
unrealistic to assume that obstetric competence could have been
improved at a rate which coincided with the remarkable reduction in
maternal mortality and which would have justified the optimistic, if
biased, judgement of a founder of the British College of Obstetricians
and Gynaecologists, W. Fletcher Shaw (page 63), who pronounced that:

... the main cause [of reduced mortality] has been the improved
training and teaching of the medical profession, both pre- and post-
graduate, and the general realisation that the care of abnormal

cases must be left to those who have had special post-graduate training. In bringing about the improvements in teaching and training, the College played a great part. Putting it no higher than that, this alone would justify the establishment of the College. [32, p. 66]

CONFIDENTIAL ENQUIRIES INTO MATERNAL DEATHS

Another claimant (or really the same claimant in a different guise) for the credit of bringing about the reduction in maternal mortality is the institution of confidential enquiries into maternal deaths in England and Wales [33–45]. These investigations had followed on from the enquiry by Dr Janet Campbell in 1924 and more specifically from an investigation carried out on behalf of the Ministry of Health's Departmental Committee on Maternal Mortality and Morbidity by two eminent obstetricians and reported in 1932 [15]. Until 1951, the Chief Medical Officer continued to collect confidential reports on maternal deaths from local Medical Officers of Health and regional assessors and published the findings in his successive *Annual Reports*. After 1951, the responsibility for the final assessment and classification of the information was transferred to the Ministry's Consultant Advisers on Obstetrics, which body continued thereafter to produce triennial reports. Its most influential members have, of course, been Fellows of the Royal College of Obstetricians and Gynaecologists, though it has also included high ranking official statisticians over some periods, but it was not until the 1980s that their moderating influence could be discerned. The body of assessors was widened to include pathologists and anaesthetists, but never a representative of professional midwives who, having been denied final responsibility for births, were also absolved from the responsibility of adjudicating the reasons for deaths.

Method of enquiry

The method of enquiry was, as before, to identify factors present in the deaths under review and judge which of these were avoidable. They never claimed that in the absence of avoidable factors death would certainly have been prevented, but the risk, they believed, would have been materially lessened. They intended that by drawing public and professional attention to them, these factors would be avoided in future practice. They showed no undue modesty in proclaiming the value of their work:

There can be little doubt that the publication of these reports and the careful assessment of each death by the doctors concerned and the regional assessors has contributed in no small measure to the reduction in maternal mortality. [37, p. 8]

This view was repeated in their next report [38, p. 11] and was later offered with hardly less confidence by the Department of Health as explanation of the subsequent spectacular continuation of the downward trend illustrated in Figure 7.1:

The maternal death rate in the United Kingdom has fallen from 100 per 100 000 total births in 1951 to six per 100 000 in 1988. It is possible that an important factor in this fall was action taken in the light of confidential enquiries into maternal deaths. [46, p. 184]

In reality, their method of enquiry is too unscientific to justify such optimism and betrays a superficial understanding of the complex causes of mortality. The procedure of professional self-audit by obstetricians is constantly held up as a model of disinterested virtue to other branches of the medical profession and is widely, but uncritically, accepted as such. As a method of bringing to light inefficiencies in the service, and in so far as these are corrected, it is certainly useful. But for impartially evaluating the achievements of treatment and directing policy towards providing the best option for clients it is not at all useful, as the results, if scrutinized, clearly show.

One flaw in this strategy for reducing mortality is that it looks only at one side of experience: it looks at the deaths but not at the survivors. A hint that this defect was at last becoming recognized appeared in the Chief Medical Officer's foreword to the report of 1979–81 [42], but the biased system of enquiry had proved too useful to their profession for the obstetrician members of the reporting body to be willing to abandon it.

Despite the problem that the investigation of obstetric practice limited to maternal deaths inevitably provides an unbalanced view of the field as a whole, a committee of representatives of the Royal College of Obstetricians and Gynaecologists has recommended to me that the Confidential Enquiries should be continued as they provide an invaluable and continuing audit of the working of the maternity services. [42, p. iv]

Without investigation it cannot be known whether the same 'avoidable' factors were present also in cases of survival and, indeed, whether they were associated at least as strongly with survival as with death. Hence it cannot be known that avoiding the identified 'avoidable' factors contributed materially to reducing the death rate.

A second flaw lies in the criterion for judging a factor to be both harmful and avoidable. This was defined as 'a departure from the then accepted standards of satisfactory care, from which ensued the train of events resulting in the death' [33, p. 1]. Accepted standards of satisfactory obstetric care were themselves never based on impartial evaluation of results, but were grossly biased in favour of practices serving the interests of obstetricians. The investigating body expressed its unwillingness to assess failures in diagnosis or clinical management as avoidable factors [37, p. 7, 38, p. 10]. Their criticism of clinical practices was likewise restrained. The increasing use of surgical induction and the higher rate which followed of instrumental delivery and dangerous complications such as pulmonary embolisms, puerperal sepsis and amniotic fluid embolisms were observed, but not considered avoidable factors. The underlying philosophy was sacrosanct, that care by specialist obstetricians, however interventive, was beneficial.

The system of collecting data only about the occurrence of death inevitably gives rise to further flaws in that it seriously limits the conclusions which can be inferred from the statistical data. The total can be divided into specific subgroups and the *proportions* in each can be calculated and compared. Further understanding can only be gained if the absolute number of deaths can be related to the number at risk of dying, so that a death *rate* can be calculated. The correct denominator should be the number of related pregnancies, but no record can be kept of all pregnancies, since many of them do not finish with registrable births or stillbirths and mothers can die before this stage is reached. The conventional denominator used is the officially recorded number of total births, which obviously understates the number of mothers at risk of early death while at the same time overstates the number of pregnancies in that some of these result in multiple births. This latter difficulty is met if deaths are related to *maternities* or mothers delivered, as has been done in some cases. Estimates of the number of pregnancies have been made but these must inevitably be very imprecise and unreliable.

If the number of deaths in subgroups of specific morbid conditions is related to the number of total births or pregnancies, the resulting *rates* would give some qualified indication of the relative incidence of these conditions in the childbearing population and changes through time could be traced. However, more significant information would be derived if the number of deaths from a specific condition could be related to the total number of mothers having this condition, in other words if case-fatality rates could be calculated. The confidential enquiries are not designed to gather this information nor is it readily available from other sources, but without this knowledge one cannot tell whether, when the *proportion* of deaths in a specific subgroup has fallen over time, this has resulted from improved treatment or decreased incidence of the condition or because some other condition has become more frequent, for arithmetically a decrease in one *proportion* must be balanced by an increase in another. For example, if the *proportion* of all deaths due to hypertensive disorders does not decline over time, is this because there has been no improvement in the case-fatality rate or because any improvement in treatment has been offset by a greater prevalence of hypertension, or is it simply the residual of changes in other subgroups? Unlike *proportions*, death *rates* in specific subgroups can all move in the same direction at the same time, all showing improvement or otherwise.

Because for decades the number of maternal deaths in specific subgroups has been small, fluctuations in the triennial *proportions* are likely to be due to chance and not to indicate trends. This limits still further the possibilities of making plausible inferences from the statistical data in the Confidential Enquiries Reports.

The purpose of identifying avoidable factors is to direct action to prevent their repetition. Up until 1935, any action to this end had been singularly unsuccessful in reducing mortality. After 1935, avoidable factors continued to be present in a similar proportion of a rapidly diminishing number of deaths. The method of enquiry prevents it from being known in what proportion the same avoidable factors were present in the increasing number of survivors. It prevents it from being known to what extent the avoidable factors were eliminated and whether, and to what extent, such elimination contributed to the reduction in deaths. It prevents any confirmation of the assumption that the factors identified as avoidable, in particular those concerned with the maternity service as provided and utilized, were indeed critical determinants of death, or that obstetrically directed care, if competently provided and obediently complied with, is indeed capable of overcoming most of nature's deficiencies. It prevents any evaluation of the relative contributions to the safety of birth of medical treatment on the one hand and the mother's general fitness on the other.

Avoidable factors

Factors which from 1924 onwards were regularly identified as avoidable fall into two broad groups: inefficiencies in carrying out accepted procedures on the part of the professionals providing maternity care and unsatisfactory co-operation with the professionals by the mothers using the service. Blame was laid on hospital doctors for delegating care to inexperienced staff, on general practitioners, who did not refer to hospital cases with complications, and on midwives who delayed in obtaining medical help. Often there was confusion of responsibility which prevented or delayed an appropriate response to a clinical condition.

Women were repeatedly blamed for not obtaining sufficient antenatal care and for not following the advice they received. Providers of antenatal care, in turn, were not sufficiently thorough in following up irregular attenders at clinics or defaulters as they were pejoratively labelled. Sometimes care, it was conceded, was misdirected: 'undue concentration on the mechanical aspects of obstetrics seemed to divert attention from the patient's general health' [34, p. 51]. The avoidable factor most greatly deplored was the mother's failure to be delivered in hospital, either because of her own choice or because of the ineffective persuasion of her professional advisers. 'In some cases it appeared that doctors and midwives too readily acceded to the patient's wish to be confined at home' [36, p. 58]. 'Too often the patient's family doctor failed to exert his authority and acquiesced weakly in the requests of the patient' [37, p. 66].

Validating accepted standards

Steps taken to reduce practical incompetence in carrying out accepted procedures must always be in the right direction. But did the confidential enquiries system produce information to confirm that the accepted procedures were themselves beneficial? It did not make good the lack of objective evidence that many aspects of antenatal care succeeded in making birth safer or that the setting in which the care is given makes a material difference to its success. It did, in due course, produce evidence that the hospital setting for intranatal care, contrary to all claims and beliefs, did not make birth safer.

Whatever the likelihood that any particular mother would not have died if she had delivered in hospital (and it can never be known what the outcome in a single case would have been if the circumstances had been other than they were), there was no evidence before 1964 that the risk of death for mothers in general was lower for those who booked for hospital delivery. When relevant data were at last published, they indicated the reverse.

Over the four triennia 1964–75, the only years for which the data were published, mortality per 1000 maternities was shown to average 0.190 for mothers booked for hospital delivery, compared with 0.165 for mothers booked for home delivery, statistically a highly significant difference ($p < 0.0001$). The disparity would almost certainly be even greater if the published data had referred to actual, not booked, deliveries at each place.

Older mothers and mothers who have already borne more than three children have death rates above average and they were especially condemned again and again for preferring to deliver at home. Total absence of supporting data did not deter confident assertions like:

. . . there can be little doubt that arrangements should be made for these women to receive their antenatal care and be confined under circumstances where the best facilities are available to deal with the difficulties and emergencies that must arise relatively more frequently than in other age and parity groups. [33, p. 47]

And

There is nothing in this Report to suggest that all women need to be confined in hospital, but there is strong evidence of the wisdom of arranging hospital care for women in groups at higher risk. [33, p. 50]

But the published results for 1964 to 1975 did not support the official condemnation, for the specific death rates for these higher risk subgroups as booked were also higher in hospital. For mothers aged 35 and over the respective annual average rates over the twelve years were 0.55 for hospital and 0.45 for home bookings; for mothers having their fourth or later child the rates were 0.39 in hospital and 0.29 at home. Continuous pressure by obstetricians to have women in these risk groups delivered in hospital was increasingly successful. The ratio of hospital to home bookings changed from 78:22 in 1964–6 to 97:3 in 1973–5 for the older mothers and from 67:33 in 1964–6 to 93:7 in 1973–5 for the mothers of high parity. If hospital care was especially beneficial for these higher risk groups, it should have caused their mortality rate (all birth places) to fall when it was given to a greater proportion of the maternities. In fact, the rate rose from 0.48 to 0.73 for the older and from 0.33 to 0.40 for the high parous mothers. This increase was in contrast to the decrease in the rate for all risk groups from 0.185 to 0.166. Most of this decrease was attributable to births booked for home where the rate fell by 40%, compared with a fall of 9% for hospital booked births.

Correlations between maternal mortality and hospitalization

Further reason to doubt that care in obstetric hospitals was generally life-saving, or at least that it was an important determinant of reduced mortality, could have been found if any attempt had been made to correlate mortality rates from direct maternal causes and the proportion of births in hospital for each of the fifteen Regional Health Authorities of England and Wales, for which both sets of figures were published only in the 1973–5 report. But these showed that the regions with the greatest proportion of births in hospital were not the ones with the lowest mortality rates. Because the annual number of deaths in each region was very small, a more reliable picture from larger numbers is obtained by relating the average mortality results over three triennia, 1973–81, to hospitalization data averaged from another official source [47]. Calculation yields a correlation coefficient between these variables of +0.16, which means that the association between hospitalization and maternal mortality was so small that very little of the variance in regional mortality rates could be explained by differences in the proportions of deliveries in obstetric hospitals. If anything, hospitalization was associated with higher mortality, the regions with more hospital births being rather more often the regions with higher mortality.

Certainly, the national maternal mortality rate was falling as the rate of hospitalization increased. But, over the period 1969 to 1979 for which there are usable data [47–49], the greater proportional increases in hospitalization and decreases in mortality did not occur between the same years. Once again, the value of the calculated correlation coefficient (+0.05) was far too low to give grounds for claiming a cause and effect relationship. Little or none of the decrease in maternal mortality could possibly be attributed to the increase in the proportion of births in obstetric hospitals.

Avoiding avoidable factors

In 1937, the Chief Medical Officer of the Ministry of Health had listed the factors which contributed to death and judged 40% of them to be avoidable. By 1950, the number of actual deaths had fallen by three-quarters, but the percentage with avoidable factors did not fall. Nor was it to do so. The similar relationship persisted throughout the spectacular decline in maternal mortality that was to follow (Figure 7.1). By 1971, the death rate at 0.21 per 1000 births was less than one-quarter of what it had been in 1950 (0.99) and about one-twenty-fifth of its level in 1935 (5.3). By 1984, it had fallen further to 0.08 [45]. But the percentage of avoidable factors continued to hover around 40 until 1966 and then rose to 57 between 1967 and 1978. The defensive, if inaccurate and illogical, explanation given was that

> . . . inevitably the generally accepted standard of satisfactory care has improved to some extent as a consequence of this publication and it is not surprising therefore to find that the proportion of avoidable factors has not decreased as has the numbers of deaths and the mortality rates. [39, p. 10]

Yet although precise criteria might have changed, the avoidable factors continued to be comprised in the same general groups – inefficiencies in the services provided and unsatisfactory co-operation by the mother. In the 1976–8 report, 41% of the avoidable factors were attributed to obstetric staff in the consultant unit with a further 15% to anaesthetists, 23% to patients, 13% to general practitioners and less than 2% to midwives.

Of the avoidable factors, 54% occurred antenatally, of which 30% were attributed to patients, 33% to obstetric staff and 20% to general practitioners; 38% occurred intranatally, of which 48% were attributed to obstetric staff and 32% to anaesthetists; and 17% postnatally, of which 44% were attributed to obstetric staff, 23% to patients and 13% to general practitioners. It is noteworthy how seldom the midwives could be blamed, yet the report, the writing of which was dominated by obstetricians, did not draw attention to the safe record of the rival profession.

In the 1979–81 report, the concept of avoidable factors was replaced with the concept of substandard care

> . . . to take into account failures in clinical care and also some of the underlying factors which may have produced a low standard of care for the patient. These include . . . shortage of resources for staffing facilities and administrative failure in the maternity services and back-up facilities such as anaesthetic, radiological and pathology services. [42, p. 2]

Substandard care is no more constructive an analytical instrument than are avoidable factors in evaluating the effectiveness of care.

Although by the mid-1980s the maternal mortality rate per 1000 births had fallen further to around 0.08, care was judged to have been substandard in 52% of the direct deaths in England and Wales in 1982–4 [43, p. 133] and stayed as high for those in the United Kingdom in 1985–90 when the Reports gave this extended coverage [44, 45]. As in the case of avoidable factors, the fault was often that care was allowed to be given by inexperienced staff or staff insufficiently aware of the dangers of certain aspects of the interventions, dangers which were now more likely to be acknowledged [43, pp. 133–8]. Since substandard care was so common in fatal outcomes, it was probably common also in non-fatal outcomes but counteracted by other factors, including the human resilience of basically healthy subjects. This probability is supported by women's accounts, reported elsewhere, of their personal experiences. Nevertheless women continued to be castigated for their irrational wilfulness in not availing themselves of the obstetric services provided and so condemning themselves to substandard care, which non-obstetric care is always assumed by obstetricians to be.

Since in successive triennial Reports care was judged to be unsatisfactory in 40–60% of deaths, and in most cases attributed to the same kind of human failing, it is unrealistic to infer that spreading awareness of a relatively small number of specific tragic events was sufficient to prevent equivalent commissions of unsatisfactory care in later years. For example, in 1982–4 three deaths after Caesarean section were attributed

to requiring junior staff to accept responsibility beyond their capabilities; in 1985–7 this was the reason for nine and in 1988–90 for
eighteen such deaths [44, 45, p. 137].

Some substandard care by junior obstetric staff was attributed to the
inadequate numbers of senior obstetricians to whom they could call for
intervention and advice. In anaesthetics there was not only a shortage
of well-trained anaesthetists, but also of facilities and equipment.

To support their claims about shortage of resources – the universal
scapegoat – obstetricians were involved in mounting, in 1984, a national
survey [50], again funded by the National Birthday Trust, of the facilities, staff and equipment, at all places of birth (page 186). On this
occasion the survey did not collect information on the outcome of
maternity for mother or child, which could have been related to the use
of the various facilities (including senior staffing) and so enabled their
effectiveness to be evaluated. The danger of embarrassing findings was
thus avoided. This deplorable omission made it clear that the survey
was intended, not to make a contribution to scientific understanding,
but to produce an inventory which could be used by obstetricians in
campaigns to obtain more resources, professedly in the interests of
patients but actually in the interests of themselves.

Changes in the causes of death

Avoidable factors may have been similar in the decades after 1950, but
there were changes in the relative frequency of the principal causes of
the diminishing total of maternal deaths: in 1952–4, toxaemia was the
cause of 22%, haemorrhage of 17%, abortion of 14% and pulmonary
embolism of 13%. By 1961–3, these were still the major causes, but their
rank order had changed: abortion and pulmonary embolism leading
with 19% and 18% respectively, followed by toxaemia and haemorrhage
with 14% and 13%. By 1970–2, the first three were the same, but haemorrhage (9%) had been superseded by the consequences of anaesthesia
(11%) and ectopic pregnancy (10%), while the frequency of amniotic
fluid embolism had increased to 4% [44, Table 1.11 (corrected figures in
the official source)].

After abortion was legalized in 1968, deaths from criminal abortion
were reduced to very small numbers. By 1985–7 abortions in total, like
sepsis, caused only 5% of the deaths. After 1970–2 the leading causes
had become hypertensive disorders (formerly toxaemia) and pulmonary
embolism, rising respectively to 18% and 17% by 1988–90. The proportions due to other named causes fluctuated; the residual group of miscellaneous causes, which includes liver disease and air embolism,
together accounted in 1988–90 for 17% of deaths, compared with only
6% in 1970–2.

The percentage of deaths due directly to anaesthesia, which had risen slowly to thirteen in 1982–4, fell sharply to four in 1985–7 and to two in 1988–90. This decline, however, may reflect a change in decisions of diagnosis, for anaesthesia contributed also to deaths with other primary causes, including adult respiratory distress syndrome, to which the deaths from anaesthesia may formerly have been assigned. By 1985–90 the relative frequency of amniotic fluid embolism had increased to 7%. All embolisms, as also intra- and postpartum haemorrhage and sepsis, are more likely to follow pregnancies and deliveries with obstetric interventions, including amniocentesis, while anaesthetic complications follow only such assisted deliveries.

No randomized controlled trial has established that the sum of the risks following intervention is less, for mother or child, than the sum of the risks associated with the conditions to relieve which the interventions are undertaken. The higher mortality rates in total and at specific risk levels, and the lack of association between increased hospitalization and reduced mortality, are strong indications that obstetric interventions as a whole have not made birth safer for most mothers.

Hypertension untreated can be dangerous; hypertension treated can also be dangerous. No randomized controlled trial has established how beneficial treatment is; it is not known how much of the declining death *rate* per million maternities [45, Table 2.1] (not *proportion* of all maternal deaths), has been due to increased efficacy of treatment for the severest hypertensive disorders (including eclampsia), or to efficacious treatment being given to more affected women, or to the improved health of mothers overcoming this particular threat to life. The secular decline in the incidence of eclampsia and pre-eclampsia has already been noted, as has the pessimistic appraisal by expert obstetricians of the efficacy of existing treatments (pages 98, 113). A multi-centre research programme has recently been conducted in several countries to assess the effectiveness of low-dose aspirin therapy in improving mortality and morbidity from hypertension (page 113).

The stifling limitations of the method of confidential enquiry are further acknowledged in the setting up of the methodologically superior British Eclampsia Survey 1992 to measure the incidence of eclampsia, as well as maternal and perinatal case-fatality and morbidity rates, and to document current methods of management and treatment [51]. Analysis of the data gathered should make possible a theoretical gain in a clearer understanding of the pathological processes associated with hypertension. But in so far as the objective is the practical one of further reducing maternal mortality, there is little gain to be made in the United Kingdom. The problem here has largely solved itself without this understanding: the death rate from eclampsia per million maternity fell from 54 in 1952–4 to only seven in 1988–90 [45, Table 2.1]. The new knowledge, however, may be of significant practical benefit in the less developed countries where severe hypertension is still an important cause of mortality.

Caesarean section is not judged to be the primary cause of death but it is involved in deaths attributed to other incidental and underlying causes, such as anaesthesia, hypertensive disorders and pulmonary embolisms. Between 1970–2 and 1988–90 the estimated case-fatality rate per 1000 sections fell from 0.78 to 0.25 [45, Table 13.4].

There may be an analogy between the experience of decreasing maternal mortality and the earlier experience of decreasing mortality from infectious diseases. Death rates from tuberculosis, diphtheria, whooping cough and measles were already falling fast thanks to improving host resistance and the pace of decline was hastened only slightly when programmes of immunization were introduced. Thus effective medical treatments made only a small extra contribution to reduced mortality. In the case of maternal mortality, the timing of events makes interpretation less clear. The first sign in the decline in the death rate only just preceded the introduction of antibiotic drugs. These were so effective that they masked any further decline in mortality due to increased host resistance to infection. A similar coincidence in the introduction of effective treatment for haemorrhage on the one hand and improving maternal fitness on the other obscured the contribution of the latter to declining mortality from this cause. Treatments introduced for the other causes of maternal death were less certainly effective and some, as was even observed in the confidential enquiries, brought their own dangers. Yet falling death rates from every single cause, including criminal abortion before 1968, contributed to the overall cascade of mortality rates for the increasingly well-formed, well-nourished cohorts of women who reached their childbearing years after 1950. It is not plausible that new obstetric treatments were being introduced or avoidable factors avoided to such effect as to sustain such a decline in the maternal mortality rate that it halved every eight or nine years (Figure 7.1).

Contrary to the claim that the authors have continued to make (page 293), there must be the greatest doubt that publicizing the avoidable factors in the reports on confidential enquiries could have contributed in more than very small measure to the reduction in maternal mortality. On the contrary, the successful implementation of the constantly repeated recommendation that delivery outside an obstetric hospital must be avoided, especially by women at higher predicted risk, exposed more of them to care associated with higher mortality.

The system of confidential enquiries, of identifying avoidable factors based on unjustifiable criteria, has served well the interests of the professional judges to set the criteria to suit their own ambitions, at the expense of the interests of childbearing women whose trust they have manifestly secured by deception. Realization of its severe limitations as an analytical tool in the field of maternal mortality should deter the propagation by its biased advocates of the method of confidential enquiry in other fields, in particular perinatal mortality, unless supplementation by sounder, more informative techniques of analysis can be ensured.

Before 1950 maternal mortality was not only the overriding obstetric problem but also a serious social problem. In 1921 deaths due to maternal causes amounted to 29.5% of all deaths of women aged 15–44. To seek a solution justified urgent and costly efforts. Thanks more to social than to medical advances, the problem has since become numerically much less important. Yet making the confidential enquiries and preparing the Reports has continued to absorb a great deal of hard work, time and money. At the same time the problems of morbidity, before and after delivery, have been relatively neglected. Some of these are self-limiting and short-term, but recent research has found that an unsuspectedly large number of others can have long-term disabling consequences. 'Childbirth must be far and away the major cause of chronic health problems among women in their child-rearing years' [52] and the General Household Survey in 1990 found 25% of women aged 16–44 reporting long-standing illness for which 19% had recently consulted a doctor [53]. In so far as the objective is to make birth safer for mothers, expenditure on research using methods other than confidential enquiry and addressing the problems not only of mortality, but also of morbidity before and after childbearing, would certainly be more fruitful.

The death rate per 1000 women in the childbearing age-group from all causes halved between 1950 and 1987 [54], but as happened between 1935 and 1950, the maternal mortality rate per 1000 total births fell in even greater proportion – by as much as 91%. This greater proportionate fall was due partly to favourable demographic changes. Since 1950 problems of childbearing have affected a decreasing proportion of women in the childbearing age-group. In England and Wales the general fertility rate – number of births per 1000 women aged 15–44 years – fell from 81 in 1951–5 to 62 in 1985–7 [54]. Fewer of the births have been to women at the upper end of the age range and fewer have been fourth or subsequent births, and though latterly there has been an increase in multiple births, these have affected only a very small proportion of fertile women. Early legal terminations of potentially high-risk pregnancies may have forestalled later dangers.

Part of the greater fall in mortality was due to the lower incidence of life-threatening morbidity specific to maternity, like eclampsia/pre-eclampsia and haemorrhage, and to lower case-fatality rates. How much of this reduced susceptibility was the result of the improved general health of the mothers and how much the result of more effective medical care and obstetric intervention, either preventive or curative, cannot be discerned from the availabie data. The comments already made (page 302) on experience up to 1950 apply to experience since then.

In England the deaths due to maternal causes, which had accounted for nearly 30% of all deaths in the childbearing age-group in the 1920s, accounted for less than 1% in the 1980s. The English experience was shared by the other economically prosperous countries and for whatever reasons, deaths of mothers in childbirth have ceased to be the medical shame and social scourge they once were.

MATERNAL MORTALITY IN THE THIRD WORLD

This good fortune was not shared by women in the poorer countries where 99% of the world's half-million maternal deaths every year in the 1980s took place:

> Women in developing countries run 100 to 200 times the risk of dying in pregnancy and childbirth than do women in an affluent country. . . . The lifetime risk of a woman in a developing country dying in pregnancy or from pregnancy-related illness may be 1 in 50 or as high as 1 in 14; this contrasts sharply with the 1 in several thousand women in the developed world. [55]

The primary reason for the high mortality is the women's poor physical condition, the result of a long history of undernourishment (even starvation) over many generations. In many of their cultures women are condemned, more thoroughly than in more prosperous countries, to inferior social status which permeates every aspect of their lives. Marriage frequently takes place at a very young age, before skeletal development is complete; contracted pelves, and hence obstructed labours, are common. In some places, for example Bangladesh, up to 90% of girls are married by the age of 18; by 17 about half have become mothers and by 19 about one-third have had two children. In developing countries in general some 10–20% of births are to girls in their teens. The younger the mother, the higher the risk of death; the mortality rate can be more than twice as high for those aged 15–19 as for those aged 20–24, but it can be between three and seven times as high for those aged 10–14. About half of all deaths in the age-group 15–19 can be due to maternal causes. For those who survive, life is made one long series of pregnancies, too often in quick succession and each one after the third becoming more dangerous [56]. Yet, despite the extra demands of frequent pregnancy and breastfeeding, when food is scarce, women get less than their fair share of it. They are required to carry out hard manual work without remission.

The provision of maternity care varies very widely in quality and quantity within and across the continents: prenatal facilities are available for from 2% to 99% of mothers, much more in the richer than in the poorer areas, much more in the urban than in the rural districts. Where facilities do exist mortality rates are usually lower, but this may reflect lesser poverty rather than effectiveness of services. Moreover, it does not always happen. For example, Gambia has levels of prenatal care coverage of 80–90%, yet it also has some of the highest mortality rates recorded [57].

The quality of prenatal care can be good and certain high risk conditions, like anaemia which is endemic and compounds mortality from other primary causes, can be diagnosed and much can be done to treat it. Likewise, prevalent vaginal infections can be detected and effectively controlled, so probably reducing the ultimate death toll and postpartum morbidity from puerperal sepsis and genito-urinary diseases. Signs of hypertension predicting pre-eclampsia or eclampsia, frequent causes of death, can also be detected, and though no specific treatment has been validated in any country as surely effective, mortality rates are found to be lower for those who have had prenatal care. But prenatal care is often poor, sometimes because sensible advice and serviceable diagnostic equipment are both lacking. When an obstetric problem is detected, the policy is to refer the mother to hospital for specialist intervention, but the transfer may be frustrated by difficulties in transport over long distances and sometimes by family or other social problems.

Whether, indeed, transfer to hospital for specialist treatment is in most cases beneficial is, like the assumed benefit from most prenatal practices, at best unproven (Chapter 3, and pages 338–41). This uncertainty limits the scope for prenatal care to prevent the most frequent causes of maternal death in the Third World and, therefore, the authority of recommendations proposed for providing the services [58].

Availability of facilities for intranatal care likewise varies widely: coverage ranges from 2% of mothers in Somalia to 90% of mothers in the richer countries of South America. Many women needing emergency treatment have no access to transfusions with uncontaminated blood or to operative delivery. Some, however, are unwilling to accept hospital care because the staff make them feel inferior (a reaction not unfamiliar in the developed countries) [57].

Many women do not have access to a competent birth attendant wherever they deliver. Incompetent intranatal care leads to more deaths in the postpartum than in the antepartum and intrapartum periods combined, haemorrhage and sepsis being the most frequent causes [59]. It can also leave the women with permanent damage and future ill health, which has been estimated to affect sixteen survivors for every woman who dies. This postpartum morbidity, which is of a more serious nature than that recently uncovered in England [52], commonly follows puerperal infections and haemorrhages and, most strikingly, unskilled efforts to deal with obstructed labour. These can leave the woman with a fistula, a false passage between the vagina and bladder or possibly rectum through which urine or faeces flow uncontrollably, causing her serious discomfort and skin irritation and, even more dreaded, an offensive smell which leads to her being ostracized and completely losing such social status as she had. Facilities for gynaecological repair are often not readily available to affected women [56].

Relatively few women, particularly in Africa, have access to sound family planning advice or the means to practise the recommended contraception. In any case cultural barriers would often prevent this, for the fathering of many children testifies to a man's virility and earns the social esteem of his peers. When child mortality is high, many children have to be born to ensure that enough will survive to adulthood to look after the parents in their old age. The *raison d'être* of women is seen to be to breed and satisfy the desires of men. This puts them at constant risk of acquiring sexually transmitted diseases, including AIDS (acquired immune deficiency syndrome), the devastating epidemic of the 1980s and 1990s.

That women would appreciate contraception was confirmed in a survey which compared actual with wanted fertility in 48 populations and found that 22% of births were unwanted.

If all women who said they wanted no more children were actually able to stop childbearing, the number of births would be reduced by an average of 35% in Latin America, 33% in Asia and 17% in Africa. Mortality would fall by an even higher proportion since the births that would be averted would tend to the high-parity/high-risk births . . . [57]

Mortality would be even more reduced if it were socially acceptable for contraception to postpone childbearing for the teenage mothers and to lengthen the intervals between pregnancies for all mothers. The same result would be achieved if early legal termination by qualified staff were made available to more than the small proportion of the world's women who already have access to it. For them the risk from abortion is much lower than the risk of birth if it is carried out before eight weeks of pregnancy, but the risk rises with each week thereafter.

Without contraception or legalized termination, the only prospect of escape from the harrowing treadmill of repeated pregnancies involves risking the greatly increased dangers of procuring an illegal abortion. But this is a desperate remedy, for 25–50% of the maternal deaths are so related.

The problem of maternal mortality has many roots – cultural, economic, social and political – and its solution will require many changes. The changes are likely to be interactive and their effects on mortality hard to separate. It has been observed in Africa and in India [60] that maternal mortality is lower in communities where women have had opportunities for secondary education, although these are unlikely to be the poorest, and the better mortality results may stem rather from better diet made possible by less poverty than from the cultural repercussions of more schooling. But more schooling might be the first effective step in raising women's social status with the incidental benefits which that implies. If longer years in school became more socially accepted, so also might an older age at marriage and reduced fertility, with knowledge of how to achieve this.

In many ways the plight of the women in poor countries replicates the plight in earlier centuries of women in the now prosperous countries. Analogy with past experience makes it certain that if improvement is to be achieved, much the greater part of it will be through raising the standard of living, especially the standard of nutrition of the mothers and their baby girls, the mothers of the future. With better maternal health and better control of fertility, many of the dangers of childbirth would not arise, while many others could be satisfactorily treated by low-technology care. Certainly there is at present an immense need for emergency rescue which obstetric treatment in large expensively equipped hospitals could provide. But this would not be to tackle the problem at its roots. It would be an unjustifiable misdirection of their limited resources if ambition to emulate their richer neighbours were to entice the poorer countries to make more than a very modest investment in costly facilities for high-technology prenatal screening and interventive intranatal obstetrics. Better results would come more basically from providing mothers with better nutrition and knowledge about family planning.

REFERENCES

1. *Genesis*, 3:16.
2. *Genesis*, 35:16, 18.
3. Donnison, J. (1977) *Midwives and Medical Men*, Heinemann, London.
4. Registrar General, *Statistical Review for 1929*, HMSO, London, Text, Table LVIII.
5. Towler, J. and Bramall, J. (1986) *Midwives in History and Society*, Croom Helm, London.

6. Wertz, R.W. and Wertz, D.C. (1977) *Lying-in: A History of Childbirth in America*, The Free Press, New York.
7. Holland, E. (1935) Maternal mortality. *Lancet*, 27 April, 973–6.
8. Macfarlane, A. and Mugford, M. (1984) *Birth Counts: Statistics of Pregnancy and Childbirth*, Vol. 1, National Perinatal Epidemiology Unit in Association with the Office of Population Censuses and Surveys, HMSO, London, Chap. 10.
9. Baird, D. (1960) The evolution of modern obstetrics. *Lancet*, 17 September, 609.
10. Registrar General, *Statistical Review for 1937*, HMSO, London, Text, Table LXXXVI.
11. Douglas, C. (1955) Trends in the risks of childbearing and in the mortalities of infancy during the last thirty years. *J. Obstet. Gynaecol. Br. Emp.*, **62**, 216–31.
12. Commonwealth Bureau of Statistics (1910 and 1940) *Demography*, Canberra.
13. Loudon, I. (1990) Obstetrics and the general practitioner. *Br. Med. J.*, **301**, 703–7.
14. Campbell, J.M. (1924) *Maternal Mortality*, Reports on Public Health and Medical Subjects No. 25, HMSO, London.
15. Ministry of Health (1932) *Final Report of the Departmental Committee* (Chairman G. Newman), HMSO, London, p. 134.
16. New York Academy of Medicine Committee on Public Health Relations (1933) *Maternal Mortality in New York City 1930–32*, The Commonwealth Fund, New York, p. 215.
17. Wertz and Wertz, *Lying-in*, pp. 161–2 (Quoting White House Conference on Child Health and Protection (1933) *Fetal, Newborn and Maternal Mortality and Morbidity*, New York, pp. 215–17.)
18. Browne, F.J. (1934) Are we satisfied with the results of antenatal care? *Br. Med. J.*, **2**, 194–7.
19. Registrar General, *Statistical Review for the Years 1940–45*, HMSO, London, Text, Table CXVI.
20. Donnison, J. (1977) *Midwives and Medical Men*, p. 189 (Quoting Hansard (1936), 5th Series, vol. 311 (Commons), cols 1117–19.).
21. Report of the Task Force on the Implementation of Midwifery in Ontario 1987 (Chairperson M. Eberts) *Appendix 1: A History of Midwifery in Canada*, Ontario Government, Ontario, p. 203.
22. Registrar General (1938) *Decennial Supplement to the Census of Population, England and Wales, 1931, Part IIa Occupational Mortality*, HMSO, London, Table 11.
23. Colebrook, L. (1954) Puerperal infection, in *Historical Review of British Obstetrics and Gynaecology, 1800–1850* (eds J.M.M. Kerr, R.W. Johnstone and M.H. Phillips), Livingstone, Edinburgh, Chap. XXVI.
24. Registrar General, *Statistical Review for 1950*, HMSO, London, Text, Medical, Table XIX.
25. Wrigley, A.J. (1934) A criticism of antenatal work. *Br. Med. J.*, **1**, 891–4.
26. Registrar General, *Annual Report Statistical Review for 1919*, HMSO, London, Text, Table LXXXI.

27. Registrar General (1931) *Statistical Review for 1929*, HMSO, London, Text, Tables LVIII, LXII.

28. Colebrook, L. and Kenny, M. (1936) Treatment with Prontosil of puerperal infections due to haemolytic streptococci. *Lancet*, **ii**, 1319.

29. Chief Medical Officer of the Ministry of Health (1946) *On the State of the Public Health during Six Years of War*, HMSO, London.

30. Registrar General (1959) *Decennial Supplement to the Census of Population, England and Wales, 1951, Part II, Occupational Mortality*, HMSO, London, Table 88.

31. Registrar General, *Statistical Review for 1951*, Part 1, HMSO, London, Table 4.

32. Shaw, W.F. (1954) *Twenty-Five Years. The Story of the Royal College of Obstetricians and Gynaecologists 1929–54*, Churchill, London, p. 66.

33. Ministry of Health (1957) *Report on Confidential Enquiries into Maternal Deaths*, Reports on Public Health and Medical Subjects No. 97, 1952–54, HMSO, London.

34. *Report on Confidential Enquiries into Maternal Deaths* (1960) Reports on Public Health and Medical Subjects No. 103, 1955–57, HMSO, London.

35. *Report on Confidential Enquiries into Maternal Deaths* (1963) Reports on Public Health and Medical Subjects No. 108, 1958–60, HMSO, London.

36. *Report on Confidential Enquiries into Maternal Deaths* (1966) Reports on Public Health and Medical Subjects No. 115, 1961–63, HMSO, London.

37. *Report on Confidential Enquiries into Maternal Deaths* (1969) Reports on Public Health and Medical Subjects No. 119, 1964–66, HMSO, London.

38. *Report on Confidential Enquiries into Maternal Deaths* (1972) Reports on Health and Social Subjects No. 1, 1967–69, HMSO, London.

39. *Report on Confidential Enquiries into Maternal Deaths* (1975) Reports on Health and Social Subjects No. 11, 1970–72, HMSO, London.

40. *Report on Confidential Enquiries into Maternal Deaths* (1979) Reports on Health and Social Subjects No. 14, 1973–75, HMSO, London.

41. *Report on Confidential Enquiries into Maternal Deaths* (1982) Reports on Health and Social Subjects No. 26, 1976–78, HMSO, London.

42. *Report on Confidential Enquiries into Maternal Deaths* (1986) Reports on Health and Social Subjects No. 29, 1979–81, HMSO, London.

43. *Report on Confidential Enquiries into Maternal Deaths* (1989) Reports on Health and Social Subjects No. 34, 1982–84, HMSO, London.

44. *Report on Confidential Enquiries into Maternal Deaths in the United Kingdom 1985–87* (1991) Department of Health, Welsh Office, Scottish Office Home and Health Department, Department of Health and Social Security, Northern Ireland, HMSO, London.

45. *Report on Confidential Enquiries into Maternal Deaths in the United Kingdom 1988–90* (1994) Department of Health, Welsh Office, Scottish Office Home and Health Department, Department of Health and Social Security, Northern Ireland, HMSO, London.

46. House of Commons Health Committee (1991) *Maternity Services: Preconception, vol. II, Minutes of Evidence*, HMSO, London, pp. 1–291.

47. Office of Population Censuses and Surveys, *Birth Statistics for the years 1974–81*, Series FM1, HMSO, London, Table 8.4.

48. Registrar General, *Statistical Reviews for the Years 1969–73*, Part II, HMSO, London, Appendix B1.
49. Office of Population Censuses and Surveys (1979) *Mortality Statistics, Childhood and Maternity, 1979*, HMSO, London, Table 18.
50. Chamberlain, G. and Gunn, P. (1987) *Birthplace*, John Wiley, Chichester.
51. Douglas, K. and Redman, C. (1992) Eclampsia in the United Kingdom. The 'Best' way forward. *Br. J. Obstet. Gynaecol.*, **99**, 335–9.
52. MacArthur, C., Lewis, M., Knox, E. *et al.* (1991) *Health After Childbirth*, HMSO, London.
53. Office of Population Censuses and Surveys (1990) *General Household Survey*, HMSO, London.
54. Office of Population Censuses and Surveys (1991) *Birth Statistics. Fertility Trends in England and Wales, 1981–91*, HMSO, London.
55. Mahler, Halfdan, Director-General, World Health Organization (1987) The safe motherhood initiative: a call to action. *Lancet*, **1**, 668–70.
56. Royston, E. and Armstrong, S. (eds) (1989) *Preventing Maternal Deaths*, World Health Organization, Geneva.
57. World Health Organization (1992) *World Health Statistics 1991. Coverage of Maternity Care*, World Health Organization, Geneva, pp. 11–14.
58. Rooney, C. (1992) *Antenatal Care and Maternal Health: How Effective is it? A Review of the Evidence*, Division of Family Health, World Health Organization, Geneva.
59. Kwast, B. (1991) Puerperal sepsis: its contribution to maternal mortality. *Midwifery*, **7**, 102–6.
60. Editorial (1987) Maternal Health in sub-Saharan Africa. *Lancet*, **i**, 255–7.

8

It is impossible to find evidence that medical care raised the safety of birth for mother or child before 1935. It is impossible to find evidence which supports the claim that improvements in the education and technical efficiency of doctors or midwives, or indeed in other elements of maternity care, were responsible for the major contribution to the spectacular and sustained improvement after 1936 in the survival of mothers in childbirth. It is just as difficult to show that these were the factors responsible for the markedly improved survival of postneonatal infants after 1900 and of neonatal infants and fetuses after 1939.

Until 1870, when fertility was high, stillbirths and neonatal deaths were accepted as inevitable. They were sometimes welcomed as a form of birth control or natural selection. In difficult deliveries doctors deliberately sacrificed the life of the fetus, if necessary to save that of the mother. Records were not kept of the extent of perinatal mortality. But after 1870, when the birth rate started to decline, the survival of infants became a matter of concern and their persistently high mortality rate ceased to be acceptable. The early years of the 20th century saw the introduction of official measures to improve maternity care, for the sake of the babies as well as their mothers (Chapters 3 and 5).

But before any of the measures adopted could have had an appreciable effect, infant mortality started to fall steeply. From around 156 per 1000 live births in 1896–1900, as high as it had ever been since 1841, the rate in England and Wales had fallen to around 138 by 1901–6; it went on to reach 62 by 1930–5 and 36 by 1946–50 [1, 2].

It was, however, the older infants who benefited most from this decline. The mortality of the newborn reflects mainly the conditions present during fetal life or events occurring at the birth, at least some of which maternity care is intended to improve. These influences on mortality are progressively outweighed after one week by influences in the baby's social environment. In the 19th century, the babies' environment exposed them to the then prevalent infectious diseases which were the chief cause of their high mortality. From 1870, the death rate for older children had been falling, as their improving nutrition made them more resistant to the infections, the incidence of which was being reduced by improved sanitation and hygiene. As the 20th century advanced, the older infants began to show the same resistance.

Data are available from 1906 for deaths at different infant ages: up to one week (early neonatal), from two to four weeks (late neonatal) and over four weeks (post-neonatal) [2]. These show that in 1906–10, 66% of the deaths were post-neonatal and 21% early neonatal; by 1931–5 these percentages were 49 and 36 respectively; by 1946–50 they were 42 and 45. Thus most of the reduced mortality took place at the post-neonatal stage and may well have been contributed to by the influence of infant welfare services and the instruction given to mothers on infant management. Post-neonatal and late neonatal mortality rates per 1000 births fell continuously between 1906 and 1950: the post-neonatal rate from 76.9 to 11.1, a fall of 86%, while the late neonatal rate fell from 15.7 to 3.3, a fall of 79%.

In contrast, it was not until after 1940 that the early neonatal rate really started to fall. Despite the increased input of resources into maternity care, it was higher in 1937 than it had been in 1921–5. It eventually fell from 24.5 in 1906 to 15.2 in 1950, a fall of 38% [2].

If infants older than one week were becoming healthier and more resistant to dangers in their environment, infants under one week should also have been becoming healthier and more resistant to the dangers of birth. It might have been expected that early neonatal mortality would decline in step with mortality at later stages. Something was happening to prevent this expected improvement. Was it that the dangers of birth were being increased, not reduced, by 'advances' in maternity care?

In Scotland maternity services were similar to those in England and so was the pattern of neonatal mortality. The rate was higher in 1941 than it had been in 1921–5 but then started to fall sharply [3]. In the USA the rate fell slowly throughout the 1930s, although somewhat erratically for the non-white population, but there too the pace of decline quickened markedly in the early 1940s [4].

The recorded history of stillbirths (from 28 weeks of gestation) is shorter but similar to that of early neonatal mortality. After stillbirths became registrable in England and Wales in 1928, the rate per 1000 births (live plus still) remained virtually constant around 41 until 1935, fell slowly to 38 in 1939, then rapidly to 22.6 in 1950 [2]. In Scotland stillbirths were first registered in 1939; the rate started falling after 1940 and by 1950 was only 64% of the 1939 level [3]. In the USA the stillbirth rate had been falling throughout the 1930s, much faster than the early neonatal death rate and much faster for the non-white population. There too the decline speeded up in the 1940s [4].

CAUSES OF PERINATAL DEATH

Attributing stillbirths and early neonatal deaths to specific causes is not always a simple and straightforward medical exercise, so that the results have to be interpreted with some reserve. From analyses of Scottish data [3, 4] it is apparent that the stillbirth rates from the four principal defined causes all fell between 1940 and 1950. The drop in the intrauterine death rate associated with maternal toxaemia, from 4.4 to 2.3, and with antepartum haemorrhage, from 5.0 to 3.9, indicates directly improved health of mothers; the drop in deaths associated with difficult labour, from 8.9 to 5.4, indicates a lower prevalence of deformed maternal pelves; the smaller drop in deaths from congenital malformation, 6.1 to 4.8, indicates less directly improved health of both parents.

There was, however, an even greater decline in stillbirths from 'ill-defined and unknown' causes, from 13.7 to 4.7, and also in first-week deaths from 'congenital debility' and 'premature birth', only part of which decline could be attributed to more precise certification in the later years. In so far as these categories could not be defined, they could not be the targets for specific remedial measures offered by maternity care. They were, rather, considered to indicate 'the efficiency of the physiological mechanisms which govern the growth and vitality of the foetus' [4, p. 186]. Death rates from all causes were higher in the lower social classes, but the excess was most striking in the categories difficult to define, which suggests that these conditions were the most sensitive to poverty. Thus poverty, particularly when it means inadequate nutrition, is shown to be the critical determinant of reproductive efficiency.

After the onset of economic recovery, the stillbirth rate declined most in the regions of England and Wales which had earlier suffered the severest depression [5]. The sudden and widespread change in mortality experience in the 1940s coincided with a sudden and widespread change in economic experience. The war effort of many countries had drawn back into employment the considerable numbers who had been idle during the world economic depression of the 1930s. Family incomes were increased and in Britain at least, food rationing and price controls enabled a far greater proportion of the population to obtain an adequate diet. Analysts were agreed that this improvement had a significant effect on the trends in mortality:

The fall in stillbirth and infant mortality rates from the 1938 level during the war period is of the order of magnitude to be expected from the levelling up of nutritional standards among the worst off section of the population [6, p. 124]

And

. . . the elimination of the grosser forms of poverty, with all that they implied, together with the provision of assured supplies of inexpensive and nourishing foods to expectant mothers in the United Kingdom was accompanied by a remarkable reduction in obstetric (stillbirths plus early neonatal) deaths, mainly from those ill-defined causes. It is difficult to believe that this was not cause and effect. [4, p. 195]

This hypothesis is consistent with American experience. In the USA, the stillbirth and early neonatal death rates for the non-white population were always much higher than for the white, but they fell much faster, particularly in the early 1940s. Poverty was always greater among the non-whites, but they benefited relatively more from the increased employment generated by the war. This probably reduced the disparity between the nutritional standards of the racial groups and accounted for the reduced disparity in the mortality of their babies [4].

Better nutrition of pregnant women clearly contributed to their own and their babies' survival. In addition, the brief period of rest and release from domestic obligations before delivery, which the evacuated British mothers enjoyed, may have contributed to their exceptionally low rates of stillbirths and neonatal deaths as well as of maternal mortality. The stillbirth rate per 1000 births in the Scottish emergency hospitals was 18, compared with the Scottish average of 36 and the death rate per 1000 live births for infants in the first two weeks of life was 10, compared with the Scottish average of 27.5 [3].

But these short-term advantages did not affect the mothers' skeletal development or the prevalence of deformities. The reduction in stillbirths caused by difficult labour was more likely due to fewer pelves being contracted than to more successful rescues by forceps or caesarean section. This suggests that a generation of women was coming to childbearing who, as infants themselves, had been less exposed to the severe malnutrition which prevents the healthy growth of bone and leads to rickets. Food supplements provided for expectant and nursing mothers in the early antenatal and infant welfare clinics probably contributed to this amelioration.

It is less easy to identify probable benefits from the medical elements of maternity care. The services provided had been expanding steadily throughout the century without any sign that they were reducing mortality. The first innovation to make a big difference to maternity mortality was pharmacological, not obstetric. But

> No new advance in medical knowledge – comparable in effect to the introduction of the antibiotics – came into use in 1941 and 1942 suddenly and markedly to improve the chances of survival of the foetus. [4, p. 195]

And

> . . . the types of death which showed the greatest decrease are among the most difficult to influence by routine antenatal practice and in any case 'the quality of antenatal supervision did not improve suddenly at the height of the war.' [4, p. 186]

THE CONTRIBUTION OF OBSTETRIC CARE

The percipient and painstaking Scottish Professor of Midwifery at Aberdeen University, Dugald Baird, whose pioneering work appreciated the necessity of considering obstetrics in a social setting, demonstrated convincingly the close association between high obstetric mortality and low social class, with supporting evidence that the material causal factor was poor nutrition [7]. Further improvements in the nutrition of the poor should lead to further improvements in mortality. Yet, as a conscientious obstetrician, he had to believe that good obstetric care was also beneficial and that the downward trend in mortality in the 1940s was also due to 'the great increase in the proportion of women confined in hospital, to improvements in the management of pregnancy and labour and in the improved care of babies' [8, p. 21].

He could not demonstrate this from national statistics, but he sought to do so from other sources. He collected results relating to their private, and hence well-to-do, patients from six obstetric specialists of high repute working in British cities and, comparing them with the average results relating to mothers of social classes I and II in England and Wales in 1939, who received care of variable quality (data supplied privately by the Registrar General), found that the selected group of private patients had much lower stillbirth rates. He made a second comparison between the stillbirth rates achieved by Aberdeen obstetric specialists treating mothers of social classes III, IV and V in hospital with the average results for these classes, however and wherever treated, in England and Wales, but found that the Aberdeen obstetricians achieved only slightly better results [7].

Professor Baird could not explain these contrasting findings. The six selected obstetric specialists carried out relatively more caesarean sections on their private patients than did the Aberdeen specialists on their hospital patients, but careful scrutiny of the causes of death confirmed that the Aberdeen specialists could not have reduced mortality by carrying out more caesarean sections, for their excess of deaths was due to conditions like prematurity which could not then have been remedied by advancing delivery.

Professor Baird did not attempt to explain in what ways the treatment given by the six selected specialists made it so much more successful than the English average for social classes I and II, but he was confirmed in his appreciation of the value of obstetric care. He considered that 'the low foetal mortality in the practices of obstetric specialists is therefore a great tribute to their skill and judgement, but it is obtained at great cost in time and nervous energy' [7, p. 535]. It was probably obtained at considerable financial cost to the women concerned. Perhaps the value of the service they bought of their specialist was not so much his obstetric skill but his personal attention, the confidence he inspired in them and the continuity of his care – fundamental factors in good midwifery, but factors which were to be neglected in future obstetric education and practice.

FURTHER INVESTIGATIONS

With his colleagues, Professor Baird assembled more data on stillbirths and early neonatal deaths between 1943 and 1951 in Aberdeen, an area with a long history of social and economic deprivation [8]. They were able to show a considerable reduction in stillbirths from birth trauma and unknown causes in mature fetuses, which together caused most fetal deaths at that time. He attributed the reduction partly to the effect of better nutrition: '. . . infants of better vitality should withstand the stress of difficult labour with less danger from trauma or anoxia' [8, p. 22], and partly to the immediate availability of skilled attention. Stillbirths from birth trauma had declined more in Aberdeen than in the rest of Scotland. Hospital facilities had expanded more in Aberdeen than nationally 'so that more patients came under specialists' supervision' [8, p. 29].; Moreover, the incidence of and stillbirth rate from birth trauma were lower for hospital booked cases than for home bookings (including transfers).

Professor Baird had already identified poverty and malnutrition as the most important causes of mortality and indicated that, although it was 'difficult to get strictly comparable groups from which to assess the risks of hospital and domiciliary confinement' [8, p. 26], he found reason to believe that these conditions were overrepresented among home bookings, which included an excess of women in poor health after having had many children, while 'most intelligent and educated mothers . . . prefer to go to hospital even when they have every reason to hope that confinement will be normal' [8, p. 27].

The stillbirth rate in 1949–51 for all pregnancies except the third was found to be much higher for home than for hospital booked cases, although in contrast the early neonatal mortality rate was always much lower for the home booked cases except for first births where it was slightly higher. Despite the inconsistency of these results and despite their admitted difficulty of getting strictly comparable groups for assessing risks at home and in hospital, Professor Baird and his colleagues made the extraordinary claim that their figures made 'it difficult to avoid the conclusion that hospital confinement is preferable' [8, p. 27]. Ignoring both their previous findings of poverty as the critical determinant of mortality and its predominance in home births, they completely abandoned logic and the need for valid evidence and concluded that 'If it is accepted that confinement in hospital is safer for certain types of patient, where the risks are high, it must also be safer for cases where the risks are less. There can be little doubt that if all women were confined in good maternity hospitals there would be fewer deaths' [8, p. 27].

This ill-considered conclusion gave much valued comfort and reassurance to the obstetric profession world-wide and was to have profound and lasting influence on the organization and conduct of maternity care. But despite his lapse in logic, Professor Baird pursued his researches methodically and was responsible for setting up the Medical Research Council Obstetric Medicine Research Unit at Aberdeen, pioneers in the field who recognized the social as well as the biological and mechanical factors affecting the outcome of childbirth.

OBSTETRICAL AND ENVIRONMENTAL CAUSES OF PERINATAL DEATH

After careful epidemiological and laboratory research, Professor Baird's next step was to categorize the causes of perinatal death into two broad groups: obstetrical and environmental [9]. He concentrated his attention on causes in the former group which, he considered, were amenable to correction by clinical intervention. In this category he included deaths due to maternal toxaemia (hypertensive complications in pregnancy), to 'mechanical' causes like birth trauma, asphyxia and cord compression, and to Rhesus factor incompatibility, as well as the deaths of mature infants weighing over 2500 grams for which the cause was uncertain but happened, he hypothesized, because the placenta had latterly become insufficient to supply the needs of the growing fetus.

The risks of perinatal death from birth trauma, asphyxia and placental insufficiency were found to increase with maternal age, particularly in first pregnancies and in pregnancies lasting longer than 40 weeks. These risks might be reduced if labours were induced to prevent prolonged pregnancy and if caesarean section was used more liberally in the hope of avoiding undue stress to the baby in labour. This policy was put into practice in Aberdeen after 1952.

By the period 1953–7, most of the first-time mothers (primiparae) aged 35 and over were induced when their pregnancy passed 41 weeks and 32% of them were delivered by caesarean section; most of the younger mothers were induced when their pregnancy passed 42 weeks and the average caesarean section rate for all primiparae was raised to 4.6%, compared with 2.8% between 1948 and 1952 [5, p. 562]. The policy appeared to be vindicated for the perinatal mortality rate from toxaemia and the mechanical and uncertain causes in mature babies was much lower in 1953–7 than in 1948–52, and the overall perinatal mortality in Aberdeen, which had been higher than in England and Wales throughout the 1940s, fell considerably below it in the 1950s [10, p. 256].

After the end of the war and the inception of the NHS, resources were allocated more liberally to maternity care, but disappointingly the sudden and dramatic decline in perinatal mortality of the war years was not maintained. Current social conditions did not worsen, but some of the childbearing women had been infants in the worst years of economic depression in the early 1930s and still bore marks of their deprivation.

Between 1931 and 1938, the perinatal mortality rate in England and Wales had fallen by 6%, between 1939 and 1948 by 34%, but between 1949 and 1958 the decline was back to 8%. In 1954 the rate, at 38.1, was as high as it had been in 1949 [2]. Existing medical resources seemed as impotent in bringing down perinatal mortality as they had been in bringing down maternal mortality before 1935. If this failure was to be reversed by medical care, new knowledge, obstetric, paediatric, sociological, pathological and administrative, was needed, not only about the babies who were dying, but also about those who survived.

To obtain this information an ambitious epidemiological survey, the first of its kind in the world, was sponsored by a charity, the National Birthday Trust, and carried out in 1958 with the active support and co-operation of the professions whose members provide maternity care. Of these, the chairman and several members of the Steering Committee were drawn from the Royal College of Obstetricians and Gynaecologists. The authors of the first report in 1963 [11] were a paediatrician (N.R. Butler) and an obstetrician (D.G. Bonham).

THE 1958 PERINATAL MORTALITY SURVEY

The method of enquiry in this survey [11], as was described above in Chapter 1 (pages 29–31), was to collect a great deal of information about every birth which took place in Britain in one week in March 1958 and, in order to obtain sufficient numbers to permit instructive statistical analyses, about every perinatal death which occurred in the next three months. The births and deaths surveyed provided a representative sample of all births in Britain at that period. The method of analysis was to cross-classify some of the categories of the births and associated deaths and so quantify relationships between them; to quantify the risk of perinatal death associated with the age, parity and social class of the mother, with the region of the country she lived in, with her obstetric history, with certain aspects of her antenatal care, with complications experienced in pregnancy, with the duration of gestation and the birthweight of the child, and with certain aspects of labour and delivery; to quantify also the risk of death before, during or after delivery and the association between several of these characteristics and the post-mortem findings of the cause of death.

In many respects, the survey produced an invaluable storehouse of information, much of it of universal relevance, and it was appropriately acclaimed. But by 1958, thirty years after the establishment of their College, obstetricians had become firmly convinced that their philosophy of interventive maternity care was correct and their practical interventions beneficial. Of course they needed to believe this, it was their *raison d'être*. Not only had they convinced themselves, they had deeply committed themselves to convincing all others concerned in providing or using the maternity service.

Because of the survey's excellence in many respects, it was assumed to be equally excellent in all respects and its findings as reported were accorded great authority in Britain and abroad. Precisely because of its wide and powerful influence, it is necessary to give some detailed consideration to the unsound foundations on which its message – the alleged confirmation of obstetricians' philosophy – rested.

Clearly obstetricians expected that their survey would vindicate their claim, that treatment under their control in obstetric hospitals did make birth safer, and would powerfully support their aspirations in securing for themselves a monopoly of the service.

The terms of reference of the Steering Committee included collecting data about the place of confinement, in order to measure its possible effect on the safety and health of the infant. This could be assessed by comparing mortality rates at the different places, which stand as proxies for the different kinds of care given at each. In fact, although they are the nearest available, they are imperfect proxies. Not all deliveries which take place in obstetric hospitals have interventive obstetric care, either because the mothers are too far advanced in labour when they are admitted, or because some obstetricians are less orthodox and intervene as little as possible. If mortality in the untreated subgroup is higher than in the treated subgroup, the hospitals' overall mortality rate will overestimate the fatal results of obstetric care, and in the opposite case underestimate them.

Likewise, not all deliveries at home have normal midwifery care. Some women choose to have no professional care at all, although for medical and social reasons their pregnancies may be at high risk and result in high mortality. This causes the overall mortality rate for home births to overestimate the fatal results of midwifery care. The effect on rates of changing proportions in subgroups having different kinds of care was explained in Chapter 6 above (pages 254–5).

The survey collected data about place of confinement, both actual and booked, and these showed, to obstetricians' understandable disappointment and apparent disbelief, that perinatal mortality was highest by far in obstetric hospitals. The actual rate per 1000 births was 50.0 in hospital, compared with 20.3 in general practitioner units (GPUs) and 19.8 at home. They had to find a reason for this disconcertingly large discrepancy. Two explanations were offered, but no attempt was made to show that either was satisfactory.

One explanation was that the actual births in hospital included some which had been transferred from GPUs or home because of serious complications in late pregnancy or labour. The mortality associated with the transferred births was very high – over three times the survey average. Obstetricians argued that adding these to the births and deaths of cases booked for hospital delivery unfairly raised the mortality rate there, and conversely unfairly lowered the mortality rates in GPUs and home. The proper comparison should be between places of booking and not places of actual delivery.

This is the same technique of analysis as was used in the Confidential Enquiries into Maternal Deaths between 1964 and 1975 and it has become accepted as obligatory in studies where general practitioners compare the results of maternity under their care and in hospital. The technique is logical, however, only so long as the objective is to compare the risks of *booking* for different places, including the risks associated with possible transfer. It is not logical if the objective is to compare the results of the different methods of intranatal care *actually practised* at each place. It is not logical to compare, on the one hand, the results of high interventive obstetric care given in hospital to a group made up of booked subjects and, on the other hand, the average results of both high and low interventive care given respectively to the group transferred and the group actually delivered in GPUs and home. Patently, like is not being compared with like as obstetricians rightly demand should be done. The method leads to the same useless conclusion as the randomized controlled trial in which the subjects do not actually receive the treatments to which they have been randomized (page 258).

Women are transferred because their attendants, observing the rules of procedure, apprehend increasing risk from a developing complication and the intention in transfer is to reduce that risk. The resulting excessive mortality does not immediately suggest that the intention was realized in 1958 and later data give strong reason to doubt that it usually is (pages 338–41). If the risk for the transferred group is actually increased by the move and the mortality rate is higher after transfer than it would have been without transfer, then the mortality rate for cases booked for delivery in GPUs or at home unfairly exaggerates the risk of intranatal care actually given at these places. In so far as it is the obstetric care the transfers eventually receive which contributes to their excessive mortality, then this is properly attributable to the hospital.

On the other hand, it can be argued that including the high mortality rate of the transfers unfairly exaggerates the risk of hospital care, if the transferred cases have been allowed to develop more serious complications than they would have done if they had been cared for throughout in hospital. Risks attributable to the physical or emotional consequences of the move itself do not measure directly the safety of intranatal care actually given anywhere, but they do reflect the possibility that implementing obstetric policy in this way may create new, additional dangers.

When the objective is to evaluate different systems of care actually given, the existence of transfers with exceptionally high mortality certainly presents an awkward analytical problem, which cannot be solved without an impartial assessment of the predicted risk of the births concerned and whether or not that risk is reduced by transfer (page 341). Analysis of mortality by place of booking only serves to obscure the issue.

In the context of the 1958 survey, the explanation it offered was unsatisfactory on logical grounds. It was also unsatisfactory on statistical grounds, for the perinatal mortality rate for booked hospital births, at 35.8, was still substantially higher than for births booked for GPUs (30.6) or home (30.9). This unexplained disparity, which was never specifically referred to, was apparently brushed aside as being more than accounted for by the other explanation, the claim that hospital births included an excess proportion at above average predicted risk.

THE PREDICTED RISK STATUS OF BIRTHS IN HOSPITAL, GPU AND HOME

It was certainly obstetric policy that all women with high risk characteristics should be delivered in hospital where the facilities were available to deal promptly with the complications of which they were in greater than average danger. It was, however, the constant lament of obstetricians, as in their Confidential Enquiries into Maternal Deaths and Professor Baird's routine experience in Aberdeen, that the mothers at greatest risk, those of higher age, lower social class and with large families, were the ones least willing to give birth in hospital.

Despite the survey's terms of reference to investigate the possible effects of place of confinement, only three predicting risk factors, maternal parity, social class and toxaemia, were cross-classified with place of birth in the published report. Of these, hospital births were not heavily biased with excessive numbers in the high risk subgroups (Table 8.1). They had more than their fair share of first births (parity 0), which overall are at slightly above average risk, but less than their fair share of fourth (parity 3) and later births, which are at considerably above average risk. Home births, by contrast, included far more than their fair share of these later high-risk births. Relatively fewer births in hospital than at home were to mothers of lower social class and this deficit was only just compensated by the hospitals' excess of births to mothers who were unmarried or whose civil state was unknown, subgroups also at high risk. Relatively more births in hospital than at home were to mothers at higher risk from toxaemia, but even in hospital less than one-fifth of all births came into this category. The figures shown in Table 8.1 relate to actual births. The proportion of births at higher risk booked for hospital was even lower.

If hospital deliveries were heavily biased with births at high risk on account of other factors, it is incredible that the data have never been published in support of the bald assertions repeatedly made. For example, in the section on gestation the report dared to comment [11, p. 131]:

> ... the Survey Mortality Ratio in both mature and prolonged pregnancies among women booked and delivered in hospital is approximately the same as average for the whole Survey. This finding is remarkable in *view of the excess of high risk mothers booked for hospital* (This author's italics.)

But even if the hospitals had had an excess *proportion* of births at high risk, this could never, for reasons of arithmetic whose rules apply with the same certainty to obstetrics as to other issues, completely explain an

Table 8.1 Births and perinatal mortality rates (PNMR) at places of birth and different levels of risk in Britain, 1958

Risk factor	Level of risk	Percentage of births		PNMR/1000 births	
		Hospital	GPU/home	Hospital	GPU/home
Maternal parity					
1 and 2	low	38.1	54.3	47.6	15.8(a)
0 and 3	moderate	54.5	35.0	46.6	23.5(a)
4 and over	high	7.4	10.7	88.0	29.2(a)
Social class					
I and II	low	16.3	15.5	38.8	15.2(a)
III and IV	moderate	67.9	70.7	49.3	19.4(a)
V, unmarried, no information	high	15.8	13.8	65.0	30.2(a)
Maternal toxaemia					
None or mild	low	75.8	85.7	38.4	16.3(a)
Moderate	moderate	6.6	3.9	51.9	26.3(b)
Severe and unknown	high	17.6	10.4	97.6	37.2(a)
Fetal gestation					
38–41 weeks	low	74.8	80.0	22.1	11.3(a)
>41 weeks	moderate	12.7	12.2	34.0	17.6(a)
<38 weeks	high	12.5	7.8	205.3	75.3(a)
Infant birthweight					
>2500 grams	low	91.1	95.5	22.6	12.1(a)
2500 grams and under	high	8.9	4.5	327.6	161.2(a)

Source: reference [11], Tables 13A, 14A, 30, 41 and 46.
Significance of difference between PNMRs: (a) p < 0.005; (b) not significant.

excess *overall mortality rate* there, as long as the specific mortality rates in each of the subgroups of risk were higher in hospital and this they always were. The rules of arithmetic, which make it impossible, were explained above in Chapter 6 (pages 252–5). It was illustrated there that less than 12% of the disparity between the overall mortality rates in hospital and in GPUs/home was due to the excess in hospital of births at high risk on account of maternal toxaemia. Even less of the excess mortality in hospital is explained by a corresponding analysis of the data relating place of birth to the other predicting risk factors, maternal parity and social class. In both cases, any excess in hospital of births at higher predicted risk was slight, but of overriding importance was the fact that their specific mortality rates at all grades of risk were considerably higher (Table 8.1).

Risk factors which have a much stronger association with outcome are the duration of fetal gestation and infant birthweight: the shorter the gestation or the lower the birthweight, the higher the mortality. These, however, are coincidental rather than predicting risk factors. Very few live births in the survey were of less than 28 weeks' gestation, but hospitals had a greater proportion at less than 38 weeks. Most of this was due to the transfer to hospital of cases with symptoms of spontaneous premature labour or with complications, such as toxaemia, for which induced premature delivery was thought to be the lesser risk. For the babies, results show that premature delivery in hospital was indeed the greater risk, for their mortality rates were two and a half times as high there as in GPUs/home. At longer gestations the rates were twice as high.

The proportion of low-weight births, those of 2500 grams or less, was nearly twice as high in hospital, an excess contributed to largely by the inductions carried out there and by the transfers. But whatever the weight, the treatment received in hospital did not make birth safer, for their specific mortality rates at all weights were far higher.

There was thus no possibility that the excess overall mortality rate in hospitals could be accounted for by any excess of births there at high predicted or coincidental risk. But the obstetricians' facile assertion that it could seemed plausible and it was widely accepted without further question by the trusting public. It was the excuse that was to be constantly pleaded and constantly accepted after 1958 for the next thirty years. Yet it is an excuse the validity of which can be tested, as has been shown here, by simple arithmetic, whenever the numerical values of the relevant specific proportions and mortality rates are known. And whenever the relevant data are available, the excuse is shown to be completely bogus, as further examples to be presented later will confirm (page 333–8).

COVERING UP UNWELCOME FACTS

By 1958, the obstetric profession, despite its much publicized conduct of self-audit, as in its Confidential Enquiries into Maternal Deaths, had already become totally impervious to evidence which discredited the success of its practices and its philosophy. Interpretation of results had to be blatantly reversed to accord with their expectations. Obstetricians' expectations must surely have been that at least the specific mortality rates would be lower in hospital for conditions associated with the high-risk characteristics for which they particularly urged hospital confinement. The public was most easily convinced of the need for obstetricians to deal with complications or potential complications beyond the competence of other birth attendants and shared their expectations. But these were not fulfilled.

Doubtless in some particular cases the facilities for immediate intervention averted disaster and made these births safer. But this advantage obviously did not apply to most births in the high-risk groups or was far outweighed by other, unspoken, disadvantages in hospital care. Not only were the specific mortality rates for the high-risk groups always higher in hospital, but they were higher by a larger margin in conditions for which obstetricians particularly canvassed the benefits of hospital treatment, high multiparity, severe toxaemia and prematurity. The survey produced no evidence to confirm that obstetric care was beneficial for any births, far less than it was beneficial for births at higher predicted risk. Rather, in the majority of cases, the high predicted risk was compounded by the iatrogenic (treatment-induced) risks of obstetric intranatal care.

No comments about these alarming results were made in the reports of the survey, nor for nearly twenty years did any critic use the statistics to carry out calculations which revealed the most significant discovery of the survey, that the place of confinement does indeed have a most important effect on the safety of birth for the infant, but in the opposite sense to what the obstetricians wanted. This inescapable conclusion was not undermined by any of the further analyses of the raw data on several aspects of the subject, the results of which were published [12–15]. But if the profession was to survive without loss of face, the conclusion had to be denied and this obstetricians did with such enthusiasm and unanimity that their propaganda was never seriously challenged. As has been already described, there had been many other examples of the strategy of covering up in the past. There were to be many more in the future.

PROFESSOR BAIRD'S ANALYSES OF THE 1958 SURVEY DATA

The survey results which showed up the lack of success achieved by hospitals in general were at variance with Professor Baird's experience in the Aberdeen hospitals, but they in no way diminished his confidence in the advantages of obstetric care, with more liberal use of induction of labour and caesarean section [10, 16–20]. Commenting on the national perinatal mortality rate which had resumed its downward trend after 1958, Baird wrote

It may well be that the current rapid fall in perinatal mortality rates is due in large measure to the cumulative effect of 25 years of relative economic prosperity, leading to a better grown and healthier generation of mothers, who are having their babies at an earlier age and planning them much more sensibly. [16, p. 8]

He qualified the relative importance of this by adding 'Such changes may be at least as important as improvements in the scope and quality of the maternity services', and later wrote

Ideally, all women should be supervised throughout pregnancy and labour by experienced specialists who have at their disposal all the resources needed to deal promptly and effectively with any emergency that may arise. An approximation to that ideal can be achieved only in a well-equipped and well-staffed hospital, in which the staff are organised and trained to work as a team. [17, p. 20]

He realized that good personal relationships between the mother and her attendants, such as were likely to prevail in the more intimate setting of a GPU or a family home, were also necessary. He had to concede in the face of the actual results that the ideal organization was not always attained, but he was intent on finding in the survey data further support for his hypothesis that, while hospital care could do little to influence the 'environmental' causes of perinatal death, it could substantially reduce the 'obstetrical' causes.

With his colleagues he undertook the onerous task of reclassifying the survey's perinatal deaths into these groups and analysing the resulting distribution according to geographic zones and place of confinement. However, he jeopardized the validity of his conclusions about the effect of care actually given in hospital by falling into the logical trap of using data relating to place of booking. He favoured the urban and rural division of zones as being most instructive because, while the rural environment was healthier, urban areas enjoyed better maternity services, including obstetric hospitals. Considering perinatal mortality from all causes he found that

The superior physique and health of women in the rural areas apparently more than compensate for any disadvantages they incur as a result of being at a distance from the main centres [of obstetric care]. [20, p. 227]

His detailed analysis [20] of perinatal mortality from obstetrical causes in deliveries booked for hospital, home or GPU in urban and rural areas respectively revealed different patterns according to maternal parity (Table 8.2). For first births (parity 0), the mortality rates for home and GPU bookings in rural zones and for GPU bookings in urban zones were rather higher than for hospital bookings. An explanation for these excesses is that first-time mothers were especially liable to be transferred from their home or GPU booking and those transferred suffered a perinatal mortality rate four times as high as did those who were not transferred. There is good reason to suspect that part of their increased mortality rate was in fact caused by the obstetric treatment they received in hospital. At all other parities in both rural and urban zones, mortality was always highest in hospital, even for booked deliveries.

His corresponding analysis of perinatal mortality from environmental causes suggests that, contrary to his expectations, the relative advantage for births *booked* for hospital was greater for those than for obstetrical causes for first births in urban, although not in rural, areas, while in all other subgroups except one the relative disadvantage of hospital booking was no less.

This confused picture was the best evidence that could be wrested from the 1958 survey data to support Baird's conclusion about the effectiveness of total hospitalization and obstetric interventions, which he drew from his experience in Aberdeen. Under his guidance and technical policies, mortality in Aberdeen, despite its history of relative deprivation, had been so reduced that it compared favourably with that in the south of England, with its history of relative prosperity. His results had been so impressive that he did not consider it necessary to carry out trials to confirm that the observed improvements were indeed the results of his obstetric interventions.

He had acknowledged that the pregnant and parturient woman needs and expects from her attendants a high level of personal attention, as well as a high level of technical skill. Results suggest that her need of the former is probably the greater. Baird was able to inspire his obstetric teams in Aberdeen to give such personal attention and, in turn, to inspire the women with confidence which overcame fear and all its damaging consequences. Ability to inspire confidence is not synonymous with ability to operate technical instruments. Baird may have undervalued his achievements in the psychological aspects of the

Table 8.2 Perinatal mortality rates per 1000 births from 'obstetrical' and 'environmental' causes by maternal parity, place of booking, and geographical area

Parity	Urban areas			Rural areas		
	Hospital	Home	GPU	Hospital	Home	GPU
Obstetrical causes						
0	14.1	13.7	14.8	15.6	18.8	18.7
1,2,3	13.1	10.5	11.0	15.1	10.5	8.7
4 +	28.8	19.0	0.6	29.0	19.4	11.0
Environmental causes						
0	17.1	20.9	19.4	16.3	14.6	13.2
1,2,3	18.4	14.4	20.6	16.0	13.8	13.2
4 +	31.5	26.0	3.6	28.6	20.9	25.7

Source: reference [20], Table 13.7.
(Data from 1958 perinatal mortality survey.)

service he offered and overvalued the usefulness of the surgical techniques he practised when he interpreted the results of his comparison between experience in Aberdeen and nationally as showing 'beyond doubt that many perinatal deaths could be prevented by a higher standard of obstetric skill. This means ready access to specialists and more beds in specialist hospitals' [20, p. 254]. This was precisely the message that fellow obstetricians wanted to hear, which encouraged their denial of the true findings of the perinatal survey and fuelled their ambition to press for total hospitalization.

THE SURVIVAL OF BABIES OF LOW WEIGHT

Baird's policy of intervention was aimed at preventing the deaths of mature fetuses. Even if successful, this would not have caused a great reduction in the overall perinatal mortality rate, for such fetal deaths made up a relatively small proportion of the total. Making up by far the largest proportion were the deaths of premature and low-weight fetuses and babies. These he attributed to environmental causes, not remediable by intranatal interventions.

Moreover, there was evidence that care in obstetric hospitals reduced their chances of survival. In the 1958 survey, the perinatal mortality rates for births with gestations of less than 38 weeks and for births weighing less than 2500 grams were much the highest for actual deliveries in hospital (Table 8.1) and were highest also for hospital-booked deliveries.

The survey evidence was consistent with that on low-weight births collected by the Chief Medical Officer of the Ministry of Health and published in his *Annual Reports* between 1954 and 1964 [21]. This showed that the rate of stillbirths plus neonatal deaths was always very significantly higher when delivery took place in NHS hospitals, in which category GPUs were then included, than when it took place at home, with which were included the small number in private nursing homes. This was so even although the home figure included the neonatal deaths of sick babies transferred to hospital.

After 1964, the Chief Medical Officer ceased publishing this information, but his office continued to collect it and copies of the raw detailed data relating to the years 1967–73 were supplied privately to the present author on her request. From these it was possible to calculate mortality rates at specific birthweights. The results showed that for births weighing up to 1500 grams, place of delivery made no significant difference to the chance of surviving the neonatal period. At all heavier weights this chance was significantly less if delivery took place in hospital (Table 8.3).

Table 8.3 Mortality of low-weight births by place of delivery, England and Wales (stillbirths plus neonatal deaths per 1000 births)

Period	Birthweight (grams)	Hospital	Home	Significance of difference
1954–58	<2500	296	181	$p < 0.00001$
1959–64	<2500	269	162	$p < 0.00001$
1967–73	<1001	898	868	not significant
	1001–1500	621	635	not significant
	1501–2000	270	242	$p < 0.01$
	2001–2250	116	99	$p < 0.02$
	2251–2500	56	40	$p < 0.001$

Source: reference [21] and unpublished data 1967–73.
Note: 'hospital' includes GPUs; 'home' includes private nursing homes and also the neonatal transfers to hospital of sick babies.

These results were publicly known until 1964 and thereafter privately known to officers in a strong position to influence the direction of policy. Supportive as they were of the true results of the 1958 survey, they should have diverted policy in the opposite direction from that being insistently urged by obstetricians in the 1960s. That they were not used in this way illustrates the degree of power and persuasion obstetricians had come to exercise over medical colleagues at the highest level. It must be a matter of speculation on what grounds publication of this enlightening but politically embarrassing material was discontinued.

However, even while it was published, its significance was ignored or dismissed and the policy of hospitalization was unwaveringly pursued. After 1970, births at home were being so drastically reduced in number that they were rapidly ceasing to be a representative cross-section of normal mothers and the associated mortality rate was rapidly ceasing to be a fair proxy for the results of low interventive midwifery care (pages 254, 344).

THE 1970 SURVEY OF BRITISH BIRTHS

In 1970 the second national survey of perinatal mortality was carried out under the same auspices and using the same method of enquiry as the survey in 1958 [22, 23]. This time it was concerned, not only to examine the associations of death at and around delivery, but also to follow up live-born children and their mothers for a week after the birth. The latter seems to have been the easier objective to achieve, for the relevant report was published in 1975 [22], but this volume contains only a little further information about the influence of the place of confinement on outcome (pages 184, 205–6). It did, however, publish the number of births and perinatal deaths at each place of delivery, and left the reader to calculate that the perinatal mortality rate was then 28.8 in consultant obstetric hospitals, compared with 9.5 in the general practitioner beds in obstetric hospitals, 5.4 in unattached GPUs and 4.3 at home. Such wide disparities surely cried out for investigation and explanation but, remarkably, none was offered either in this first report nor in the second, devoted to perinatal mortality, which was eventually published in 1978 [23]. The delay, according to the preface, was due to 'a change of authorship and editorship at a late stage of data analysis'. It was left as a matter of speculation whether there had been disagreements about how frankly the disconcerting results should be published and how much should be obscured.

Remarkable omissions from this report were explicit statements of mortality rates in total and in specific subgroups of risk at each place of birth, although they can be calculated or plausibly estimated from the data that were printed by a reader armed with a pocket calculator – not, in 1978, a ubiquitous vade-mecum. It seemed that critical appraisal of this aspect of the survey findings was to be discouraged.

If anyone had questioned the reason for the great excess mortality in hospital, they would almost certainly have been fobbed off with the perennial excuse that it was due to the excess of high-risk births which take place there, implying that the high risk lies in the predicting factors and not in the treatment given.

For maternal age and parity the proportion of births, but not the deaths, in each subgroup at each place was given. Thus it is not possible to calculate by the direct method of standardization described above in Chapter 6 (pages 254–6) whether their greater proportion of births in the higher risk subgroups was sufficient to account for the excess mortality in hospital. However, since the specific mortality rate for each risk subgroup was given for all places combined, the calculation can be carried out by the indirect method of standardization also described above in Chapter 6. The results given in Table 8.4 show that hardly any of the hospitals' excess mortality was due to their excess of births at high risk on account of maternal age and parity.

Exceptionally, both mortality rates and proportions of births in specific risk subgroups at each place of birth were published for the risk factor, toxaemia. These show that, as in the 1958 survey, mortality rates were always highest in hospital (Table 6.1) and their greater proportion of births in the subgroups at higher risk explained only a very small part of the overall excess mortality in hospital (Table 8.4).

Table 8.4 Perinatal mortality rates per 1000 births: actual and standardized for risk factors.

Risk factor	Hospital	GPU/Home*
Actual	27.8	4.9
Standardized for		
Maternal age	27.5	5.2
Maternal parity	27.3	5.1
Maternal hypertension/toxaemia	27.6	4.8
Antenatal prediction score	26.6	5.4
Labour prediction score	23.9	7.7
Method of delivery	25.8	6.2
Infant birthweight	22.9	9.6

*Excludes general practitioner beds in consultant hospitals.
Source: references [22] (Table 2.19) and [23] (Tables 2.25, 2.31, 4.17, 5.7, 5.8, 5.9, 5.11) and unpublished data.

THE USE OF RISK PREDICTION SCORES

To meet the problem that some births are at high risk from more than one factor, two composite risk scores were constructed by the authors of the survey report to assess the combined effect of the most important factors. These scores, the antenatal prediction score (APS) and the labour prediction score (LPS), their composition, the problems of giving appropriate weights to the included factors and their validation are discussed above in Chapter 6. Despite their limitations, the two scores provided a method of statistical analysis by means of which the comprehensive risks of births in hospital and outside, as assessed in pregnancy and in labour, could be measured more completely than had ever been possible before, while the survey provided a large sample (16 815), representative of singleton births in Britain around 1970, to which the analytical instruments could be applied.

Births with the same total labour prediction score were deemed to be at the same total risk. Therefore groups of births with the same score could properly be compared. Like could now be compared with like. Groups of births in hospital, whether there because of selective booking or because of later transfer in pregnancy or labour, could properly be compared with groups of births in GPUs or home with the same score, at the same level of risk at the same stage of labour. Births with complications would have appropriately high scores wherever they took place. Thus the labour prediction score presented a means of evaluating fairly reliably the claim that the higher overall mortality rate in hospital was due simply to their greater proportion of births at high overall risk resulting from selective booking and transfers; it got round the problem of making fair allowance for transferred cases.

ANALYSIS BY PREDICTION SCORE AND PATTERNS OF PERINATAL MORTALITY

Antenatal prediction score

It can be reckoned from the tariff of points making up the antenatal prediction score (Table 6.1) that a maximum score of 30 was possible. When the scoring system was applied to births in the survey, only 7% were found to have scores over 8, while 53% had scores of 0–2. In fact, few births were at high predicted risk. Less than half, even on the booking criteria set by obstetricians, needed hospital delivery.

The number of births with each antenatal prediction score at each place of delivery was published in the report and this showed that hospital births included a greater proportion at moderate and high risk. This was to be expected, especially since the factors which in obstetricians' judgement certainly needed specialist care were given the highest points. The death rates for all births in the low, moderate and high risk groups were also published and these were in the ratio 1.0 : 1.69 : 2.84. If it is assumed that the ratio between death rates at each level of risk was the same at each place of delivery, a probable estimate of the unpublished specific death rates can be made. The result is shown in Table 8.5.

It is worth noting that, not only was the rate much higher in hospital in total and at each level, but the rate for the low-risk group in hospital was far higher than for the high-risk group in GPU/home (a relationship already noted in Table 8.1 between the specific mortality rates for the three predicting risk factors in 1958). Because of this excess in specific rates, it is once again arithmetically inevitable that only a small part of the hospitals' excess mortality rate could be due to their excess proportion of births at moderate and high risk as the result of selective bookings and early transfers.

When, as in Table 8.4, the actual mortality rates are standardized, that is, recalculated to show what they would have been if each place had had the same proportion of births at each level of antenatal risk from combined factors, very little of the disparity between the rates is accounted for; indeed hardly more than is accounted for by allowing for a single factor, for example, maternal age or toxaemia. This reflects the interdependence of the factors. Allowing for the risk from one factor allows for most of the risk from the others. This makes it improbable that including yet other factors, like height or smoking, which are

Table 8.5 Proportion of births and perinatal mortality rates (PNMR/1000 births) by antenatal prediction scores (APS)

APS	Level of risk	Survey PNMR		Proportion of births		Estimated PNMR*	
		Actual	(ratio)	Hospital	GPU/home	Hospital	GPU/home
0–2	Low	15.3	(1.0)	0.47	0.67	19.3	3.9
3–7	Moderate	25.9	(1.69)	0.44	0.30	32.6	6.5
8 and over	High	43.4	(2.84)	0.08	0.03	54.8	11.0
All		21.4		1.00	1.00	27.8	4.9

*For hospital: $(0.47x) + (0.44x \times 1.69) + (0.08x \times 2.84) = 27.8$, therefore $x = 19.3$.
For GPU/home: $(0.67y) + (0.30y \times 1.69) + (0.03y \times 2.84) = 4.9$, therefore $y = 3.9$.
Source: reference [23] (Tables 2.25, 2.31).

known to be related directly or indirectly to the included factors, would explain appreciably more of the disparity between mortality rates.

Labour prediction score

From the tariff of points making up the labour prediction score (see Table 6.4) it can be reckoned that a maximum score of 23 was possible, but the highest actual score was 12 and only 2.6% of births had scores over 8, while nearly 70% had scores of 0–2. Only a small minority were at very high risk; the substantial majority were at low risk.

Apart from previous caesarean section, the factors known early in pregnancy were deemed to constitute only a small proportion of the potential total risk at delivery, although it is precisely on the predictive reliability of these factors that obstetricians justify the booking rules on which they insist. In compiling the score, they deemed the greatest risk to come from adverse conditions near delivery. Although mothers with higher antenatal prediction scores were indeed *more likely* to develop complications, most of them did not in fact do so. And although mothers with low antenatal prediction scores were *less likely* to develop complications, some of them did so. But clearly, whatever the antenatal prediction score, only a minority of births could have been affected by these complications which would have given them labour prediction scores greater than 2. However, they did affect a greater proportion of the births in hospital, as would be expected from the booking and early transfer policies and the scoring weights. Nevertheless, 363 births with scores of 4 and over did take place in GPUs or at home.

When the actual mortality rates are standardized to show what they would have been if each place had had the same proportion of births at each level of risk, only a little more of the disparity between the rates is accounted for (Table 8.4). This confirms that the risks of complications are to a considerable degree interdependent with the biological and social risk factors. Thus not much more of the hospitals' excess mortality could be explained by their excess of births, whether originally booked or eventually transferred, which developed complications.

Again, this result is arithmetically inevitable for, despite obstetricians' expectations, the specific mortality rates were higher in hospital at every labour prediction score from 0 to 8 (Table 8.6). One of the three births at GPU/home with a score of 9 died, a worse ratio than the 19 out of 90 births in hospital with scores of 9–12, but the numbers are too small to support any conclusions about the relative safety of these births at highest risk.

Most noteworthy, and to orthodox thinking most unexpected, is the finding that, although the mortality rate was twice as high in hospital for the very low risk group, the disparity was wider at the low,

Table 8.6 Percentage of births and perinatal mortality rate (PNMR) by labour prediction score (LPS) and place of birth

LPS	Level of risk	Percentage of births		PNMR/1000 births	
		Hospital*	GPU/home	Hospital*	GPU/home
0–1	Very low	39.4	59.4	8.0	3.6[†]
2	Low	23.0	22.3	17.9	4.8[‡]
3	Moderate	15.6	10.6	32.2	2.0[§]
4–6	High	18.2	7.5	53.2	14.2[‡]
7–8	Very high	2.9	0.2	149.1	111.1
0–12	All	(n = 11141)	(n = 4660	27.8	4.9

*Excludes general practitioner beds.
Significance of difference in rates: [†]$p < 0.025$; [‡]$p < 0.005$; [§]$p < 0.001$.
Source: Unpublished data from the British Births 1970 survey.

moderate and high risk levels. Once again, the rate for high-risk births in GPU/home (14.2) was found to be lower than for low-risk births in hospital (17.9). And although there were only twelve births in GPU/home at very high risk (scores of 7–8), the results do not suggest that even these would have been safer in hospital.

Some complications are undoubtedly very dangerous, too dangerous by consensus for the delivery to be left in the care of midwives. Urgent life-threatening conditions do not provide acceptable subjects for randomized trials. The only hope of establishing which is the most effective treatment would be retrospective comparisons of different methods where alternatives were actually practised. The literature is strangely void of objective demonstrations of the proven or probable superiority of specific treatments for specific dangerous complications. It has to be assumed that aggressive obstetric intervention, the treatment of last resort, may indeed reduce the danger of certain conditions and make hospital care for these safer, but in the absence of evidence this has to remain an assumption. The results of the obstetricians' survey, however, show unequivocally that such instances were too few for the hospitals' greater safety to be reflected in any of the identified risk groups. They were always far outnumbered by cases where hospital care was less safe.

Older proponents of hospitalization never tire of recalling the dreadful complications they used to encounter in deliveries at home, but obviously relatively few of these could have ended in a fatal outcome given the actual low mortality rates achieved there.

Although in hospital and overall the mortality rate was higher, the higher the labour prediction score, in GPU/home the rate was found to be marginally lowest for moderate-risk births. This may reflect inaccuracy in the weights given to specific risks or it may be simply the statistical artefact of small numbers. There was only one death in 493 births at this risk level. One or two extra deaths would have raised the mortality rate and preserved a smooth upward progression, but they would not have made the rate for the moderate-risk group significantly higher than for the very low risk group. This may indicate that low interventive methods effectively protect against death over a range of predicted risk. Conversely, the steeply rising mortality rate in hospital seems to confirm the frequently repeated dictum of the French obstetrician, Michel Odent, that the fetus already at increased risk is less able to withstand the stresses of obstetric intervention. It would seem that obstetric intervention, contrary to intention, does not in most cases reduce the stress of difficult labour for the fetus and hence the dangers for it of trauma and hypoxia.

The completeness of the labour prediction score

The completeness of the labour prediction score, and hence the legitimacy of the conclusions arising from its application, has been challenged because it does not include cases where the fetus is already dead and hospital deaths are thought to include an excess of these as a result of cases being transferred from GPU or home booking. But even if this were true, it could not nearly explain the hospitals' excess mortality in the 1970 survey, for their mortality rate for live births was by itself more than twice the mortality rate for all births, live plus still, in GPU/home.

Nor does the labour prediction score include congenital malformations, but the official statistics show that the stillbirth rate from this cause in 1970 was only marginally higher in hospital than in GPU/home.

There may be other factors, whether or not recognized, which influence mortality besides those included in the labour prediction score. In so far as these are interdependent with the included factors, most of the risk attaching to them will already have been allowed for (Table 8.4). To explain any more of the hospitals' excess mortality, factors not included in the labour prediction score would have to be largely independent of the included factors.

The emotional states or attitudes of the mothers have a very important influence on the birth process. But they are difficult if not impossible to measure, so it is not known whether they are interrelated with factors included in the labour prediction score. They may well be independent. However, women are not selected for hospital delivery because they are expected to have feelings of apprehension, tension or

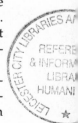

suspicion when they get there. If in fact there is an excess of these among mothers in hospital, this would explain some of the hospitals' excess mortality. But it would be a hospital-induced risk, a devastating indictment of hospital care and a strong contraindication for it.

No other independent factors have yet been recognized. If they are not recognized, they cannot possibly feature among the criteria by which booking and transfer policies are regulated. Therefore there is no mechanism through which hospital births could include an excess of births at high *predicted* risk on account of *unrecognized*, independent factors. Moreover, these unrecognized, independent factors would have to be twice as powerful as all the factors included in the labour prediction score, if they were to account for the remaining unexplained excess mortality in hospital.

It is not plausible that such powerful physiological influences on mortality should have eluded world-wide observation and research and remained unrecognized. The conclusion has to be that the hospitals' excess mortality arises, much less from their excess of births at high risk before delivery, than from their excess of births at high risk during or after delivery, consequent on the methods of intranatal and postnatal management they practise and probably also on the damaging emotional states they inspire.

If indeed the unidentified factor could be shown to lie in the emotional reactions of the women, this would be overwhelming evidence that obstetricians' concentration on the physical processes of childbirth and their neglect of the psychological processes has been seriously misguided and has led to harmful policies. Although undoubtedly some women feel confident and relaxed in hospital, there is a vast amount of anecdotal evidence from women in many countries of their personal adverse feelings provoked by care in hospitals governed by obstetricians' principles of management. In contrast, women's verdicts on their emotional reactions to the midwifery care they have received at home or in small maternity units are overwhelmingly favourable [24]. Studies which have sought to measure the preferences of women who have experienced both hospital and home confinements have found home to be much the more popular setting [25–27]. Obviously, scope for obtaining representative samples of women with first-hand experience on which to make comparisons was progressively restricted as hospitalization became more comprehensive.

TRANSFERS – WHAT DO THE DATA REALLY TELL US?

It has long been the established practice that, when complications are suspected or have developed in pregnancy or labour, the management of the births is transferred from home or GPU to hospital in the expectation that the associated dangers will thereby be mitigated. This practice is based on the assumption, in advance of supporting evidence, that complications are more likely to develop and become more serious in the absence of obstetric management at an earlier stage, or that obstetric management even at a later stage can overcome the problems. Actual results give reason to question the validity of these assumptions, for some complications are more strongly associated with specific obstetric interventions than with inaction (Chapter 4), while the perinatal mortality rates for the transferred births are typically higher than the average for all births booked and delivered in hospital, and very much higher than the average for all booked and delivered in GPUs or at home. Without any effort to investigate why this should be so, the excess mortality has always been interpreted simply as confirming the advisability of forestalling the potential need for transfer by booking all births for hospital delivery.

The increase in the proportion of births in hospital was achieved by arbitrarily widening the risk criteria by which pregnancies were judged to need obstetric management and narrowing the criteria by which they could be booked for delivery at home or in a GPU. But although the average predicted risk status of these latter births was in this way reduced, more of them apparently needed transfer, for the proportion of transfers rose from 13% in the 1958 survey to 23% in 1970. The same upward trend was observed in local studies in Newcastle-upon-Tyne [28], in Oxford [29], and also in the Netherlands, from 19.7% in 1969–73 to 33.0% in 1979–83 [30] (page 353). Recent concessions to midwives have led to units being set up in close proximity to obstetric labour wards, units ostensibly managed by midwives but with strict rules imposed by obstetricians for booking only women with characteristics predicting low risk at delivery and specifying conditions in labour necessitating transfer to obstetricians' management. Fear of disciplinary action, with possible deregulation, in the event of an unsatisfactory perinatal outcome constrains midwives to follow the rules thought to lead to the best treatment by the superior profession.

Of these already low-risk populations, considerable proportions (24% in Aberdeen in 1990–1 and 54% in Leicester in 1990–2 [31, pp. 903, 910] apparently needed transfer. The upward trend in proportions transferred surely reflected a change in criteria for transfer rather than a change in pathological condition in increasingly healthy populations. Professional propaganda was successfully eroding the confidence of general practitioners and midwives and persuading them that deviations from ever more arbitrarily defined normality qualified as complications beyond their skills to deal with safely.

When only a small proportion of non-hospital bookings is transferred, it is likely to be made up of serious complications and the mortality for these births is likely to be much higher than for the births not transferred. The greater the proportion of transfers, the more the average risk for the group is decreased by the inclusion of less serious cases, so that one would expect the mortality rate for a larger transfer group to exceed that for cases not transferred by a smaller margin. However, the larger group of transfers in 1970 had a mortality rate per 1000 births about 12 times that for those not transferred (59 versus 5), compared with less than six times in 1958 (116 versus 20). In the Newcastle study this factor in 1966–9 was seven; in the Oxford study in 1975–7 it was actually 35 and in the Netherlands in 1969–83 it was 30.

Once the professions accept the belief that transfer is beneficial, it becomes unethical, or even criminally negligent, not to transfer. The procedure is beyond the stage where a prospective randomized controlled trial is practicable. The only method of confirming or discrediting the belief is retrospective analysis of actual results and the inference from this exercise points strongly to discreditation.

The reasons given for transfer in pregnancy include most frequently maternal toxaemia and fetal postmaturity, for which the effectiveness of available medical remedies has never been proven (pages 113, 347), and much less frequently, antepartum haemorrhage, disproportion and malpresentation. Poor progress or delay at any stage relative to arbitrary criteria (which are themselves unjustifiable – pages 158–60) are the most frequent reasons for transfer in labour [29] (page 353). The mortality rate associated with severe toxaemia was quantified in the 1970 survey as just over twice that associated with no toxaemia. The rate at over 42 weeks' gestation was quantified as just over twice that at 39–42 weeks'. The rate associated with the much less frequently occurring antepartum haemorrhage was less than four times as high as that when there was no bleeding. If malpresentation, disproportion or any other condition which leads to transfer in labour results in a caesarean section, then a mortality rate about 2.5 times that for spontaneous cephalic presentation would be expected. Even if the other reasons for transfer carry a high fatality rate, they make up such a small proportion of all transfers that they have little effect on the overall average.

Thus, if these values are reasonably representative of the relative degrees of mortality risk attaching to the complications indicated, a generous forecast of the mortality rate of a group made up of such high risk cases, weighted according to the frequency of their occurrence, might be higher than that for the lower risk group not transferred by a factor of three or four, but not by the higher factors just described. The pattern that emerges is that the later the date, the smaller is the proportion of births booked for delivery outside hospital; the greater the proportion of these lower risk births which are transferred, the more the mortality rate of the transfers exceeds that of those not transferred, and the more the mortality rate of the births booked and delivered in hospital, despite including more at lower risk, exceeds that for those actually delivered out of hospital with normal midwifery care (excluding the uncared for births at home).

The frequency with which complications are recorded as developing depends on how they are defined and who is responsible for the diagnosis: obstetricians are likely to diagnose more conditions as complications requiring prompt intervention; experienced midwives are likely to wait while many potential problems resolve themselves. Nevertheless some births at home or in GPUs are transferred and those with labour prediction scores over 2 in the 1970 survey must have had the same complications for which some of their peers were transferred, but obviously they had much lower mortality (Table 8.6).

There are sound biological reasons, with many known examples from the animal kingdom, why birth is made less safe by moving the labouring mother. Telling a human mother that the birth is not progressing normally must make her anxious and damage her self-confidence. Her body generates more of the hormones biologically designed to delay delivery, the influence of which further obstetric interventions have to counter. It seems reasonable, therefore, to infer that the upset, physical and emotional, of a transfer in labour, and the subsequent treatment, increasingly interventionist, add to the risks which transfer was undertaken to reduce and explain the resulting excess mortality. The additional risk, however, seems to be even greater when the transfer takes place before labour. The detailed data of the Dutch and Oxford studies [30, 29] show that the increased mortality is greatest by far for the births transferred during pregnancy; the emotional worry caused for the women concerned about their physical problems and the corrective interventions thought necessary apparently have a greater adverse effect than any reassurance given them by the promised and actual benefits of obstetric management. Doctors have seriously underrated the importance of the contribution maternal emotions make to the physiology of childbirth, and to its efficiency and safety, and overrated the effectiveness of their physical interventions.

It now becomes clear why, if deaths are increased as a result of transfer, attributing them to the place of booking does not fairly represent the results of the midwifery methods practised at home or in GPUs, and why comparisons of mortality rates by place of booking make it impossible to reach valid conclusions about the relative safety of the methods of intranatal care actually practised in different places. Comparison by place of booking makes the results of hospital care appear less damaging. Perhaps this is why it is insisted on by obstetricians.

EVIDENCE WITHHELD

Clearly, the material gathered in the 1970 survey wholly discredited the 'avoiding the need for dangerous transfer' argument in favour of total hospitalization, as well as confirming every other piece of evidence against it, from both recent and earlier experience. But the findings were published in such a way that only the most painstaking research could unravel them; the most decisive findings were concealed until 1983, when the critical statistics were reluctantly released, after two and a half years of temporizing, in response to the private, persistent request of the present author.

No one with knowledge and authority spoke up in the name of truth to contradict the false accusations made of the dangers of birth at home or in GPUs and the false claims made for the safety of births in hospital. So the screw was allowed to go on turning inexorably until provisions for domiciliary care were all but extinguished and the number of unattached GPUs was remorselessly reduced, despite well-informed and popularly supported arguments to keep them open. Obstetricians could produce no valid evidence to substantiate their case, but they kept up their bluff and used their influence with health authorities to discredit their opponents, continuing the reproachable tactics of earlier centuries (pages 44, 377–80), so that their domination of the maternity service survived unscathed.

OFFICIAL RECORDS OF STILLBIRTHS AND PERINATAL DEATHS BY PLACE OF BIRTH

In England and Wales it has been a legal requirement since 1874 to register the births and deaths of live-born infants and since 1928 to register stillbirths. The place of death was recorded but not the place of birth. For stillbirths, however, the place of birth is the place of death, so the registration data made possible analyses of stillbirths by place of delivery. The statistics were published annually from 1965 to 1981 [32, 33], but only from 1969 were the hospitals with beds allocated for general practitioner maternity but not obstetric care – unattached GPUs – shown separately. From 1965, stillbirth rates were lowest by far for home births, but from 1969 it became clear that the wide disparity was not between home and any institution, but between places where intervention was rare and where it was common, stillbirth rates in 1969 being slightly lower in GPUs than at home. This confirmed the dichotomy found in perinatal mortality in the 1958 and 1970 surveys.

Stillbirth rates (SBRs) were analysed according to the age and parity of the mother and the legitimacy of the birth. Births in obstetric hospitals included a greater proportion at higher risk on account of these factors, but as in the 1958 and 1970 surveys and for the same reason, this excess proportion accounted for only a very small part of the hospitals' excess mortality, because at all levels of predicted risk, stillbirth rates were much higher in hospital.

Stillbirth rates in the different places in 1969 and 1981 in specific risk groups are summarized in Table 8.7(a), where for simplicity of exposition the births are divided into two groups only, the lower risk group consisting of second and third legitimate births to women aged 20–9 and the higher risk group comprising the remainder. (Births in private hospitals and 'elsewhere', which together made up 1.3% of all births at both dates, are excluded.

At both dates, at both risk levels, SBRs in hospital were much the highest. Since the rates are derived from the total population, and not a sample from it, the rules for testing the statistical significance of sample results do not apply. Unlike the survey results, the rates were

Table 8.7 Mortality in high- and low-risk groups by place of birth, England and Wales

Year	Level of risk*	Hospital	GPU/home	GPU
(a) Stillbirth rates per 1000 births				
1969	Low	13.7	3.1	3.0
	High	17.6	6.4	5.2
	All	16.6	4.9	4.9
1981	Low	5.4	2.6	1.4
	High	7.2	4.8	1.4
	All	6.7	3.9	1.4
(b) Perinatal mortality rates per 1000 births				
1985	Low	8.8	4.2	1.2
	High	11.1	10.7	2.4
	All	9.9	7.0	1.6

*Low risk is defined in the case of stillbirths, as second and third legitimate births to mothers aged 20–9 and in the case of perinatal deaths, as legitimate births to mothers aged 20–9. High risk is defined in each case as the remainder.
Sources: references [32] (Appendix Tables B2, B3), 33 (Table 8) and [34] (Tables 23a, 23b).

higher in GPU/home than in GPUs alone and the margin was wider in 1981 than in 1969, as ever fewer planned births were allowed to take place at home where the average SBR came increasingly to reflect the high mortality of the uncared-for births (page 254). At both dates, the SBR for the low-risk group in hospital was higher than for the high-risk group in GPU/home and two to three times higher than in GPUs.

From 1975, data linkage by computer made possible official records of perinatal mortality by place of birth cross-classified by maternal age and by legitimacy [34]. The results for 1985, in Table 8.7(b), show the same pattern of mortality as in earlier years, again with a wide margin between hospitals and GPUs. They give no indication that the ever more sophisticated obstetric interventions achieved relatively greater reductions in mortality for hospital births.

Direct standardization, as illustrated in Table 6.1(b) above using all the detailed data available, reduced the 1969 SBR/1000 births in hospital from 16.6 to 16.4 and raised it in GPU/home from 4.9 to 5.4, still leaving the latter rate less than one-third of the former. In 1969, 70% of all births were in hospital, but by 1985 this proportion had risen to 95%. Standardizing for maternal age and legitimacy in that year did not change the hospitals' perinatal mortality rate from 9.9, but raised the rate in GPU/home from 7.0 to 7.9, still only 80% of the rate in hospital.

Excluding the tiny proportion of births in private hospitals and 'elsewhere', 95.4% of the remainder took place in obstetric hospitals in 1981, compared with 71.6% in 1969. The arithmetic of direct standardization shows that, if this proportion had not increased, the stillbirth rate for all births would have fallen, not to 6.6 as it did, but to 5.9 ($0.716 \times 6.7 + 0.284 \times 3.9$). With other places again excluded, the proportion of births in hospital increased from 87.9% in 1975 to 96.6% in 1985. The corresponding calculation shows that if it had not done so, the perinatal mortality rate for all births would have fallen, not to 9.9 as it did, but to 9.5 ($0.879 \times 9.9 + 0.121 \times 7.0$). Right up to the last, the steps towards total hospitalization are shown to produce a net disadvantage.

CORRELATING TRENDS IN MANAGEMENT AND MORTALITY

Since all the records show that mortality rates in all subgroups of recognized risk are higher in obstetric hospitals than in other places of planned delivery, it must follow that increasing the proportion of all the nation's births which must take place in hospital cannot have been the cause of the falling national perinatal mortality rate over the same period. One arithmetical method of illustrating this has just been described. Another method is to analyse time trends in rates of hospitalization on the one hand and mortality on the other (pages 267–8).

Data available for England and Wales over the years 1969–1981 allow the proportional annual changes in each variable to be calculated, as in Table 8.8. The years when the increases in hospitalization were greatest are seen most often to be the years when decreases in mortality were least, and vice versa. Statistically the rank correlation coefficient (Spearman's rho) between the annual changes is found to be significantly negative (−0.87, $p < 0.001$), which implies with a high degree of confidence that if hospitalization had increased proportionally less, perinatal mortality would have fallen proportionally more (Fig. 8.1). This is precisely opposite to the causal correlation which obstetricians, without analysis, have mistakenly inferred and which they have used, without reservation, to persuade the public of the success of their management.

Having more births in hospital means subjecting more births to intranatal interventions, particularly induction and acceleration of labour and instrumental and operative deliveries, with the required anaesthesia. Recognized indications for these practices and trends in the frequency of their use at different times and places were described in Chapter 4 (pages 155–71). Obstetricians' interpretations of indicating criteria obviously varied widely and could have depended little on objective evaluations of the effectiveness of the interventions. Each of these, while bringing risks of its own, was intended to make a net reduction in perinatal mortality by outweighing the dangers of the complication. Of the interventions, only induction was regularly used in over 15% of births. The effect of each of the others on overall mortality would be small, too small for trends in the national rates for specific interventions to show any correlation with the national mortality rate.

However, the induction rate, rising rapidly from the mid-1960s to the mid-1970s then falling nearly as rapidly to the mid-1980s, could not have been a causal factor in the continuously declining mortality rate. Again, the larger proportional increases in the induction rate took place in the years when the proportional decreases in the mortality rate were smaller and vice versa, giving a significantly negative correlation coefficient between the annual changes in the variables (−0.61, $p < 0.01$). It can be inferred that the net effect of the other intranatal interventions was also harmful and contributed to the stronger negative correlation between hospital care as a whole and outcome.

The inverse relationship with mortality must be expected when births are induced, not to forestall a medical complication, but to serve the social convenience of the mother or the administrative convenience of the birth attendants, for a new risk is created where none existed and this often happened (pages 155–7). But confirmation is hard to find that induction reduces the danger of perinatal death even in the medical

Table 8.8 Trends in hospitalization and perinatal mortality, England and Wales

Year	Births in obstetric hospitals			Perinatal mortality/1000 births		
	% of all births	% change from year before	Rank of change	Rank of change	% change from year before	Actual
1969	69.6					23.4
1970	73.0	+4.9	1½	12	+0.4	23.5
1971	75.6	+3.6	5	7	−5.1	22.3
1972	78.8	+4.2	4	11	−2.7	21.7
1973	82.3	+4.4	3	9	−3.2	21.0
1974	86.3	+4.9	1½	10	−2.9	20.4
1975	87.9	+1.8	6½	5	−5.4	19.3
1976	88.3	+0.5	12	4	−8.3	17.7
1977	89.9	+1.8	6½	8	−4.0	17.0
1978	91.2	+1.4	8	3	−8.8	15.5
1979	92.3	+1.2	9½	6	−5.2	14.7
1980	93.4	+1.2	9½	2	−9.5	13.3
1981	94.2	+0.9	11	1	−11.3	11.8

Sources: references [32–34].

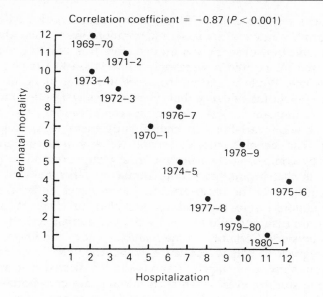

Figure 8.1 Scattergram of ranks of proportional changes in rates of hospitalization and perinatal mortality. Rank 1 denotes the greatest increase in hospitalization and the greatest decrease in perinatal mortality. Rank 12 denotes the smallest increase in hospitalization and the only increase in perinatal mortality. Drawn from data in Table 8.8.

complications for which it is advocated, principally post-maturity [35], suspected fetal growth retardation and maternal hypertension. Analysis of their own experience has led certain obstetricians to conclude that their PNMR would not have been reduced by an induction rate above 9.5% [36] or 8% [37], levels far below the then current national rates. Other studies have found no advantage, but some disadvantage, for example an increased risk of caesarean section, in inducing labour in prolonged pregnancies [38, 39]. In any case, later research into the physiology of the placenta could not find support for Baird's original hypothesis of its degeneration by term and hence dispelled his justification for intervening to end the pregnancy [40].

Diagnosis of retarded growth is still very unreliable, but even when it is correctly identified, 'interventions available to the physician . . . (for example diet supplementation, timing of delivery and choice of venue or mode of delivery) are of doubtful value' [41, p. 110]. It has never been demonstrated that growth-retarded babies, whose gestation is artificially curtailed, thrive better under the inevitably distressing conditions of neonatal intensive care than they would have done *in utero*.

Obstetricians expected their interventions to be life-saving. The perinatal surveys of 1958 and 1970 and many other studies have shown higher mortality rates when these interventions were used than when they were not, but, obstetricians argued, this was not to compare like with like: the interventions were only undertaken to prevent an even worse outcome. While in certain instances this claim is no doubt justified, there is plentiful evidence that interventions were often undertaken on slender indications of impending complications and plentiful evidence of wide variations in clinical judgement of appropriateness and need. The benefits and disbenefits of any intervention can be measured by comparing the outcome in a group exposed to the intervention with that in another group, similar in other relevant respects, but not so exposed. The necessary trials were never undertaken before the interventions were adopted as accepted practice. What causes fashions to flourish and wither, in any field of human activity, is something of a mystery. Certainly, in the management of childbirth, accepted practice is quick to follow seductive will-o'-the-wisps requiring interventions, but slow to change in response to the discrediting findings of retrospective studies, even when such findings are corroborated by the strong negative correlation demonstrated on a national scale between the use of interventions and outcome.

CONFIRMATION FROM DUTCH RESULTS

Retrospective studies can only make comparisons between practices or conditions which have been allowed to exist and the suppression of alternatives in childbirth throughout the world eliminates the sources of comparative material. Holland is the only economically developed country where a substantial number of births has continued to take place at home. As in other countries, there was a steady trend towards hospitalization but it started later than elsewhere and eventually followed a different pattern. The proportion of births at home fell from 75% in 1953 to 53% in 1970 [42] to 35% in 1978, but then rose marginally to 36% by 1986 [43]. Over the same period the national perinatal mortality rate kept falling, but as in England the two trends were not causally related. In 1953 the PNMR in hospital (65.0/1000) was three times the PNMR for home births (21.6) [42], but with only 25% of all births in hospital, it was perhaps plausible to argue that these included all at high predicted risk and that this explained all the excess mortality. In 1986, with 64% of all births, most of which could not have been at high predicted risk, it was no longer plausible to use this explanation for the hospitals' excess mortality which had widened to six times (13.9 versus 2.2) [43], thus repeating the pattern already observed in the English data (pages 340–1). When the national PNMR of 1986 is standardized – recalculated to show what it would have been if the proportions of births in hospital and at home had remained the same as they were in 1953 – it is clear that it would have been much lower (5.1) than it actually was (9.7) (0.25 × 13.9 + 0.75 × 2.2 = 5.1). Far from causing the decline in perinatal mortality, the increased hospitalization, as in England, kept mortality from falling by as much as it would otherwise have done.

Dutch hospitals are unusual in that their perinatal mortality rates do not reflect simply the results of obstetricians' methods of care, for independent midwives are able to bring in their clients and conduct deliveries according to their own principles. In 1986 the hospital PNMR was the average of care by obstetricians who attended 70% of the births and by midwives who attended 29% of the births. Likewise, the PNMR for home births measured the average results of care by general practitioners who attended 33% of these deliveries and by midwives who attended 66%. It is therefore much more informative to compare the PNMRs for the different birth attendants separately. This can be done using official material, supplementing the published data with unpublished computer print-outs to which the present author and her Dutch co-researcher, Dr Damstra-Wijmenga, were given privileged access [44, 45].

The resulting analysis, as in Table 8.9, reveals even more striking

Table 8.9 Perinatal mortality rates/1000 births by birth attendant, place of birth and risk factors, Holland 1986, with number of births in each category in parentheses

Risk factor	Obstetricians/ gynaecologists Hospital	General practitioners Home	Midwives	
			Hospital	Home
All births	18.9 (83 351)	4.5 (21 653)	2.1 (34 874)	1.0 (44 676)
Parity				
0	20.2 (41 861)	5.9 (6 088)	1.7 (17 429)	1.5 (15 031)
1 and 2	16.5 (36 739)	3.8 (13 064)	2.6 (15 532)	0.8 (26 472)
3 and over	26.1 (4 751)	4.4 (2 501)	1.6 (1 913)	0.6 (3 173)
Maternal age				
<20	20.9 (1 816)	4.8 (208)	2.2 (1 366)	1.5 (661)
20–24	23.3 (15 902)	4.0 (3 718)	1.8 (8 411)	1.4 (8 254)
25–29	17.8 (35 104)	3.9 (9 959)	2.3 (14 640)	0.7 (21 105)
30–34	17.8 (22 741)	4.9 (6 090)	2.0 (8 198)	1.1 (12 227)
>34	18.1 (7 788)	6.6 (1 678)	3.1 (2 259)	3.7 (2 429)

Sources: CBS Monthly Bulletin of Population and Health Statistics 87:11 Table 1 and CBS computer print-outs of stillbirths and 1st week deaths. Not included are the 610 births attended by both physician and midwife and the 409 without known attendant.

contrasts. The PNMR for all births was higher for doctors in hospital (18.9) than for doctors at home (4.5), which was in turn higher than for midwives in hospital (2.1), which was in turn higher than for midwives at home (1.0). The difference between each of these pairs of adjacent PNMRs is significant at a level so high as to make it virtually impossible that it could be a statistical chance. The pattern of mortality was repeated at every level of risk on account of parity and maternal age. Arithmetic necessity dictates that, even if births under obstetricians' care included a greater proportion in the subgroups at higher risk, this excess proportion could have accounted for very little of the excess mortality observed.

Overall the PNMRs in the subgroups at highest risk on account of maternal age or parity were less than twice the PNMRs in the subgroups at lowest risk. The disparity in PNMRs is vastly wider between term and preterm births. Although the official Dutch statistics record the length of gestation of the babies who die, they do not record the length of gestation of the babies who survive, so that it has not been possible to calculate specific PNMRs at each length of gestation.

This gap in vital information was effectively filled by data derived from the National Obstetrics Registration (LVR), set up in the 1980s with the close co-operation of the Royal Society for Obstetrics and Gynaecology (NVOG), the Dutch Organisation of Midwives (NOV) and the Health Inspection (GHI) in order to register nationwide data on obstetric care [46]. The system is voluntary but by 1986 covered 82% of obstetricians and 70% of independent midwives, both considered to be representative samples, but it did not then cover any general practitioners. This source reports the proportion of births cared for by obstetricians and midwives respectively which had very short (<33 week), short (33–36 week) and normal (>36 week) gestations.

By applying these proportions to the available official data on births and deaths, specific PNMRs at each of these gestations can now be estimated, as in Table 8.10. Of births with very short gestation 95% were cared for by obstetricians, but the PNMR for these (185.5) was higher than for the 5% cared for by midwives (169.8). Because of the small numbers under midwives' care, this result could be a statistical chance and the higher rate for obstetricians might reflect that they managed a greater proportion of births at the very shortest, and so most dangerous, gestations. But like the English experience shown in Table 8.3, it does not positively support the claim that obstetric management and proximity to facilities for neonatal intensive care make birth in hospital safer for the most immature babies.

For the babies with short gestation, 33–36 weeks, the PNMR for obstetricians (46.4) was much higher than for midwives (12.6) and this difference was virtually certain to be real – not due to chance. At gesta-

Table 8.10 Perinatal mortality rates/1000 births by birth attendant, place of birth and length of gestation, Holland 1986, number of births in parentheses

Weeks of gestation	Obstetricians Hospital	Midwives Hospital and home	Significance of difference
<33	185.5 (3 084)	169.8 (159)	Not significant
33–36	46.4 (7 835)	12.6 (1 273)	$p < 0.00001$
>36	8.1 (71 932)	0.8 (77 958)	$p < 0.000001$
Not known	130.0 (500)	75.5 (159)	$p < 0.05$

Sources: CBS Monthly Bulletin of Population and Health Statistics 87:11 Table 1 and CBS computer print-outs of stillbirths and 1st week deaths. Not included are the 610 births attended by both physician and midwife and the 409 without known attendant. Proportional distribution by gestation: SIG (Dutch Information Centre for the Health Care Services) 1987 5 jaar LVR 1982–6 obstetricians – Table 7; midwives – page 4.

tions in the normal range, 37 weeks and over, the difference was even wider: ten times as high for obstetricians (8.1) as for midwives (0.8).

In 1986, only 2% of all the births in Holland under the care of obstetricians or midwives were of very short gestation. Only for these few is the evidence less than certain that birth is not overwhelmingly safer when supervised by a midwife. Only 7.6% of all births had gestations of <37 weeks. A greater proportion of the births under obstetricians' care (13.1%) than under midwives' care (1.8%) were preterm. This excess was due partly to midwives, following protocol, successfully transferring mothers in early spontaneous labour, partly to previous booking by obstetricians of mothers at predicted risk of preterm labour which, as in the case of the transfers, they were unable to delay, and partly to their interventions intended to relieve diagnosed maternal or fetal distress. However, obstetricians' care achieved a PNMR for all these preterm births of 86, nearly three times as high as the PNMR (30) following midwives' care. Since it is unlikely that all of this excess was due to an excess of births at the very shortest gestations (under 30 weeks), it must be accepted that these results are far from supporting the claim that high technology obstetric and neonatal care makes birth safer for immature babies.

The great majority of births, even in hospital, were not preterm. Whatever were the high-risk conditions and dangerous complications which were diagnosed as needing care by obstetricians, they obviously did not usually cause preterm delivery and it is precisely in their propensity to do this that much of the risk of complications lies. Subgroups at the highest risk from poor obstetric history, from intercurrent diseases like severe hypertension or from haemorrhages of any kind in pregnancy could expect to have PNMRs around three times the PNMR of subgroups which do not suffer any of these conditions; for affected pregnancies which go to term nevertheless, the excess mortality rate would be less than threefold.

In any case the high-risk conditions affect only a small proportion of all mothers delivering term babies. Most of the obstetricians' deliveries could not have been at high predelivery risk. Obstetricians attended nearly as many term births as did midwives. The small proportion of their original bookings which midwives transferred to obstetricians because of late complications or intra-uterine death (and most of these would result in preterm delivery) would affect only marginally the relation between the average risk status at the start of labour of term pregnancies under obstetricians' and midwives' care respectively. Their excess of births at high predelivery risk could not possibly have been great enough to account for a PNMR ten times as high for obstetricians as for midwives.

The Dutch results confirm the suspicions already raised, not only that care by obstetricians is incapable, save in exceptional cases, of reducing predicted risk, but even that it actually provokes and adds to the dangers.

That the PNMRs in total and in most risk groups of maternal age and parity were significantly higher for midwives delivering in hospital than at home may be due to their selection for hospital of women with problems, but many women without problems elected to deliver in hospital lest an unforeseen complication should arise, not realizing that unforeseen complications have repeatedly been found to arise more frequently in the hospital setting [47, 48]. The very low PNMRs for home births, even for those in high-risk groups, may reflect not only the competence of the midwife but also the beneficial effect of emotional security for the mother in a familiar setting. Would the 15 000 first babies delivered in their unequipped homes in 1986 with a PNMR of 1.5 really have fared better if they had joined the 42 000 delivering under obstetricians' care in hospital with technological equipment ready to cope with all emergencies and a PNMR of 20.2?

This national experience was closely mirrored by the findings of a study of 8055 births originally booked for a midwifery practice near Amsterdam between 1969 and 1983 [30]. Of these births 2067 were transferred to obstetricians' care, 1430 in pregnancy and 637 in labour. The PNMR/1000 births (39.4) associated with all the births transferred (in pregnancy 51.7 and in labour 11.0) was many times higher than for the births retained by midwives (1.3).

The data were analysed in greater detail for a doctoral thesis [49] which classified the births and associated deaths both by type of carer and by degree of obstetric risk, high (judged by the principal factor) or low. The high-risk group included preterm and IUGR (intrauterine growth retarded) births, breech presentations and twins. For this group the PNMR was very significantly higher for those transferred for obstetricians' than for those retained for midwives' care, 98.8 (47/227) versus 21.9 (2/57); outcomes at less than 32 weeks' gestation cannot be compared since only one baby in this subgroup was not transferred for care by obstetricians, but the respective PNMRs for the preterm births at 32–36 weeks' gestation (excluding fetuses already dead at the time of transfer) were 138.1 (25/181) and 17.9 (1/56), and for all the growth-retarded babies the PNMRs were 53.1 and 14.7. For all the low-risk births the relative disparity between the PNMRs, 12.1 (17/1409) and 0.5 (3/5770), was even wider.

Certainly, a much greater proportion of the births under obstetricians' care (32%) than under midwives' care (4%) were in the defined high-risk groups, but if these proportions had been the same in both cases as the overall average, the PNMR under the obstetricians would have been 21.5 instead of 39.4, while under the midwives' it would have been 2.8 instead of 1.3. This standardization still leaves a large excess mortality for births under obstetricians' care, once again not explained by an excess of high-risk births.

The local experience of first birth, which is not of itself regarded as high risk in Holland, was similar to the national. Of the first births, 1429, including 1017 (71.2%) in the low-risk group (vertex presentation at term), were to transferred mothers, with 53 deaths giving a PNMR of 37.1; 2608 first births remained under midwife care, with five deaths giving a PNMR of 1.9. Stated reasons for transfer were toxaemia and postmaturity, 'threatening preterm delivery', 'suspected IUGR' and antepartum haemorrhage, conditions most unlikely to justify a PNMR 18 times as high. Of later births 638 were transferred, including 392 (61.4%) in the low-risk (vertex, term) group, with twenty-eight deaths giving a PNMR of 43.9, while 3380 remained under midwife care, with three deaths and a PNMR of 0.9. Stated reasons for transfer were malposition, poor progress, fetal distress, 'ruptured membranes no progress after 12 hours', again conditions unlikely to explain the wide disparity in mortality rates.

The most frequent reasons for transfer in pregnancy were toxaemia – nearly twice as frequent as 'threatening preterm delivery' or malposition or disproportion – and in labour 'poor progress in second stage' and 'signs of fetal distress'. Stated reasons for transfer in the low-risk group were toxaemia, postmaturity and disproportion.

In view of the wide excess in the specific PNMRs in all subgroups of risk, it is difficult for the layman to believe that in most cases birth was made safer by transfer to care by obstetricians, antenatally or intranatally. Yet the frequency of transfer at both stages increased over the fourteen years of the study, from 19.7% in the first four years (1969–72) to 33.0% in the last four (1980–83). Greater proportions were latterly transferred for all the reasons already quoted for except for malposition during delivery. Thus since no hint was given that mothers in the catchment area had become less fit for childbearing, the criteria for impending complication must have become more inclusive. The number of deaths associated with the transferred births in the first and last periods was not stated, so the opportunity was missed of showing whether greater proportions of referrals, with their higher incidence of interventions, reduced mortality in the study group but in the light of the overall results, it seems that such an outcome was very unlikely.

The obstetrician researchers did not question the rightness of transfer; indeed in their report midwives were sometimes reproved for not transferring more promptly, but praised for their ability to forecast conditions which, when transferred, would be associated with high mortality. The probability based on past results that mortality even in these cases would be lower under midwife care was disregarded.

The recent results, on the local as on the national scale, of maternity care in the Netherlands reliably confirm what might have been surmised from the earlier results there – that midwives practising their skills in human relations and without sophisticated technological aids, are the most effective guardians of childbirth and that the emotional security of a familiar setting, the home, makes a greater contribution to safety than does the equipment in hospital to facilitate obstetric interventions in cases of emergency.

EXPERIENCE IN NEW ZEALAND

In other countries the organization of the maternity service, the systems of data collection, and the lack of resources to carry out research have meant that analyses of results on a national scale are rarely available. One exception is New Zealand where, like other countries which before 1950 were settled mainly by European migrants, maternity care came early to be dominated by doctors, with nearly all births taking place in some kind of hospital.

Increasingly, the specialist doctors, sharing the universal philosophy of their profession about the conditions which make birth safer, have pressed for the concentration of deliveries in large, regionally centred obstetric hospitals equipped for technological interventions, with the inevitable closure of small hospitals which serve the many scattered rural communities. Medical policy is to refer all cases predicted to be at higher risk to the more specialized hospitals. To investigate the claims of relative safety, a visiting American Professor of Family Medicine initiated research to classify all the births and perinatal deaths in New

Zealand between 1978 and 1981 according to the different types of hospital [50].

To take account of different levels of predicted risk in these, the results were analysed by infant birthweight. Far from substantiating the alleged lack of safety in the level 1 hospitals – mostly the small rural units distant from specialist centres and staffed only by GPs and midwives – the PNMR for the births weighing 1500 grams and over (99% of the total) was found to be significantly lowest there. For the 94% weighing 2500 grams or more, the PNMR was lowest in the smallest hospitals and rose steadily to be highest in the level 3, most specialized hospitals. It is highly unlikely that similar upward grading in identified risk from predicting factors would go far towards explaining this upward trend. These best equipped units, with facilities for immediate neonatal intensive care, had the lowest PNMR for the lightest babies; nevertheless it was only marginally lower in the hospitals with an annual throughput of more than 2000 births a year than in those with fewer than 100. Whether this advantage would have been maintained had outcome been measured at a later postnatal stage is not known.

It was concluded that

The significantly lower perinatal mortality rates of normal-weight infants in level 1 hospitals by comparison with level 2 and 3 facilities may indicate that low-risk mothers fare better in low technology environments . . . [where] the level of intervention and the setting in which birth occurs are more appropriate to the medical and non-medical requirements of the mothers who go there. [50]

EXPERIENCE IN FINLAND

The rapid social and economic developments which changed Finland from being a rather backward agricultural country in the 1930s to a wealthy industrialized country in the 1970s were accompanied by equally striking changes in the organization of maternity care. In 1938, 50% of births took place at home under midwifery care, 33% were in hospital and 17% had no trained attendant. By 1950, these percentages were respectively 37, 58 and 5; by 1965 nearly all births were in hospital, and thereafter increasingly in the most specialized ones. The incidence of the common obstetric interventions increased, but not at the same rate in each of the hospitals for which detailed data were available [51].

Death rates for both mothers and babies came tumbling down, and from relatively high levels in 1950 were by the end of the 1970s among the lowest in the world. There was the familiar temptation to infer that the increased hospitalization and obstetric management had caused the improvement in mortality, but this inference could not be supported because no correlation was found to exist between the annual changes in the technological practices in hospital and the perinatal mortality rates [51].

Likewise, analysis of results in the period 1977–81 discredits the claim which might have justified the policy of concentrating births in the largest, most specialized hospitals, for the PNMR was highest in these and very significantly lowest in the least specialized, local hospitals for all births weighing over 2500 grams (95% of the total).

For low-weight births, the neonatal mortality rate was also lowest, but not significantly, in the local hospitals, despite their distance from intensive care facilities. On the other hand, the stillbirth rate was highest there [52]. The distribution between places of delivery of intra-uterine deaths which are obviously not affected by intranatal practices was not known. An earlier study in Norway had found that 90% of deaths of low-weight fetuses happened before labour [53]. The excess stillbirth rate for small fetuses in the local Finnish hospitals may have reflected an excess of intrauterine deaths and not any deficiency in the intranatal care given there.

EXPERIENCE IN THE USA

No comparable analysis of perinatal mortality by level of hospital has been carried out in the USA, but data have been collected relating to a few geographically remote or economically deprived areas where intra-natal care has been managed by midwives, some with, some without recognized training. Mortality rates at all times have been well below the corresponding State and national averages. Outstanding examples, still operating in recent decades, include the Frontier Nursing Service, founded in 1925 to bring nurse-midwifery care to poor communities in a mountainous region of Kentucky far from technological facilities; the Catholic Maternity Institute founded in 1943 to meet the needs of poor mothers in Santa Fe, New Mexico; the Su Clinica Familiar in Texas, founded in 1972 to serve the needs of Mexican migrants; the North Central Bronx Hospital, New York, where certified nurse-midwives, with appropriate medical consultation but using few intranatal inter-ventions, serve a community of mainly poor black and hispanic mothers; the Farm, a spiritual community in rural Tennessee, where all births are attended by uncertified, but highly skilled and experienced midwives [54, 55].

The success of care by different attendants could be measured by comparing the perinatal mortality rates recorded between 1959 and

1966 at different stages of a State-funded programme for nurse-midwives in Madera County, a poor agricultural area of California. Before 1960, the birth attendants were exclusively general practitioners; between mid-1960 and mid-1963, nurse-midwives were funded to practise; then the California Medical Association arranged for the midwives to be replaced by obstetricians/gynaecologists. The neonatal mortality rate/1000 births in the county was 23.9 in 1959, 10.3 from mid-1960 to mid-1963, and 32.1 from January 1974 to June 1966 (a pattern similar to that between birth attendants in Holland in 1986, depicted in Table 8.9). The percentage of premature births in the three periods was 11.0, 6.4 and 9.8 respectively.

This hierarchy of safety was borne out only in respect of morbidity in a study, unique in American annals, which compared outcomes in two groups of 1046 births well matched for predicting risk factors, which had been delivered in 1975–7 in hospital (actual) and at home (actual plus late transfers to hospital). This method of analysis measures the risk of booking for different places of delivery, but not the risk of the kind of care actually given (pages 320–1). Obstetricians attended 75% of the hospital births, general physicians attended 25% of the hospital births and 67% of the home births, the remaining 33% being attended by midwives, mostly lay. The perinatal mortality rate was the same in each group as booked, but the group which intended to and did deliver in hospital, although at the same risk when labour started, sustained many times more intranatal complications, interventions and signs of morbidity in both mothers and babies [56]. It seems that 'While hospital technology is there to be used, most of the time it is used because it is there' [54, p. 211].

More recent data confirm that very good outcomes have continued to follow low technology maternity care, even after births not always considered to be at low predelivery risk. Statistics describing the 1786 births attended by the Farm midwives in the 21 years, 1970–91, showed no maternal deaths and a PNMR of 11.2 (9.5 excluding the lethal congenital malformations); fifty-five (3%) of the births were breech presentations of which midwives safely delivered thirty-two; seventy-nine (4.4%) births were transferred to hospital, but only thirty-nine had instrumental delivery, twenty-nine (1.6%) by caesarean section, a rate far below the national average. No women were barred from initial booking on account of their age or parity, except those with certain disorders like diabetes and hypertension, and few were barred on account of adverse obstetric history. Unfortunately it is as difficult as ever to find reported outcomes over the relevant decades for a control group, evenly matched for all relevant predelivery characteristics but having orthodox obstetric management, with which the apparently excellent outcomes for this fairly small number of midwife-managed births may be fairly compared, so that unequivocal conclusions may be reached about the safest methods of maternity care [57, 58].

The North Central Bronx Hospital [59] has been organized on principles which distinguish it from most other hospitals in America or other countries, for midwives are entrusted with the sole management of a high proportion of the pregnancies and deliveries and share with obstetricians the management of the remainder, which have specific medical complications but are not transferred to other hospitals. Yet over three-quarters of the mothers served by this hospital would be assessed, according to generally acknowledged criteria, as at high risk. Many suffer the disadvantages associated with poverty, race, avoidance of antenatal care and childbirth education, addiction to drugs and alcohol, and a high prevalence of sexually transmitted infections.

Despite the potential problems and although as many as 11% of the mothers arrived for the first time when they were about to deliver, 86% of the 3287 deliveries in 1988 were conducted by the midwives on staff, who provided most care at all stages. The caesarean section rate was 11.8% (half the national average). Also notable were the low rates of induction and augmentation of labour, of episiotomy and perineal damage and the significant involvement of midwives in breech deliveries. Though 15% of the infants had meconium staining, the PNMR was only 15.2 and nearly 90% of the survivors had Apgar scores of 7 or more at one minute. It was presumably the ones with lower scores who made up the 370 (11.1%) admissions to neonatal intensive care and that these included most of the 339 (10.2%) who weighed 2500 grams or less and/or the 378 who were born by caesarean section. Of the thirty neonatal deaths, eighteen weighed 1000 grams or less; none was transferred to another hospital.

This report would have been even more informative if it had related conditions in mother or fetus to the kind of delivery they had, or related elements of intranatal care to specific outcomes. It would also have been enlightening if it had been possible to compare practices and outcomes between disadvantaged groups giving birth elsewhere under policies of active intervention, so that readers could judge for themselves the relative effectiveness of midwives' care.

Following the tradition of the 20th century, however, most American babies are born in hospitals under obstetric management and most mothers have been indoctrinated to accept claims that such provisions make childbirth safest. For the minority who have rebelled against the medicalization of a natural process, alternative options have been increased by the development of free-standing birth centres, at first in rural areas with populations too small to reward obstetricians adequately, and then from the mid-1970s in urban areas also, where their use has been discouraged by obstetricians, on the ostensible grounds of their lack of safety. To meet the implied challenge, the Maternity Center Association collected and analysed data describing the experience of 11 814 women, admitted for delivery in 1985–7 to eighty-four centres, of which sixty-three were operated solely by certificated or lay midwives [60].

Although the women were at below average predelivery risk according to many, but not all, of the recognized demographic and behavioural risk factors, 15.8% of them (29% first births, 7% later births) were transferred to hospital, including 2.4% as emergencies, but only 4.4% had caesarean sections. No mother died, but fifteen of the 11 826 infants (1.3/1000) did, including seven with lethal congenital malformations, and all but seventy-one (0.6%) survived in very good condition.

The results compared very favourably with outcomes for the low-risk births extracted from the few larger series in obstetric hospitals where this estimation had been done. It seemed fair to conclude 'that birth centers offer a safe and acceptable alternative to hospital confinement for selected pregnant women, particularly those who have previously had children, and that such care leads to relatively few caesarean sections' – a judgement which may not please obstetricians.

These and other data from America, as well as from other countries, point to the conclusion that

> in all times past and present, midwifery, as an approach to pregnancy and parturition, is sound, safe and superior . . . . when doctoring is applied wholesale as the dominant and fundamental approach to maternity care, it is not sound, it is not safe, and it achieves inferior outcomes . . . . the more highly specialised the doctoring . . . and the more highly technologic the setting . . . , the worse the results. [54, p. 128]

INTERVENTIONS AND COMPLICATIONS

The American experience mirrors exactly what has been observed in Holland and England. In a Dutch study in 1984, which compared the outcome when women at the same predelivery risk opted freely to deliver at home or in a university hospital, significantly more intranatal complications occurred in those who opted for hospital and significantly more of the babies needed special care. 'The fact that in a hospital . . . the very surroundings and equipment may give rise to iatrogenic complications is apparently overlooked' [47]. Another Dutch study found that phototherapy was more often given in the hospital than in the home setting to treat the same degrees of neonatal jaundice [61].

Similarly in England, in 1983, the experience of two well-matched groups of low-risk women, booked for delivery in a consultant unit or the attached GPU of the same Oxford hospital [48], was that the group under specialist care, even the non-induced subgroup, was exposed more frequently to various obstetric procedures, from which they and their babies derived more harm than benefit, compared with the simple and safe deliveries of the comparable low-risk women in the attached GPU, where babies were much less likely to need intubation or special care.

Whereas there are many records of births taking place away from specialist obstetric care being completed without maternal complications, for example among the evacuated mothers in war-time Britain (pages 287, 314), uncomplicated deliveries have for many years been the experience of less than half the mothers delivering in NHS hospitals in England and this proportion has shrunk as more births have taken place in the obstetric units. In 1973, when 82% of births were in obstetric hospitals, 45% of all hospital births were without maternal complication [62]. In 1985, when 95% of births were in obstetric units, only 38% escaped complication [63]. Complications for the mother inevitably mean a less smooth passage for the baby. This degeneration happened over a period when much attention was paid to antenatal care whose justifying objective is to forestall complications in labour, while at the same time, according to every other index of well-being, childbearing women were becoming ever healthier and fitter to reproduce. This is one further demonstration that, in general, intervention in maternity care, antenatally or intranatally, does not succeed in its purpose of making childbirth safer for mother or child.

THE WRONG TOOLS FOR THE JOB

It would only have been reasonable to expect the intranatal interventions most frequently used to have caused the great decline in perinatal mortality rates if they had been appropriate remedies for the most frequent causes of perinatal death. In fact this was never the case. Most perinatal deaths have always been of infants (or fetuses) of subnormal weight, especially when the low weight is compounded with immaturity, the incomplete fetal development associated with preterm birth. As was shown on page 115, over thirty years of obstetric management and neonatal care had reduced neither the incidence of low-weight births (and presumably preterm deliveries) nor their contribution to the total number of perinatal deaths.

Obstetric intranatal interventions are obviously irrelevant to reducing the incidence of spontaneous preterm delivery and the success of obstetric antenatal interventions has so far been very limited, though for hypertensive mothers whose babies are at risk of retarded growth regular treatment with low-dose aspirin has recently been associated

with higher birthweights (Chapter 3, page 113). The known causes of low-weight births, preterm and term, their association with maternal stress, social, psychological and medical, and the inappropriateness of most obstetric treatments to reduce the incidence of this high-risk state, on the contrary their capacity to increase it, were discussed at some length in Chapter 3 (pages 115–24).

Low-weight birth is not entirely dependent on the current state of the mother. One of the last studies of the indefatigable Dugald Baird, by then Sir Dugald, using the accumulated data base he had been instrumental in organizing in Aberdeen, established that the mothers of low-weight babies in one generation were especially likely to have themselves been once low-weight babies, and their mothers in turn were especially likely also to have been of low weight when they were babies [64]. The incidence of low weight thus describes the same generational pattern as does perinatal and maternal mortality. But whereas improving maternal health over the generations has led to a great decline in the proportion of births which have ended in perinatal or maternal death, it has not led to any decline in the proportion of births which are of low weight, arising either from preterm delivery or from poor fetal growth in preterm or term deliveries. One might have expected the less serious pathology to have responded more readily to more favourable conditions. Some other counteracting factor or factors must have been operating to prevent this.

Smoking in pregnancy prejudices the supply of oxygenated blood to the fetus and results in lower birthweight (page 120). Studies have suggested that 10–15% of preterm births may be attributable to smoking [65]. There has been a secular increase in smoking among women in general, but many women stop or cut down smoking in pregnancy, so it is not known to what extent, if any, increased smoking has offset the expected decreases in preterm and low-weight births from better health.

Ironically, the significant counteracting factor may rather have come from increased obstetric intranatal interventions. By definition, induction of labour and elective caesarean section shorten gestation and produce lighter babies. Of these interventions, induction affected larger numbers. Routine birth statistics do not permit their effect on prematurity to be measured, but in the 1970 perinatal survey the proportion of induced births was not much less for births up to than over 38 weeks' gestation, 22% against 28% [23, p. 171]. In both gestation groups the PNMR/1000 births was much higher following induction, 91.7 against 64.3 up to 38 weeks, 11.8 against 6.7 at 38 weeks and over [23, p. 180]. More of the births in hospital (12.1%) than in GP units and home (6.4%) took place before the 38th week of gestation [23, p. 123]. While some of this excess may have been due to hospitals booking women at risk of repeating a previous experience of preterm delivery or admitting as transfers from GPUs and home an excess of spontaneous preterm labours which they did not manage to postpone, the remaining excess was probably due to induction, much more commonly a hospital procedure. The explicit data of the 1958 survey [11, p. 131] show that gestations under 38 weeks were very significantly more frequent, and their PNMRs higher among births booked for hospital than for GPUs or home, including transfers.

The effect of induction on birthweight was not reported in the 1970 survey, but it was probably the main reason why hospital births included 36.8% weighing <3000 grams and 10.1% weighing <2500 grams, compared with 19.4% and 3.2% respectively in GPUs and home [23, p. 123]. Since 1958, these proportions had increased in hospital from 28.1% (<3000 grams) and 8.8% (<2500 grams), but decreased in GPUs and home from 21.1% (<3000 grams) and 4.5% (<2500 grams) [11, p. 141].

These results suggest that the factors which led to the decrease in the perinatal mortality rate led also, in the absence of intervention, to a decreased proportion at low weight, but that this consequence was more than offset by the increasingly frequent use of induction. They point to one of the mechanisms through which the decline in the national PNMR was kept smaller than it would otherwise have been. The hypothesis that factors which should have reduced the proportion of low birthweight babies over time were offset by the increased smoking of pregnant women requires the unlikely assumption that smoking trends moved strongly in opposite directions according to place of delivery.

Since the mid-1970s the proportion of induced labours as officially recorded has been reduced and the proportion of births by caesarean section has increased; the proportion of low-weight births, which had risen to 7.4% in 1985, had fallen back to 6.8% by 1990, but the statistics are too unspecific to justify speculating about a cause and effect relationship to explain these trends.

Although the proportion of low-weight births had not fallen between 1958 and 1990, the associated mortality had. The PNMR for babies weighing up to 1500 grams was one-third of what it had been in 1958 and obstetricians and neonatologists like to take credit for this remarkable transformation. But the PNMR for all births weighing under 2500 grams had fallen to about one-quarter of the 1958 level and for births weighing over 2500 grams to one-fifth.

While perinatal mortality has been reduced by certain elements of obstetric care, for example in the treatment and prevention of Rhesus iso-immunization, and in the prevention of rubella, the evidence is that the reduction overall and hence at most weights was due far less to obstetric or paediatric management than to the improved health status of the parents, particularly the mother. It is probable that the same health factor contributed, to a greater or lesser extent, to the improved survival of the low and very low weight babies.

The hypothesis that improved parental health made a greater contribution than technological interventions is supported by the earlier English evidence that, in the years before neonatal intensive care was developed (Table 8.3), the chance of survival for small babies was never less and usually far greater for births without interference at home. Over the years 1963 to 1971, it was the untypical practice in a large obstetric hospital, King's Mill, serving a geographically defined area in Nottinghamshire, to give only careful nursing to babies born weighing between 501 and 1500 grams and avoid technological neonatal interventions. When the survivors were followed up at school age, it was found that

> In terms of survival, handicap and intellectual capacity . . . outcome compared favourably with that of infants born over the same period in areas where intensive methods of perinatal care were used. . . . We found it difficult, therefore, to escape the conclusion that scientific and highly skilled interventions . . . made little impact on the outcome for infants of very low birthweight. [66]

This finding supports the claims made by paediatricians in Bogota, South America, that survival is as good if the very tiny infant is kept warm between the mother's breasts, with unrestricted access to their own milk supply. The reliability of the Colombian mortality statistics was found to be questionable, but the psychological benefits to mother and child were confirmed [67]. This so-called 'kangaroo care' is vastly less costly and much more widely practicable than neonatal intensive care which can only be given in suitably equipped and staffed high technology hospital units. By 1993, however, it had not proved feasible to mount a controlled trial in Britain to measure the relative merits of each method. Western paediatricians, and Western medical and public opinion, have such faith in the advantages of modern technology that they dare not risk not using it.

But neonatal intensive care does also have serious disadvantages, besides its high financial cost [68]. Most preterm babies need ventilatory support and mechanical ventilation damages their lung growth. Graduates from intensive care units have to be admitted to hospital in later childhood with above average frequency, often with respiratory illnesses [69, 70]. Necessary routine handling alone provokes problems: falls in temperature, interruption to breathing and slowing of heart rate. Protection from infection and attachment to life-support apparatus means isolation in an incubator, deprived of soothing motherly contact when comfort is needed and of the essential stimulation of a normal environment. Separation from the mother may be prolonged with possibly adverse psychological consequences. More invasive procedures have to be used to combat specific pathologies, with little relief from analgesia or sedation, which are withheld because they impair the infant's already compromised breathing, and this is sanctioned by the belief held by some neonatologists that the underdeveloped neurological system is less sensitive to pain. There is, however, evidence that the extremely immature infant is supersensitive to pain [71].

> It cannot be denied that this [intensive care] is highly distressing for the infant and their parents. . . . Whether pain is remembered is open to philosophical discussion and whether it leads to short- or long-term benefit or harm is unknown. . . . So if intensive care improves chances of survival, as neonatologists believe, this may be achieved at very high cost to the infant.

Many obstetricians share the neonatologists' belief. Rating the chances of survival as greater in an intensive care unit than in an unsatisfactory uterus, they consider it advantageous to terminate compromised pregnancies by induction of labour or elective caesarean section. A study of very immature infants born at a London hospital noted a very significant increase (p < 0.001) in the proportion delivered by caesarean section, from 10% in 1981–3 to 32% in 1984–6 [71, p. 1121]. This kind of management has been advocated in numerous small and uncontrolled studies, as beneficial to survival or quality of survivors. But 'When confounding variables were controlled for, no benefit was found even for breech presentations' [72].

In another study, the high neonatal mortality rate suffered by low-weight infants delivered by caesarean section prompted the conclusion 'In view of the maternal morbidity associated with caesarean section and the poor neonatal outcomes at birthweights < 1500 grams, the use of operative delivery for very low birthweight infants deserves further scrutiny' [73].

Intervention cannot possibly be beneficial in those cases where the diagnosis of unsatisfactory uterine development is mistaken. There is as yet no method of reliably identifying fetal growth retardation and, as has already been said, intervention has resulted in the birth of many premature but not growth-retarded infants [74]. Nor can fetal weight be reliably estimated to ensure that intervention to relieve a hypertensive mother will not result in the birth of a dangerously underweight baby. Enthusiastic experts, engaged on their own studies, are said to claim that ultrasound makes possible estimates of fetal weight accurate within 10%, though accuracy is less in smaller fetuses and when the measurement is performed as a routine by persons not involved in the study – a well recognized phenomenon (pages 259–60). In 1985–7, in the London hospital already referred to, 'weight estimates for infants at 28 weeks' gestation were frequently more than 30% out' [71, p. 112].

Nor has it been demonstrated that the growth-retarded babies correctly diagnosed survive better if their gestation is curtailed or thrive better with intensive paediatric care than *in utero*. On the contrary, 'The reported incidence of major handicap, including cerebral palsy, in preterm, small-for-dates babies, followed up for at least two years, is much higher than in their term counterparts' [75].

There is thus good reason to doubt the wisdom of interventions to cut short those pregnancies diagnosed, correctly or incorrectly, according to the theories of obstetric management as being at mortal risk, and good reason to infer that it has been this practice which has helped to prevent the incidence of low-weight birth from declining, like perinatal mortality, to reflect the effects of improved parental health. Although there has been a welcome decline in the PNMRs for low-weight births, there has been an even greater decline in the PNMRs for normal-weight births. There is good reason to expect that many of the infants, if their gestation had been allowed to continue, would have enjoyed the lower risk of death of their heavier contemporaries. Induction of labour and elective caesarean section, as commonly used, would not have been appropriate tools for reducing either perinatal mortality or morbidity.

REDUCING MORTALITY FROM CONGENITAL MALFORMATION

Congenital malformations make up the second most frequent cause of perinatal death. They go on to 'cause 25% of deaths in infancy and 18% of hospital paediatric admissions' [76, p. 163]. Obstetric intranatal interventions are clearly irrelevant to prevention or remedy. Neonatal surgery can occasionally prevent or postpone death, but in some cases this can be a doubtful benefit. Prevention takes place more effectively at the antenatal stage when, through the screening tests of alphafetoprotein estimation, amniocentesis, chorionic villus sampling and ultrasound screening, fetuses with certain kinds of impaired development, notably of the neurological tract, can be identified and affected pregnancies can be terminated if the parents so wish (Chapter 3, pages 125–6).

Since therapeutic abortion was legalized in Britain in 1968, the PNMR due to congenital malformation has fallen. In the 1958 survey [11, p. 229] it was 5.8/1000 births; in 1985 [34] it was 1.75, a fall of 70%. (From 1986 the method of collecting the raw data changed, so that later statistics may be less complete.) The PNMR from all causes also fell between 1958 and 1985 by 70% and congenital malformations continued to make up the same proportion of all perinatal deaths. The number of abortions carried out for this indication accounted for less than one-third of the decline in mortality. Some other factor must have influenced the incidence of congenital malformation.

In Britain the incidence of neurodevelopmental malformations with very high case-fatality rates, like anencephaly and spina bifida, has always been higher in areas of relative poverty with associated poor health. In other countries too, notably in the period of famine in wartime Holland [77], they have been found to be associated with poor diet and vitamin deficiencies in the mother, conditions amenable to remedy, as has now been demonstrated by vitamin supplementation [78, 79]. These congenital malformations are therefore yet another manifestation of poor parental health. The health status of parents has been improving over the century; studies in Britain and several other countries, like the Netherlands, Scandinavia, Canada, Australia and Hungary, where the standard of living has risen, and in Eire, where also the standard of living has risen but where abortion is not legal, have noted parallel declines in the incidence of these malformations, in particular anencephaly, and consequently of deaths [64, 80–83].

Unlikely to be a cause of fewer congenital malformations is the improved survival of babies of low and very low birthweight, since the risk of these anomalies is higher for such babies, especially those whose intrauterine growth has been retarded, though most malformed babies have normal birthweights.

Geneticists have established associations between chromosomal damage in both male and female genes and deficient nutrition, as well as toxins from tobacco and alcohol. Further fruitful attacks on congenital malformations as a cause of perinatal death will come from continued improvements in standards of health and life-styles, from preconceptional genetic counselling and more reliable antenatal screening. Obstetric intranatal interventions have nothing to contribute.

HYPOXIA

The third most frequent cause of perinatal death, which can, of course, be a contributory factor in the other two, is hypoxia, an insufficient supply of oxygen to the baby before, during or after birth. The fetus receives its quota of oxygen from its mother's blood through the placenta. Any impairment of the maternal–placental–fetal circulation, for example if the mother has pre-eclampsia or high or low blood pressure, prejudices the oxygen supply, but rarely does so sufficiently to endanger life. Most of the perinatal deaths due to hypoxia, or in the extreme case asphyxia, occur intranatally or postnatally [84]. The hypoxic infant will be distressed and obstetricians are always on the alert to pick up signs of distress early enough to intervene and avert the danger, relying commonly on warning signals from electronic fetal monitors (EFMs) and less commonly on analyses of fetal blood gases. Unfortunately, evaluation of results has so far failed to find that the use of EFMs has reduced perinatal mortality (page 178).

In any case, fetal distress is all too often the obstetricians' own creation. The crisis attitude to the onset of labour which their preparation for birth inculcates is apt to raise the mother's blood pressure from the start. The intermittent pressure of uterine contractions causes temporary variations in the flow of blood, natural stresses which the maternal–placental–fetal circulation is designed to cope with. Natural labour should not cause hypoxia for the baby unless the mother is unfit and becomes exhausted by the effort. But if oxytocin is used to induce or accelerate labour, this will cause abnormally severe contractions which the circulatory systems are not designed to cope with and the flow of blood may be reduced below the level necessary for fetal health. A similar effect will be produced if the mother's blood pressure is reduced as an incidental consequence of one or more aspects of obstetric management: by keeping the mother supine, with the heavy uterus pressing on the important blood vessel, the vena cava; or by restricting her mobility in order to permit electronic fetal monitoring or the administration of oxytocin by drip; or if a managed labour is nevertheless prolonged and the mother becomes exhausted, especially if she is denied sustaining food and drink; or if she is given epidural anaesthesia; or if overenthusiastic attendants exhort her to hold her breath and push down before she feels the involuntary urge to do so [85, pp. 65, 115, 126–7]. Or premature artificial rupture of the membranes may allow the umbilical cord to prolapse or to be compressed between the baby and the wall of the uterus, so that the blood supply to the baby is dangerously interrupted [85, pp. 84–5].

Once the baby is born, it should be alert and its lungs should be ready to take over responsibility for the oxygen supply. Its need to do so is the more urgent, the earlier the cord has been clamped and this source of oxygen cut off. But if the mother has been given pharmacological pain relief, the baby may be too sedated to want to start independent breathing and the longer it delays doing so, the more serious the danger of hypoxia. The immature baby whose lungs are not yet adequately developed for their new role is in extreme danger. Heroic efforts at neonatal resuscitation often save lives, but at a price. It was widely assumed that intranatal or postnatal hypoxia caused neurological damage which could lead to deficits, like neonatal fits or cerebral palsy, and that obstetric interventions, most reliably caesarean section, would reduce such danger. This argument was accepted in Courts of Law, thus encouraging the practice of interventions, despite contradicting evidence. One study covering births between 1960 and 1975 found that

Babies born at home or small maternity units without resident medical staff [GPUs] have lower cerebral palsy rates than babies born in consultant units (especially teaching hospitals), even when 'imported' births from outside the survey area are discounted and differences in birthweight are allowed for [86].

Continuous electronic intrapartum monitoring, which had been found in a large study to result in fewer neonatal seizures, was not found to have reduced the incidence of cerebral palsy in the childhood follow-up study, a finding which destroyed the last remaining hope of benefit from this invasive procedure [87]. These results are supported by more recent research which finds that most cerebral palsies are not in fact caused by perinatal hypoxia. Most are thought to originate in early fetal development and to be caused by inadequate nutrition when brain cell division is at its maximum intensity. Failures at this stage can never be reversed by medical care of any kind, so that intranatal interventions in most cases cannot be helpful. The incidence of cerebral palsy is known to have increased in those countries, like Sweden and Western Australia, which have kept reliable records of the condition; it may reflect the increased survival of babies for low weight, for it is certainly the higher, the lower the birthweight [88–90].

It is obvious that, if hypoxic babies are to survive, they urgently need to be given extra oxygen, how much depending on the maturity and competence of their lungs. Dispensing the right amount of oxygen for the individual infants requires delicate judgement. Overdosing damages the eyes and causes the condition retinopathy of prematurity (formerly retrolental fibroplasia), which means total blindness as the price the child has to pay for the saving of its life. It took several years of enthusiastic resuscitation and many blinded children before the causal connection between treatment and outcome was realized and dosages were modified to secure a less dangerous balance, so that the incidence of retinopathy was much reduced [91]. It was not however eliminated and further research has shown that several factors intrinsic to prematurity are involved in injuring the retinal vessels [92]. This is another of the possible morbid outcomes which detract from the apparent advantages of facilitating the birth of preterm and underweight babies, now that their chances of survival are so much greater.

OBSTETRIC INTRANATAL CARE: WEIGHED IN THE BALANCE AND FOUND WANTING

The pathological conditions, such as rhesus iso-immunization, in which obstetric intranatal interventions have unquestionably saved lives, have

been the numerically less important causes of perinatal death. Obstetric treatments in such cases have made a small but welcome contribution to the overall reduction in perinatal mortality. But for the conditions which have continued to be the most frequent causes of perinatal death, there are sound physiological reasons why the most frequent interventions could not reduce mortality from these causes. There is abundant and consistent statistical evidence that they have not in practice done so, that on balance they have made birth less, not more, safe and that the declining trends in perinatal and maternal mortality could not have depended on the coincidental increase in the practice of the obstetric management of childbirth.

REFERENCES

1. Registrar General, *Statistical Review for the Year 1960, Part 1 Medical*, HMSO, London, Table 4.
2. Registrar General, *Statistical Review for the Year 1973, Part 1B Medical, Supplement*, HMSO, London, Table 24.
3. Douglas, C. (1955) Trends in the risks of childbearing and in the mortalities of infants during the last thirty years. *J. Obstet. Gynaecol. Br. Emp.*, **62**, 216–31.
4. Duncan, E., Baird, D. and Thomson, A. (1952) The causes and prevention of stillbirths and first week deaths; Part I: The evidence of vital statistics. *J. Obstet. Gynaecol. Br. Emp.*, **59**, 183–96.
5. Baird, D. (1960) The evolution of modern obstetrics. *Lancet*, 10 September, 557–64.
6. Woolf, B. (1947) Studies in infant mortality. *Br. J. Soc. Med.*, **2**, 73–125.
7. Baird, D. (1947) Social class and foetal mortality. *Lancet*, 11 October, 531–5.
8. Baird, D., Thomson, A. and Duncan, E. (1953) The causes and prevention of stillbirths and first week deaths; Part II: Evidence from Aberdeen clinical records. *J. Obstet. Gynaecol. Br. Emp.*, **60**, 17–30.
9. Baird, D., Walker, J. and Thomson, A. (1954) The causes and prevention of stillbirths and first week deaths; Part III: A classification of deaths by clinical cause; the effect of age, parity and length of gestation on death rates by cause. *J. Obstet. Gynaecol. Br. Emp.*, **61**, 433–48.
10. Baird, D. and Thomson, A. (1969) Reduction of perinatal mortality by improving standards of obstetric care, in *Perinatal Problems* (eds N. Butler and E. Alberman), Churchill Livingstone, Edinburgh, Chap. 14.
11. Butler, N. and Bonham, D. (1963) *Perinatal Mortality*, Churchill Livingstone, Edinburgh.
12. Tew, M. (1977) Obstetric hospitals and general practitioner units – the statistical record. *J. R. Coll. Gen. Pract.*, **27**, 689–94.
13. Tew, M. (1978) The case against hospital deliveries: the statistical evidence, in *The Place of Birth* (eds S. Kitzinger and J. Davis), Oxford University Press, Oxford, pp. 55–65.

14. Tew, M. (1985) Safety in intranatal care: the statistics, in *Modern Obstetrics in General Practice* (ed. G.N. Marsh), Oxford University Press, Oxford, pp. 203–23.

15. Tew, M. (1986) Do obstetric intranatal interventions make birth safer? *Br. J. Obstet. Gynaecol.*, **93**, 659–74.

16. Baird, D. and Thomson, A. (1969) Background to the perinatal mortality survey, in *Perinatal Problems* (eds N. Butler and E. Alberman), Churchill Livingstone, Edinburgh, Chap. 1.

17. Baird, D. and Thomson, A. (1969) General factors underlying perinatal mortality rates, in *Perinatal Problems* (eds N. Butler and E. Alberman), Churchill Livingstone, Edinburgh, Chap. 2.

18. Baird, D. and Thomson, A. (1969) The survey perinatal deaths reclassified by special clinico-pathological assessment, in *Perinatal Problems* (eds N. Butler and E. Alberman), Churchill Livingstone, Edinburgh, Chap. 11.

19. Baird, D. and Thomson, A. (1969) The effects of obstetric and environmental factors on perinatal mortality by clinico-pathological causes, in *Perinatal Problems* (eds N. Butler and E. Alberman), Churchill Livingstone, Edinburgh, Chap. 12.

20. Baird, D. and Thomson, A. (1969) Geographical differences in perinatal mortality by clinico-pathological cause, in *Perinatal Problems* (eds N. Butler and E. Alberman), Churchill Livingstone, Edinburgh, Chap. 13.

21. Chief Medical Officer of the Ministry of Health, On the state of the public health, *Annual Reports for the years 1954 to 1964, Maternal and Child Health*, HMSO, London.

22. Chamberlain, R., Chamberlain, G., Howlett, B. *et al.* (1975) *British Births 1970 Vol. 1, The First Week of Life*, Heinemann, London.

23. Chamberlain, G., Philipp, E., Howlett, B. *et al.* (1978) *British Births 1970 Vol. 2, Obstetric Care*, Heinemann, London.

24. Kitzinger, S. (1978) Women's experiences of birth at home, in *The Place of Birth* (eds S. Kitzinger and J. Davis), Oxford University Press, Oxford, pp. 135–56.

25. Alment, E., Barr, A., Reid, M. *et al.* (1967) Normal confinement: a domiciliary and hospital study. *Br. Med. J.*, **2**, 530–5.

26. Goldthorpe, W. and Richman, J. (1974) Maternal attitudes to unintended home confinement. A case study of the effects of the hospital strike upon domiciliary confinements. *Practitioner*, **212**, 845–53.

27. O'Brien, M. (1978) Home and hospital confinement: a comparison of the experiences of mothers having home and hospital confinements. *J. R. Coll. Gen. Pract.*, **28**, 460–6.

28. Barron, S., Thomson, A. and Philips, P. (1977) Home and hospital confinement in Newcastle-upon-Tyne 1960–1969. *Br. J. Obstet. Gynaecol.*, **84**, 401–11.

29. Bull, M. (1980) Ten years' experience in a general practice obstetric unit. *J. R. Coll. Gen. Pract.*, **30**, 208–15.

30. Van Alten, D., Eskes, M. and Treffers, P. (1989) Midwifery in the Netherlands. The Wormerveer study. *Br. J. Obstet. Gynaecol.*, **96**, 656–62.

31. House of Commons Health Committee (1992) *Maternity Services, vol. III, Appendices to the Minutes of Evidence*, HMSO, London, pp. 651–922.

32. Registrar General. *Statistical Reviews for the Years 1965–1973, Part II Population*, HMSO, London, Appendix B.
33. Office of Population Censuses and Surveys. *Birth Statistics, 1974–1981, Series FM1, nos 1–8, Place of Confinement*, HMSO, London, Table 8.
34. Office of Population Censuses and Surveys. *Mortality Statistics: Perinatal and Infant: Social and Biological Factors*, Series DH3, no. 18, HMSO, London, Tables 23a, 23b, 14a.
35. Steer, P. (1986) Postmaturity – much ado about nothing? *Br. J. Obstet. Gynaecol.*, **93**, 105–8.
36. O'Driscoll, K., Carroll, C. and Coughlan, M. (1975) Selective induction of labour. *Br. Med. J.*, **2**, 727–9.
37. Williams, R. and Studd, J. (1980) Induction of labour. *J. Matern. Child Health*, **5**, 16–21.
38. Gibb, D., Cardozo, L., Studd, J. *et al.* (1982) Prolonged pregnancy: is induction of labour indicated? *Br. J. Obstet. Gynaecol.*, **89**, 292–5.
39. Cardozo, L., Fysh, J. and Pearce, J. (1986) Prolonged pregnancy: the management debate. *Br. Med. J.*, **293**, 1059–63.
40. Fox, H. (1985) Placental structure, in *Scientific Basis of Obstetrics and Gynaecology*, 3rd edn (ed. R. Macdonald), Churchill Livingstone, Edinburgh.
41. Hall, M., MacIntyre, S. and Porter, M. (1985) *Antenatal Care Assessed*, Aberdeen University Press, Aberdeen, p. 110.
42. Huygen, F. (1976) Home deliveries in Holland: Dutch maternity care and home confinements. *J. R. Coll. Gen. Pract.*, **26**, 244–8.
43. Tew, M. and Damstra-Wijmenga, S. (1989) Safest birth attendants: recent Dutch evidence. *Midwifery*, **7**, 55–63.
44. Centraal Bureau voor de Statistiek (1987) Birth by Obstetric Assistance and Place of Delivery, 1986. *Month. Bull. Popul. Health. Stat.*, **11**, 22–31.
45. Centraal Bureau voor de Statistiek (1986) Computer print-outs of raw data on birth by obstetric assistance and place of delivery, unpublished, private access granted.
46. SIG (Dutch Information Centre for the Health Care Services) (1987) *5 jaar LVR 1982–86*, Utrecht.
47. Damstra-Wijmenga, S. (1984) Home confinement: the positive results in Holland. *J. R. Coll. Gen. Pract.*, **34**, 425–30.
48. Klein, M., Lloyd, I., Redman, C. *et al.* (1983) A comparison of low-risk pregnant women booked for delivery in two systems of care: shared-care (consultant) and integrated general practice unit. I. Obstetrical procedures and neonatal outcome – II. Labour and delivery management and neonatal outcome. *Br. J. Obstet. Gynaecol.*, **90**, 118–22, 123–8.
49. Eskes, M. (1989) Het Wormerveer Onderzoek, doctoral thesis (unpublished English translation of summary), Amsterdam, University of Amsterdam.
50. Rosenblatt, R., Reinken, J. and Schoemack, P. (1985) Is obstetrics safe in small hospitals? *Lancet*, **ii**, 429–31.
51. Hemminki, E. (1983) Obstetric practice in Finland, 1950–1980: changes in technology and its relation to health. *Med. Care*, **21**, 1131–43.
52. Hemminki, E. (1985) Perinatal mortality distributed by type of hospital in

the central hospital district of Helsinki, Finland. *Scand. J. Soc. Med.*, **13**, 113–18.

53. Hoffman, H., Meirik, O. and Bakketeig, L. (1984) Methodological considerations in the analysis of perinatal mortality rates, in *Perinatal Epidemiology* (ed. M. Bracken), Oxford University Press, Oxford.

54. Stewart, D. (1981) *The Five Standards for Safe Childbearing* (ed. D. Stewart), Napsac Reproductions, Marble Hill.

55. Gaskin, I. (1981) The Farm: a living example of the five standards, in *The Five Standards for Safe Childbearing* (ed. D. Stewart), Napsac Reproductions, Marble Hill, pp. 327–44.

56. Mehl, L. (1978) Research on alternatives: what it tells us about hospitals, in *Twenty-First Century Obstetrics Now!* (eds D. Stewart and L. Stewart), Napsac International, Marble Hill.

57. Durand, A.M. (1992) The safety of home birth: the Farm study. *Am. J. Public Health*, **82**, 450–2.

58. Gaskin, I. (1993) Personal communication.

59. Haire, D. and Elsberry, C. (1991) Maternity care and outcomes in a high-risk service: the North Central Bronx Hospital experience. *Birth*, **18**, 33–7.

60. Rooks, J., Weatherby, N., Ernst, E. *et al.* (1989) Outcomes of care in Birth Centers. *N. Engl. J. Med.*, **321**, 1804–10.

61. Van Enk, A. and De Leeuw, R. (1987) Phototherapy: the hospital as risk factor. *Br. Med. J.*, **294**, 747–8.

62. Department of Health and Social Security/Office of Population Censuses and Surveys (1980) *Hospital Inpatient Enquiry Maternity Tables 1973–76*, Series MB4 No. 8, HMSO, London, Table 18.

63. Department of Health and Social Security/Office of Population Censuses and Surveys (1988) *Hospital Inpatient Enquiry Maternity Tables 1982–85*, Series MB4 No. 28, HMSO, London, Table 6.4.

64. Baird, D. (1985) Changing problems and priorities in obstetrics. *Br. J. Obstet. Gynaecol.*, **92**, 115–21.

65. Lumley, J. (1987) Epidemiology of prematurity, in *Prematurity* (eds V. Yu and E. Wood), Churchill Livingstone, Edinburgh.

66. Steiner, E., Sanders, E. Phillips, E. *et al.* (1980) Very low birthweight children at school: comparison of neonatal management methods. *Br. Med. J.*, **281**, 1237–40.

67. Whitelaw, A. and Sleath, K. (1985) Myth of the marsupial mother: home care of very low birthweight babies in Bogota, Colombia. *Lancet*, **i**, 1206–7.,

68. Sandhu, B., Stevenson, R., Cooke, R. *et al.* (1986) Cost of neonatal intensive care for very low-birth-weight infants. *Lancet*, **i**, 600–3.

69. Skeoch, C., Rosenberg, K., Turner, T. *et al.* (1987) Very low-birthweight survivors: illness and readmission to hospital in the first 15 months of life. *Br. Med. J.*, **2**, 579–80.

70. McIlwaine, G., Mutch, L. *et al.* (1992) The Scottish low birthweight study. *Arch. Dis. Child.*, **67**, 675–708.

71. McIntosh, N. (1988) Clinical issues, in *The Very Immature Infant* (eds A. Whitelaw and R. Cooke). *Br. Med. Bull.*, **44**, 1126.

72. Sinclair, J., Torrance, G., Boyle, M. *et al.* (1981) Evaluation of neonatal intensive care programs. *N. Engl. J. Med.*, **305**, 489–93.
73. Pinion, S. and Mowatt, J. (1988) Pre-term caesarean section. *Br. J. Obstet. Gynaecol.*, **95**, 277–80.
74. Hall, M., Chng, P. and Macgillivray, I. (1980) Is routine antenatal care worth while? *Lancet*, **ii**, 78–80.
75. Chiswick, M. (1985) Intrauterine growth retardation. *Br. Med. J.*, **291**, 845–8.
76. House of Commons Health Committee (1991) *Maternity Services: Preconception vol. II Minutes of Evidence*, HMSO, London, pp. 1–291.
77. Stein, Z., Susser, M., Saenger, G. *et al.* (1975) *Famine and Human Development: The Dutch Hunger Winter of 1944/45*, Oxford University Press, New York.
78. Smithells, R., Nevin, N. *et al.* (1983) Further experience of vitamin supplementation for prevention of neural tube defect recurrences. *Lancet*, **i**, 1027–31.
79. MRC Vitamin Research Group (1991) Prevention of neural tube defects: Results of the Medical Research Council Vitamin Study. *Lancet*, **338**, 131.
80. Carstairs, V. and Cole, S. (1984) Spina bifida and anencephaly in Scotland. *Br. Med. J.*, **289**, 1182–4.
81. Owens, J., Harris, F., McAlister, E. and West, I. (1981) Nineteen year incidence of neural tube defects in area under constant surveillance. *Lancet*, **ii**, 1032–5.
82. Office of Population Censuses and Surveys (1990) *Congenital Malformation Statistics, England and Wales*, MB3 no. 6, HMSO, London.
83. Kloosterman, G. (1978) Organisation of obstetric care in The Netherlands. *Ned. Tijdschr. Geneesk.*, 1161–71.
84. Chamberlain, G. (1985) The fetal hazards in pregnancy, in *Modern Obstetrics in General Practice* (ed. G. Marsh), Oxford University Press, Oxford, pp. 132–51.
85. Inch, S. (1982) *Birthrights*, Hutchinson, London.
86. Jarvis, S., Holloway, J. and Hey, E. (1985) Increase in cerebral palsy in normal birthweight babies. *Arch. Dis. Child.*, **60**, 1113–21.
87. Grant, A., O'Brien, N., Joy, M. *et al.* (1989) Cerebral palsy among children born during the Dublin randomized controlled trial of intrapartum monitoring. *Lancet*, **ii**, 1233–6.
88. Bryce, R., Stanley, F. and Blair, E. (1989) The effects of intrapartum care on the risk of impairments in childhood, in *Effective Care in Pregnancy and Childbirth* (eds I. Chalmers, M. Enkin and M. Keirse), Oxford University Press, Oxford.
89. Pharoah, P., Cooke, T. *et al.* (1990) Birthweight specific trends in cerebral palsy. *Arch. Dis. Child.*, **65**, 602–6.
90 Hagberg, B., Hagberg, G. *et al.* (1989) The changing panorama of cerebral palsy in Sweden. *Acta Paediatr. Scand.*, 283–90.
91. Silverman, W. (1980) *Retrolental Fibroplasia: A Modern Parable*, Grune and Stratton, New York.
92. Phelps, D. (1992) Retinopathy of prematurity. *N. Engl. J. Med.*, **326**, 1078–80.

9

Epilogue: drawing fair conclusions from factual evidence

Two opposing theories underlie the management of childbirth. Enough practical experience has now been accumulated for it to be judged which of the theories is vindicated. When the history is told, it becomes very clear that at no time in the past or present and in no country have medical interventions made childbirth safer for most mothers and babies. No evidence can be found to support theories that, in general, applying the methods of physical science can evolve obstetric procedures which improve the natural birth process. A few interventions are undoubtedly beneficial, and these are sincerely appreciated, but they are appropriate in only a small proportion of births and so have only a marginal influence on mortality and morbidity. (The pathology of infertility and the marvels of *in vitro* fertilization are beyond the scope of this book.) By contrast, many interventions undoubtedly cause positive harm; further interventions have to be devised in the hope of counteracting this harm, but often succeed only in compounding it. The research findings of the distinguished chronicler, William Silverman, of the disaster of iatrogenic retrolental fibroplasia were succinctly summed up by a fellow paediatrician in these words, as true in 1993 as when they were written in 1987:

> The recent history of perinatal medicine abounds with instances in which belated controlled trials eventually revealed that the apparent benefits of some widely acclaimed treatment had merely disguised the real extent of its tragic consequences. [1]

On the other hand, plenty of evidence can be found to support the theory that childbirth manages best without direct human intervention and that successful reproduction depends, first and foremost, on the good health of parents, the same dependent relationship that exists in all other living species. Human intervention is best restricted to creating conditions which conduce to good health. Impaired health of mothers may be caused by deficiencies in their current environment, in particular the quality of their nutrition, but it is more damaging to their childbearing function if they have suffered deficiencies all their lives, from conception onwards. This was the fate of many generations of poorer women in the industrializing countries, especially those brought up in the towns. Their cumulative physiological deficits took many decades to outgrow. Downward trends in maternal and perinatal mortality are explained by the gradual spread of prosperity, leaving a diminishing proportion of mothers malnourished and reproductively inefficient. In countries like Finland and Japan, the sudden attainment of economic prosperity after 1950 was matched by an equally sudden drop in perinatal mortality. This suggests that their previous relative poverty had not resulted in a diet deficient in the essential elements of nutrition for healthy skeletal development and so did not hinder the mothers' favourable reaction when better conditions arrived.

Why has obstetric treatment failed to make most births safer? All medical treatments carry a greater or lesser degree of risk and only bring benefit when used to cure or prevent conditions carrying even greater degrees of risk. A healthy person does not need curative medical treatment. Most childbearing women are healthy and do not need curative obstetric treatment, but obstetricians, ensuring a constant high demand for their services, have redefined pregnancy and labour as a state of illness, always needing treatment at some level, preventive if not curative. Their scope for doing this has been widened by the rapidly developing techniques for prenatal diagnosis. For births predicted to be at lower risk of complications, obstetricians agree that their supervision may be necessary only so that they are ready to act in the very few cases where the unpredicted complication actually does occur. For births predicted on their own increasingly comprehensive definition to be at higher risk of complications, obstetricians insist that their supervision is always necessary, so that they may intervene promptly in the few cases where a predicted complication does actually occur, even although they have never had evidence that for most complications the risk is thereby reduced, and much evidence that it is increased. Such outcomes, unsupportive to their arguments, arise because obstetricians have failed to weigh correctly the risks of treatment against the imputed risks of maternity related illness.

That their treatment usually turns out to be the greater risk is because it rests on a fundamentally unsound basis. Modern obstetric interventions have been devised in the light of the findings of research into the biochemistry and biophysics of the reproductive processes and the bio-chemistry and biophysics of their pathology, as though a complete understanding of the processes is to be found within these disciplines. The problems have been reduced to ones of physical science and are to be tackled by applying the impressive range of techniques now at the command of physical science. That this approach has for the most part been unsuccessful in solving the principal problem of how to make childbirth safer is *prima facie* evidence that the approach is misdirected. Proper cognizance has not been taken of the fact that the physical aspect of reproduction is inextricably involved with its emotional and social aspects. The efficient functioning of the physical processes is absolutely dependent on appropriate stimuli from the emotional processes which in turn are governed by social stimuli. Messages are transmitted from mind to body via the endocrine system. Too little attention has been paid to the mediating science of endocrinology.

The obstetric environment, obstetric methods and obstetric propa-ganda have saturated childbirth with an atmosphere of danger and fear, which are diametrically opposite to the appropriate emotional stimuli for the physical processes – the feelings of confidence and relaxation, engendered by familiar, reassuring surroundings. Obstetric propaganda has made the optimal conditions difficult to provide in any modern setting, but results show that these are most nearly achieved by con-fidence-inspiring, emotionally supportive, non-interventive midwifery, practised in an environment protected from the menace of high tech-nology.

LESSONS FOR THE FUTURE FROM THE PAST

Any policies for reform have to be based on an understanding of the forces which moulded the present situation and an appreciation of the formidable obstacles which would have to be overcome.

Action to reduce losses in childbirth still further would have to con-centrate on improving the health of the neediest mothers. In the light of past performance, there is not the slightest reason to believe that the desired objective would be achieved by increasing the medical input into maternity care. On the contrary, fewer losses would result if the medical input into maternity care were greatly restricted, while access to, and uptake of, healthy diets and social support became universal. 'Health policy is indivisible from social policy. A greater difference will be made to the lives of mothers and babies by a coherent social policy aimed at mitigating the effects of and abolishing poverty than any tech-nological advance.' [2]

But the forces inspiring and implementing the principles of healthy

life-styles are feeble, compared with the powers of the champions of obstetric management whose singleness of purpose and political skills have won for them the domination of maternity care. The former attract the support of few commercial interests. The latter attract the allegiance of many bodies who identify their professional or commercial interest with the proliferation of obstetric care. At the centre of the contest, obstetricians at all times have played their cards very cleverly.

From the 17th century, captivating bluff and dishonest disparagement of the rival midwives secured the man-midwives' entry to the field by enticing clients to transfer their custom. These tactics served their successors in good stead to widen the bridgehead and consolidate their gains. Already in the 1830s, American medical students were being taught that 'If females can be induced to believe that their sufferings will be diminished or shortened and their lives and those of their offspring be safer in the hands of the profession, there would be no difficulty in establishing the universal practice of obstetrics.' [3].

By then doctors had, ironically, appealed to science to assist in the task of mystification. Science was an intellectual discipline dominated by men and beyond the understanding of women. Science, pursued by thinking men, aspired to explain how nature worked and so was respected; instinct, experienced by women, inspired unthinking behaviour prompted by nature actually working, and so was despised. That science was making poor progress in explaining how the natural process of reproduction did work and could provide no evidence that it improved on nature did not matter. Doctors' experience being predominantly of complicated deliveries, it seemed obvious to them that reproduction was essentially pathological and where the presence of pathology could not actually be identified, the foreknowledge of science could threaten it. In 1892, British doctors argued before the House of Commons Select Committee enquiring into the need for midwives' registration that 'as a result of civilisation, childbirth could no longer be regarded as a natural process. . . . Every birth should, therefore, be attended by a medical practitioner who should "guide" and "control" it [4, p. 130], an ideal reiterated in 1969 by a leading obstetrician of his day (page 326). Throughout the 20th century, the incessant stream of propaganda, with no more valid foundation, has continued to capture public opinion, to make everyone believe that childbirth is fraught with dangers against which only care by obstetricians can protect.

But further complementary strategies were needed to make obstetricians' conquest impregnable and these were devised and carried out in due course with outstanding thoroughness: the effective downgrading and intimidation of the midwifery profession; the ensuring of compliance in future doctors by appropriately indoctrinating medical students, as in 19th century America, and stifling their criticism of authority; the distortion and suppression of evidence and the misrepresentation of results; the elimination of places of birth practising less interventive methods of care to prevent the possibility of discrediting comparisons of results; the gradual ousting of general practitioners; the fostering of academic research in directions of 'scientific' interest but irrelevant to making most births safer; the enlisting of allies with professional or commercial interests in the propagation of obstetric methods; a discreet influence on the press, medical and lay, to discourage the publication of criticism. That such a complete and effective range of policies to prevent competition should develop spontaneously, without direction and co-ordination, does indeed seem remarkable.

It would, of course, be wrong to suggest that the obstetric profession has not always had forthright critics within its ranks, obstetricians whose observations and trials point to conclusions at variance with accepted practice, or that the medical press has always been unwilling to publish their reports. Such reports after all make up the material from which much of this book has been drawn. The reasons for distrusting the propaganda should be widely known in the profession. Yet these contradictory revelations have had surprisingly little effect on orthodox thinking and behaviour. They seem to be received with blind eyes and deaf ears – an ostrich-like hope that if unpalatable facts are ignored or denied, they will go away or be forgotten and criticism will disappear. This reaction was illustrated with regard to the safety of home birth in a belated acknowledgement by the Professor representing the British Paediatric Association when he told the Winterton committee: '. . . it was a misunderstanding of the original statistics of the 1958 study [shown in Table 8.1] that led to babies all being delivered in hospital. The data was there and was not scrutinised clearly enough. . . . my view would be that babies can be safely delivered at home', a view with which two Professors from the British Association of Perinatal Medicine then agreed [5, para. 27] (page 325).

Experience so far has fortified this attitude. Although they have masqueraded under the cloak of science, obstetricians have paid remarkably little regard to scientific evidence. They were undeterred by the judgement in 1921 of an honest American practitioner [6]:

The fact that modern maternity hospitals, where is centered the obstetric skill and knowledge of our profession, have been unable to decrease the dangers of birth to mother and child over the figures in the early part of the nineteenth century is *prima facie* evidence that modern obstetric surgery is ineffectual in combating those dangers.

As in Britain (pages 58–9, 60–3), the most the profession felt obliged to do was to improve the competence of the practitioners in carrying out the practices, not to question whether it was the practices themselves which were ineffectual.

Examples abound of practices pursued in defiance of evidence of their harm. The dangers of the recumbent posture for delivery were being written about in the USA in the 1880s [7]. But this was the posture enforced by most obstetricians in all countries for the next century. And when concessions were made, allowing alternative postures if supervised by midwives, this was done less in response to scientific evidence than to satisfy consumer demand; it was good policy to improve relationships with a captive, but often protesting, clientele, and perhaps improve outcome, so long as obstetricians' convenience and dignity were not compromised (pages 187–8). Much higher maternal morbidity following episiotomy was already reported in 1935 [8], and studies have confirmed this finding ever since (pages 164–5), but episiotomy continues to be widely practised. Routine electronic monitoring of the fetal heart, in pregnancy or in labour, boosts the obstetricians' scientific image without, as evaluative studies now show, bringing any benefit to the baby or mother (pages 123, 178). Exposure of its very limited benefits did not limit its use. Obstetricians can exercise their power over mothers by making them believe that electronic monitoring, like ultrasound scanning, reveals knowledge essential to the future safe conduct of the pregnancy and birth; obstetricians prey on mothers' instinctive concern for the welfare of their babies (and themselves) to ensure their compliance with obstetric management.

Scientific research in recent years has shown that most of the medical elements of antenatal care are ineffective [9], yet regimens in most antenatal clinics have not been changed. Antenatal clinics are, however, very effective in inculcating the rightness of, and necessity for, obstetric intranatal care and so maintaining control of the maternity service by obstetricians (pages 107–8, 133). And this control has not been shaken by the publication of the results of the statistical comparisons of outcomes following interventive care by obstetricians and less interventive care by midwives and general practitioners. These analyses are as scientific an exercise as is possible with the available data (Chapters 7 and 8) and as such should have carried great weight with a scientifically-based discipline, allegedly searching for the truth. They were, however, dismissed with apparent disbelief and feigned incomprehension. They were not allowed to influence obstetricians' thought, for in 1993, even after the considered judgement of the Winterton Report, the President of the RCOG wrote defiantly, 'We believe, in the present state of knowledge, that the hospital is the only place where expertise and emergency services are immediately available; this is the safest place for delivery and we make no apologies for that.'[10]

Others of the many examples of obstetricians' disregard for the findings of scientific research, which consistently discredit their philosophy and undermine their authority, have been alluded to earlier in this book. Their proclaimed professional objective is to make birth safer for mother and child, but they pay no heed, and abuse their undeserved authority to exhort everyone else to pay no heed, to any research finding, however decisive, which shows that their methods do not achieve this objective.

ETHICS: ANOTHER ALLY FOR OBSTETRICIANS

Obstetricians appealed to physical science to uncover the physiological mysteries of safe childbirth and, when it failed to do so, they misused science to mystify the mothers and the public. They are as ready to harness ethics to advance their cause. They appeal to ethics to sanction practising orthodox, untested, therapies and to abstain from trials to test the effectiveness of alternatives. But ethics is not an objective discipline; absolute rightness is not known. Standards can always be adjusted to suit different points of view. Obstetricians claim to understand what action is in the best interests of mothers and babies, but they have no right or competence to do so, for their claim has always rested on a foundation of physiology which is susceptible to scientific evaluation but which has failed in the test. A gentle general practitioner critic has written:

> Having based their whole argument on one of safety, the reluctance of the profession to consider this evidence objectively – without refuting it by statistical argument – suggests that their decision has been made on preconceived assumptions which they are not willing to reconsider in the light of available evidence. The fact that this reluctance might cast doubt in some minds as to whether the reasons for it stem principally from a concern for patient care, or principally from intra-professional self-interest, has ethical implications of considerable significance. . . . Is it appropriate or even ethical to allow this [decision making about obstetric care] to remain almost solely in the hands of those who, by virtue of making obstetrics their specialty, have acquired a perspective that, although highly advanced scientifically, has restricted their view of the human experience of childbirth? [11]

(The description 'highly advanced scientifically' is only accurate in a very partial sense, as has just been demonstrated.)

It is in no way unusual for workers in any field to fight for the advancement and continuation of their occupation, to argue that this serves best the interests of their customers in particular and society in general, that their cause is in fact 'ethical'. The strength of evidence brought in support of their arguments, and the extent of distortions, varies but the common sense and knowledge of the public is often sufficient to see through hypocrisy and judge who are really the intended beneficiaries. Obstetricians pose as saviours of life, of new life. There could hardly be a more moving and popular ideal whose sincerity the public are least likely to question. But to defend their profession, they have to withhold and pervert knowledge in order to maintain public ignorance and delusion – hardly an example of ethical practice.

Even with a strong case against their occupation, no workers willingly consent to its destruction. The harmful consequences of smoking tobacco are now undisputed. Tobacco manufacture is an important source of employment in the city of Nottingham. Pay and conditions in the industry are good, so good that the trade unions concerned, representing decent men and women, 'have even rejected proposals from the local labour movement to press the company . . . for a policy of diversification into other products using the Nottingham workforce. Instead the unions have strongly backed the company in opposing attempts to reduce smoking in public places' [12]. It is no more realistic to expect organized obstetricians, also decent men and (the few) women, to admit their shortcomings and so to give up absorbing, satisfying jobs with the accompanying high prestige and high incomes (albeit slightly offset by high premiums for defending law-suits). Yet this is the self-sacrificing behaviour that would be required of obstetricians and conforming general practitioners if they were to give the honest, unbiased advice, based on the evidence of actual results, called for by the Winterton and *Changing Childbirth* Reports [5, 13]. Strategies which would bring about the necessary reform of medical attitudes without too much pain have still to be developed.

THE TRIUMPH OF BLUFF

Reality is, however, that obstetricians have been able to maintain their bluff over several centuries and wherever Western medicine is respected. It has suited the wider medical profession to acquiesce in obstetricians' bluff because it is in some measure the same kind of bluff that medicine, pre-scientific and scientific, has practised and continues to practise on people in general. Certainly scientific medicine has won deep admiration for its many conquests of distressing pathological conditions, successes which the profession has advertised enthusiastically to a receptive public. Yet

> The proportion of deaths in the UK today which are regarded as potentially preventable through good medical treatment is small – about five per cent. While many other diseases are partly treatable, it is generally accepted that medical care has had little impact so far on the overall death rate from some of the most important diseases, such as cancers and heart disease [14, p. 112].

Understandably, the medical profession has responded coolly to well-researched demonstrations [14–16] that poor health is most strongly associated with poverty, and that the general level of health in a community depends far more on the quality of its environment, present and past, than on the quality of its medical services (Chapter 1). Further evidence of the persistent effect of poverty and maternal malnutrition in the past lies in the association now being demonstrated between on the one hand low birthweight and retarded fetal growth, as manifested in subnormal body measurements at birth, and on the other hand adult cardiovascular and possibly other diseases [17, 18]. It is now being discovered that maternal welfare in one generation determines the welfare of the entire population in the next. This must be a fundamental and lasting concern to society as a whole. Doctors' organizations expend more effort in pleading for more resources for medical treatments, and teaching people to rely on these, than in educating the public to accept responsibility for maintaining their own health and encouraging them to follow a life-style that will keep them well and much less often in need of medical treatments. In contrast, any threatened restriction on medical services is opposed vociferously, nominally 'in the interests of patients'.

Obstetrics is only an extreme example of the general case. Its continued success suggests that the bluff is something that people want very deeply – some promised certainty in an uncertain world, a desire to be spared the burden of personal responsibility, the same recognition of human insufficiency that looks to religion to make good. To judge by the composition of church congregations in Western cultures, women seem to be particularly conscious of human insufficiency. Whether for reasons of biology or social indoctrination, women have a very long history of submitting to male domination. When males claimed a surgical competence, in due course bolstered by pseudo-science, to make the process of childbirth safer and pleasanter, the claim must have seemed congruous with the normal expectations of submissive women. This was just another sphere in which men had to be acknowledged as superior. Undoubtedly, men were superior when it came to exploiting an opportunity for their own benefit and in the management of childbirth they excelled, wearing down any opposition from their clients, from their professional rivals, the midwives, and from critics within their own ranks.

The opposition was never accurately informed. Although there is a long history of women disliking the procedures of obstetric management, their objections could always be overridden by assurances, albeit untruthful, that these were in the best interests of their babies. But even after 1978, when they were offered impartial and valid analyses of results which openly challenged the comfortable conspiracy between obstetricians and their allies, even the active protesters were hesitant about accepting this irrefutable evidence in their favour. The news was too good to be believed; so thorough was their indoctrination with obstetricians' propaganda that the majority of women, as clients or midwives, clung to the false beliefs they had been taught. More accurately, limited publicity for the news kept the majority of women from knowing how false their beliefs actually were.

A second reason for success in the wearing down process was the much poorer organization of the opposition, for women are notoriously reluctant to band together to fight for their own advantage and when they do so, they show much less skill than men. They are uninspired chess players and do not emulate men's ability to visualize possible attacking moves by their opponent and protect all the loop-holes in their own defence. In so far as women win conflicts, they are more likely to do so by passive resistance and by enlisting the active support of sympathetic males. In their fight to break the obstetricians' monopolistic stranglehold of the management of childbirth, crusading women have been greatly helped by the support of a few courageous doctors, both specialists and general practitioners.

However, until the medical profession as a whole can bring itself to assess the results of different methods of maternity and neonatal care impartially and, putting the interests of its practitioners and commercial allies second to the interests of mothers and babies, change its advice to everyone, to those involved in providing care and to those involved in using it, in accordance with the facts it finds, policies and practice will be hard to alter.

Yet it is unrealistic to expect the impetus for change to come from those who will not benefit from it. If maternity care is to be organized in accordance with facts, not delusions, the onus for reform has to come from the users of the service, and from society as a whole, its political leaders and its social policy makers. Rational argument based on research evidence needs political support if it is to influence practical organization. By 1992 the House of Commons Health Committee took up the challenge [5] and its widely advertised inquiry into the maternity services drew evidence from many sources and many points of view representing both users and providers. Its carefully weighed verdict on how the organization of the services should be reformed to focus on the welfare of the users instead of on the professional interests of medical providers as hitherto was endorsed in 1993 by the Department of Health's Expert Maternity Group [13]. Now at last in one country, maternity care has an authoritative basis for its organization; rational argument and research evidence have won the necessary political support.

Unlearning deeply ingrained beliefs, skilfully implanted, is never a quick or painless process. Recent experience in several countries has shown that profound changes in previously entrenched political attitudes can take place. Change is not impossible if motivation is there. If, fully informed about the true risks and released from the influence of false propaganda, some women nevertheless prefer obstetric management for their pregnancies and deliveries, this option should not be withdrawn as long as whoever pays for it agrees. But adequate provisions should be made, at much less cost, for all those women who would prefer the proven advantages of physically non-interventive, and emotionally supportive, midwifery to enjoy this option. This is what all the investigations of the World Health Organization have led it to recommend. It is this advice its member nations would be wise to follow.

In a period of political re-appraisal of the vested interests of the providers of goods and services, the time is ripe for a counter-revolution in maternity care, for the end of a harmful professional monopoly and the restoration of choice to mothers in carrying out their natural, and socially essential, function.

REFERENCES

1. Maddock, C.R. (1987) A population-based evaluation of sustained mechanical ventilation of newborn babies. *Lancet*, ii, 1254–8.
2. House of Commons Health Committee (1992) *Maternity Services. Vol. III, Appendices to the Minutes of Evidence*, pp. 651–922 (memorandum by Medical Practitioners' Union, HMSO, London.
3. Hodge, H. (1838) *Introductory Lecture to the Course on Obstetrics and the Diseases of Women and Children*, University of Pennsylvania (T.G. Auner), Philadelphia.
4. Donnison, J. (1977) *Midwives and Medical Men*, Heinemann, London, p. 130.
5. House of Commons Health Committee (1992) *Maternity Services*. Vol. I (The Winterton Report), HMSO, London, paras 1–453.
6. Holmes, R.W. (1921) The fads and fancies of obstetrics: a comment on the pseudoscientific trend of modern obstetrics. *Am. J. Obstet. Gynecol.*, 2, 233.

7. Arney, W.R. (1982) *Power and the Profession of Obstetrics*, University of Chicago Press, Chicago, p. 63.
8. Nugent, F. (1935) The primiparous perineum after forceps delivery: a follow-up comparison of results with and without episiotomy. *Am. J. Obstet. Gynecol.*, **2**, 249–56.
9. Enkin, M. and Chalmers, I. (eds) (1982) *Effectiveness and Satisfaction in Antenatal Care*, William Heinemann, London.
10. Simmons, S. (1993) The present status of the Royal College of Obstetricians and Gynaecologists. *Br. J. Obstet. Gynaecol.*, **100**, 5–6.
11. Zander, L. (1981) The place of confinement – a question of statistics or ethics? *J. Med. Ethics*, **7**(3), 123–7.
12. Lee, N. (1989) *Health for All in Nottingham?* Nottingham Health Strategy Group, 51 Braidwood Court, Nottingham.
13. Department of Health (1993) *Changing Childbirth*, Report of the Expert Maternity Group, HMSO, London.
14. Smith, A. and Jacobson, B. (eds) (1988) *The Nation's Health: A Strategy for the 1990s*, King Edward's Hospital Fund for London, London.
15. Black, D., Morris, J., Smith, C. *et al.* (1980) *Inequalities in Health. The Black Report*, Penguin Books, Middlesex.
16. Whitehead, M. (1988) The health divide, in *Inequalities in Health*, Penguin Books, London.
17. Barker, D. (1990) The fetal and infant origins of adult disease. *Br. Med. J.*, **301**, 1111.
18. Barker, D., Osmond, C., Simmonds, S. *et al.* (1993) The relation of small head circumference and thinness at birth to death from cardiovascular disease in adult life. *Br. Med. J.*, **306**, 422–5.

Author index

Numbers in square brackets are those of the reference numbers appearing on the page(s) shown. Numbers in *italics* refer to entries in the reference lists at the end of each chapter.

Subject index

Page numbers in *italics* refer to tables and those in Roman numerals refer to the glossary.

OPIUM AND THE PEOPLE Revised edition
Opiate Use and Policy in 19th and early 20th Century Britain

Virginia Berridge

At the beginning of the nineteenth century, opium was widely used as an everyday remedy for common ailments. By the 1920s, it was classified as a 'dangerous drug' and its use was severely restricted. In an examination of the social context of drug taking in Victorian England (morphine, cannabis and cocaine, as well as opium) the book explains this decisive change in attitude. This revised edition analyses how and why restrictive policies were put in place in the early decades of the twentieth century, and how the 'British system' of drug control accommodating both legal and medical controls was first established. It surveys the ways in which that balance has operated for the rest of the century. This study sheds fresh perspectives on the motivations which survive in the formation of current drug policies.

Reviews of the first edition

"A simultaneous and significant contribution to the history of medicine, to the understanding of nineteenth-century English society, and to the analysis of present-day addiction problems."   **Brian Harrison, THES**

"Current concern with the proliferating misuse of psychoactive drugs reverberates with echoes of the past. This is emphasized and lucidly placed into a detached historical perspective by this excellent book"   **Martin Plant, BMJ**

A DOCTOR'S DILEMMA
Stress and the Role of the Carer

John W. Holland

"There are not many books that successfully weave psychological theories of this sort into a convincing account of the everyday pressures of general practice without seeming too theoretical. John Holland succeeds in this. This book is most welcome."   **Andrew Elder, British Medical Journal**

"Full of vivid clinical examples and lively stories...discussions are in everyday language, practical, thoughtful and without jargon. Holland addresses difficult ideas in clear writing which is free from jargon."
Newsletter, Royal College of General Practitioners

"It is well enough written to make it hard to put down, which cleverly ensures that the 'stressed' professional will feel compelled to finish it."
Journal of the Balint Society

Also published by Free Association Books

THROUGH THE NIGHT
Helping Parents and Sleepless Infants - With a new preface
Dilys Daws

"Absorbing and instructive reading for many professionals."
British Journal of Psychiatry

"A clearly written book which will be easily digested by both parents and professionals...(it) will enable all workers to have greater insight."
The Psychologist

"An easy introduction for medical students, nurses, midwives, health visitors, social workers, paediatricians, and psychologists to the breadth of the current thinking on early child development."
Tavistock Gazette

"Through the Night is the most interesting, readable and memorable book on human infant development I have ever read."
James McKenna PhD, Univ. of California Irvine School of Medicine.

"(A) beautifully recounted and carefully conceptualized account of sleeping difficulties in small children. This book will be read with profit by parents and paediatricians, by child and family psychotherapists."
International Review of Psycho-Analysis

"Child psychotherapists have a lot to learn from this book."
Journal of Child Psychotherapy

"A valuable tool for therapists...it provides an excellent introduction to the therapeutic issues about parenting young children."
Jo Douglas, Health Visitor

Through the Night describes pioneering work in the baby clinic of a General Practice by a child psychotherapist from the Tavistock Clinic. Sleep problems can tear a family apart. Since it was first published in 1989, *Through the Night* has been helping parents to understand their sleepless infants - and themselves. Dilys Daws listens to the 'cries' of the family as a whole. Her approach - based on meeting the parents and baby together a few times - is proving to be of great practical help to parents. *Through the Night* is the first book on the technique of parent-infant psychotherapy to be published in the UK.

SAFER CHILDBIRTH?

A Critical History of Maternity Care   Third Edition
Marjorie Tew

'Every now and again a book is published that breaks established moulds of thinking and challenges preconceptions and prejudices. This is such a book.'   – *Sheila Kitzinger*

1998 saw the fiftieth anniversary of the founding of Britain's National Health Service. In view of its high cost, the need for changes in the provision of the services it comprised was realised. Doctors were enjoined to concentrate on those treatments which can be shown, not only to be clinically effective, but also cost-effective in that they achieve more satisfactory results than those which are more expensive.

In the field of maternity care, much evidence has by now been compiled on the clinical effectiveness of treatments, but so far no system has been found to require those who provide the service, at any level, to follow the evidence thus established.

The first edition of *Safer Childbirth?* in 1990 showed that actual results have never supported the widely-held belief that today's reduced rates of death or sickness for mother or child were *caused* by increased hospitalisation or obstetric interventions, and the second edition in 1995 added the further compelling evidence gathered by the House of Commons Health Committee in their thorough inquiry from 1990-1992 into the maternity services, including the scientific evaluations, by then completed, of obstetric practices. The recommendations of the Parliamentary Report in 1992, followed in 1993 by the Government Report, *Changing Childbirth*, should have revolutionized the direction of maternity care; mothers, not doctors, should henceforth have the dominant role in deciding what sort of care best served their and their babies' interests. With a foreword by Sheila Kitzinger and a new introduction by the author, this edition of *Safer Childbirth?* tells how the hopes were dashed that the maternity service would be reformed and become an outstanding example of evidence-based medicine, as it was ready to do.

This important, original work is essential reading, not only for all providers and users of maternity care, but also for students of social policy.

Marjorie Tew was until her recent retirement a Research Statistician at Nottingham University Medical School, Nottingham, UK.

Cover design: Alan Forster

Free Association Books
Please send for a free catalogue

ISBN 1-85343-426-4

9 781853 434266